Inaba Katsu Bunrei's 稲葉克文禮

腹證奇覽

Extraordinary Views of Abdominal Patterns

Fukushō-Kiran

AF716916

Jay Kageyama

The Chinese Medicine Database
www.cm-db.com
Portland, Oregon

Extraordinary Views of Abdominal Patterns

腹證奇覽

Fukushō-Kiran

Jay Kageyama

Copyright © 2018 The Chinese Medicine Database

1017 SW Morrison #307A
Portland, OR 97205 USA

COMP designation original Chinese work and English translation

Cover Design by Jonathan Schell L.Ac.
Library of Congress Cataloging-in-Publication Data:

Inaba Bunrei, fl. - 1805
[Extraordinary Views of Abdominal Patterns. English]
Fukushō-Kiran = Extraordinary Views of Abdominal Patterns.
/ translation Jay Kageyama
p. cm.
Includes Index.
ISBN 978-0-9906029-5-8 (alk. paper)
Medicine, Japanese I. Kageyama, Jay. II. Title: Extraordinary Views of Abdominal Patterns.

All rights reserved. No part of this publication may be reproduced, stored in a retrieval system or transmitted in any form by any means, electronic, mechanical, photocopying, recording or otherwise, without prior written permission of the publisher.

International Standard Book Number (ISBN): 978-0-9906029-5-8
Printed in the United States of America

Contents

Illustrations

Indices

Foreword to the Fukushō-Kiran

The *Fukushō-Kiran,* is the 18th century record of the lifelong clinical experience of the practically illiterate folk physician Inaba Katsu Bunrei. A ruffian by all accounts, Inaba was born into poverty and orphaned since childhood. He traveled the Japanese countryside, per his own account, 'engaging in vulgar acts unbefitting of a proper gentleman'. But upon the urging of an auspicious friend, he decided to take on the study of medicine. A study which proved arduous, none the least due to his illiteracy and lack of prior formal education. His journey was further beset by adversity in the form of rejection by all teachers he beseeched. Until his ultimate sensei Kaku Taiei, took pity on the ambitious Inaba and compassionately trained him in the prescription of *Hàn* canonical herbal formulas through the palpatory diagnosis of the abdomen, a skill not recorded in books, nor requiring particular academic wherewithal.

After years of training, Inaba set off on the road again as an itinerant physician, and examined and treated every possible patient he encountered. Echoing the journey of an Edo samurai who must put on his helmet ten thousand times to test his skill in battle, Inaba commenced the fulfillment of his practical training by treating thousands of patients on his path.

But it is said that old dogs cannot learn new tricks, and that old ways are hard to change. Later in life, Inaba's continued alcoholism caught up with him as he suffered stroke after stroke. And while each time, he was cured through the expert herbal care of his disciples, his condition worsened with each event. Though he originally never considered his own knowledge worthy of recording, it was due to his failing health and upon the urgent requests of his disciples that Inaba finally agreed to impart his body of knowledge to be committed to writing and preserved for posterity. It is said that Inaba himself never witnessed the completion of the manuscript. But his chief disciple Wakuda Yoshitora ensured the success of the project and in later years further elaborated on his sensei's knowledge by authoring the *Addendum to the Fukushō-Kiran.*

Distilling detailed information on the ins and outs of abdominal diagnosis by reading the original writings of Zhāng Zhòngjǐng is difficult to say the least. And we owe it to the wisdom and diligence of generations upon generations of formidable Kampo masters such as Tōdō Yoshimasu and the aforementioned Inaba Katsu Bunrei, to have synthesized a clear and practical system for investigating a patient's abdomen as a guide for the selection of the exact canonical herbal formula. While Zhāng Zhòngjǐng primarily emphasized pulse diagnosis, he secondarily corroborated his finding with abdominal palpation. Therefore, Fukushin is an indispensable skill for anybody wishing to practice exactly the way Zhāng Zhòngjǐng practiced.

At the Institute of Classics of East Asian Medicine, we have been using both Japanese and Chinese versions of the *Fukushō-Kiran* as our abdominal diagnosis textbook since the inception of our curriculum a decade ago. So, it is with great elation that we welcome this excellent translation and publication by the indefatigable translators and editors of the Chinese Medicine Database. Congratulations not only on the translation of the text, but also on the cleaning up and reproducing of the many old abdominal drawings. This book is both a parable for the journey of the study of classical medicine, as well as it is a practical hands-on instruction in the typically pragmatic style of the folk physicians of yore. I cannot recommend this work strongly enough to anybody wishing to study and emulate the practice style of the Zhāng Zhòngjǐng.

Arnaud Versluys, PhD, MD (China), L.Ac.
Director, Institute of Classics in East Asian Medicine

The Background and Significance of the Work

Palpation of the abdomen (Ch: *fù zhěn* 腹診; Jp: *fukushin*; literally, "abdominal examination") has existed as a diagnostic examination method in China since ancient times. In recent years, it has gradually become popular among practitioners of Oriental medicine in the West and is sometimes known as "*hara* diagnosis" (*hara* is the native Japanese reading of the character for abdomen [i.e., *fù* 腹]). Although the history of the practice dates back to at least the *Nàn Jīng* 《難經》 (Jp: *Nan-kyō*; The Classic of Difficult Issues), which is thought to have been written or compiled near the end of the Eastern *Hàn* (Ch: *Dōng Hàn* 東漢; Jp: *Tō-Kan*) dynasty (25–220 CE), the practice seems to have developed little in China due to the increasing popularity of pulse diagnosis/tongue diagnosis, etc. and instead flourished in Japan during the *Edo* 江戸 period (1603–1868 CE).

It was during this period that *Kampō* 漢方 (literally, "Chinese method"), the native Japanese system of medicine, began to evolve separately from traditional Chinese medicine (TCM), and abdominal diagnosis became more widely utilized among Japanese physicians in comparison with pulse diagnosis. Although there are several factors that led to the increased popularity of the practice during this period, perhaps the most important reason is that Japanese-style abdominal examination was found to be much simpler to learn in comparison with the subtleties of TCM diagnostic techniques such as pulse diagnosis/tongue diagnosis. Moreover, abdominal examination requires little to no knowledge of traditional Chinese medical theory, as each abdominal pattern is thought to correspond to a single formula under a theory known as formula-pattern matching or formula-pattern correspondence (Ch: *fāng zhèng xiāng duì* 方症相對; Jp: *hō-shō-sōtai*). For this reason, it was relatively easy for physicians to adapt abdominal examination into clinical practice, as even uneducated persons could become adept at diagnosing and treating conditions without the need to understand the complex dialectic classification of syndrome diagnosis in TCM.

The popularity of the practice can be seen by the number of works published on the subject: According to the *Classification of Reference Books on the Abdominal Diagnostics* (Jp: *Fukushinsho No Bunrui* 腹診書の分類) by Ōtsuka Keisetsu 大塚敬節, at least fifty works on abdominal examination from authors belonging to various schools of Kampō were published during the Edo and Meiji 明治 (1868–1912 CE) periods. Of these, the works of Yoshimasu Tōdō 吉益東洞 (1702–1773 CE), perhaps the most influential physician of the Ancient (Antiquity) School (Jp: *kohō-ha* 古方派) of Kampō medicine, and Inaba Bunrei 稲葉文禮 (date of birth unknown–1805 CE), the author of the present work, have been considered to be the most authoritative works on abdominal diagnosis in Japan. Whereas Yoshimasu was a prolific writer and his life is well documented, the life of Inaba is shrouded in mystery, and most of the information that we have concerning his life comes from the author's own introduction to the present work. For this reason, I will omit the details concerning his life in this prolegomenon.

Concerning the Translation, Text, and Commentary

With regard to the translation of the present work, I have followed the three-facet theory of translation of the influential translator Yán Fù 嚴復 (1854 – 1921 CE) to improve the accessibility of Chinese/Japanese cultural concepts to Western audiences. That is, I have aimed for a translation that is faithful (Ch: *xìn* 信), expressive (Ch: *dá* 達), and elegant (Ch: *yǎ* 雅). Because it is impossible to always maintain a perfect balance among these three elements, I have generally erred on the side of literal translation instead of dynamic equivalence. Furthermore, although most traditional Chinese/Japanese medical terms have been translated into English by a number of excellent scholars, there is still no consensus concerning which translation set is the most appropriate, and many translated classical works are inconsistent in the use of terminology. Therefore, in order to ensure the uniform translation of these medical terms, I have generally followed the translations found in Nigel Wiseman's *A Practical Dictionary of Chinese Medicine*, with supplements from various sources such as Zhu-fan Xie's *Classified Dictionary of Traditional Chinese Medicine* and the works of eminent sinologists such as James Legge and Paul Unschuld. Finally, for transliteration of proper nouns and so-called "untranslatable" concepts, I have a utilized a modified Hepburn Romanization scheme for Japanese and pinyin Romanization for Chinese.

Concerning the original text itself, with the exception of the author's preface, which was written in literary Chinese (Ch: *wén yán wén* 文言文; Jp: *kambun* 漢文), this work was originally written in classical/literary Japanese (Jp: *bungotai* 文語體), the standard written language of premodern Japan. This language is largely based on literary Chinese, and due to the high number of Chinese characters that are used, readers familiar with Chinese should be able to follow the original text to a certain extent. The author occasionally quotes some phrases in classical Chinese in the main text, but these phrases have been written in *kakikudashibun* 書き下し文 as they were intended to be read by Japanese speakers and the original Chinese phrases are noted in the commentary.

As is common with all pre-modern East Asian texts, the original text of this work contains many nonstandard, variant, and simplified characters (*zokuji* 俗字, *itaiji* 異體字, and *ryakuji* 略字, respectively), which I have changed to standard traditional characters (*seiji* 正字) as necessary in order to facilitate the understanding of modern readers and due to the limitations of modern fonts. Although it is common in Japan to use Japanese simplified characters (*shinjitai* 新字體) in modern reprintings of classical texts, I have purposely maintained the original traditional Chinese characters, so that students of Chinese medicine who are familiar with the traditional characters will be able to follow the Japanese text. Moreover, I have left the traditional *kana* usage (Jp: *kana-zukai* 假名遣ひ) intact, while making minor formatting changes such as changing the *katakana* 片假名 to *hiragana* 平假名 and adding *okurigana* 送り假名 and punctuation marks where necessary to improve the overall readability. The text appears to include a number of erroneous characters, which I have generally left unchanged in order to preserve the integrity of the original text so that specialists make decide for themselves the proper reading. Unfortunately, due to certain limitations, I was unable to attach *furigana* 振り假名 to the Japanese text. While it is understandable that many students and native speakers of Japanese would appreciate a pronunciation guide of uncommon Chinese characters used in the work, it is my sincere hope that the copious notes on relevant medical, linguistic, historical, and cultural information in the commentary will assist readers with no knowledge of the history of Kampō medicine to understand the appropriate reading and usage of such difficult terms.

It should also be noted that because the work was originally designed to be an easy-to-use clinical manual for medical practitioners to select an appropriate formula for treatment of a given condition presented by a patient, little reference is made to classical Chinese/Japanese medical theory, and there is little discussion regarding exact anatomical landmarks. Therefore, I have included the modern drug indications established by the Japanese Ministry of Health, Labor and Welfare (MHLW), many of which were influenced by the abdominal findings of Yoshimasu, Inaba, and Wakuda, so that the reader can better understand the influence of this work on modern Kampō medicine and select appropriate formulae that have stood the test of time with regard to efficacy, safety, etc.

It is my sincerest hope that this book will be useful to many Western practitioners of traditional Oriental medicine and those interested in the history of Japanese medicine.

To my knowledge, this is the first translation of the work into a Western language, and the first modern reprinting in which the original text is presented in its entirety without any edit of the content. Therefore, I take full responsibility if the work contains any mistakes in the Japanese text or mistranslations and await a more experienced translator to improve upon the rough translation provided here.

All questions, comments, and suggestions from readers are welcomed so that the follow-up work will be even more useful to clinicians who wish to incorporate Japanese abdominal examination in clinical practice.

Without the support of a number of individuals and organizations, including the Chinese Medicine Database, the completion of this translation project would not have been possible. I am especially indebted to Dr. San-pao Li 李三寶, who shared with me the joy of classical Chinese language and culture, and Dr. Ikeda Shūzō 池田秀三, who for better or worse, instilled in me a respect for the importance of an empirical approach to textual criticism (Ch: *kǎo zhèng xué* 考證學; Jp: *kōshōgaku*).

Jay Kageyama
(影山慈英)

自序
Author's Preface[1]

Chinese: 古人有言曰、短綆不可以汲深井、信矣、如不佞、何以足知此道之深底乎、雖然、歲月之所畜、日夜之所積、與門人二三子復言之、

Japanese: 古人、言有りて曰く、「短綆は以て深井を汲む可からず」と、信なり。不佞が如き、何を以てか此の道の深底を知るに足らんや。然りと雖も、歲月のふる所、日夜の積む所、門人二三子のために復た之れを言はん。

An ancient person once said, "One cannot draw [spring water] from a deep well by using a short rope." This saying is indeed true.[2] How could someone as unskilled as I hope to understand the profundities of this way [of abdominal examination]? Being that as it may, I shall once again pass on to you, my pupils, what I have learned during my training day and night over many years.

Ch: 克幼而孤、及長放蕩無賴、常徘徊于京攝之間、鄙夫野人之所爲、大人君子之所惡、無一所不爲焉、

Jp: 克、幼にして孤なり、長ずるに及びて放蕩無頼、常に京・攝の間に徘徊し、鄙夫野人の爲す所、大人君子の惡む所、一も爲さざる所無し。

---

1. The preface was written in literary Chinese (Ch: *wén yán wén* 文言文, Jp: *kambun* 漢文), a practice that was common until the middle of the 20th century. The text included *kunten* 訓點 (guiding marks for rendering Chinese into Japanese), written to the side of the original Chinese text. Therefore, I have added the Japanese text (Jp: *kakikudashibun* 書き下し文) indicating how it was to be read by Japanese speakers.

2. This is found in "Chapter IV: On Honor and Disgrace [Ch: *Róng Rǔ* 榮辱; Jp: *Eijoku*]" of *Xún Zǐ*《荀子》(Jp: *Junshi*). The original text and translation are as follows: "短綆不可以汲深井之泉、知不幾者不可與及聖人之言" (One who has a rope that is too short cannot draw [spring water] from a deep well. One who has insufficient knowledge cannot plumb [the profundity] of the sages' words).

I, Katsu, was orphaned as a small child. As I grew up, I became more and more dissolute and unruly, ruining myself by leading a wanton life. I spent my days wandering the region stretching from the capital [i.e., Kyōto] to Settsu and performing all manner of vulgar and unrefined deeds, ones that any gentlemen would find contemptible.[3]

Ch:適有感於友人之言、而欲學醫、然素目不知書、耳不聞文、唯周流于四方、踵名家高門以求得其方法、曩游于浪萃、師事鶴泰榮先生、

Jp:たまたま友人の言に感ずる有りて、醫を學ばんと欲す。然かれどももと目、書を知らず。耳、文を聞かず。唯だ四方に周流して、名家高門にいたり、以て其の方法を得ることを求むるのみ。さきに浪華に游び、鶴泰榮先生に師事す。

One day, I was inspired by the advice of my friend and decided to study medicine. However, my eyes had never read any type of book. My ears had never heard any sort of teaching.[4] I traveled far and wide in every direction [across Japan], searching out the most renowned and talented [physicians] to learn the techniques [of medicine]. I finally traveled to Naniwa,[5] where I studied as an apprentice under my sensei, Kaku Taiei.[6]

Ch:先生曰、汝性頑愚、頗愶鄙倍、且年已長、欲教以文字、令讀古人之書、恐不可終以期其成、我教汝以診腹之事乎、汝亦不顧佗、夙夜講明以爲治療、

Jp:先生曰く、「汝が性、頑愚にして頗る鄙倍なるを愶り、且つ年すでに長ず。教ふるに文字を以てし、古人の書を讀ましめんと欲するも、恐らくは終に以てその成るを期すべからざらん。我、汝

3. Settsu Province, located next to Kyōto, (Jp: *Settsu-No-Kuni* 攝津國) today comprises the eastern part of Hyōgo Prefecture and the northern part of Ōsaka Prefecture.

4. Based on this passage and comments made by Wakuda Yoshitora 和久田叔虎 in *Fukushō-Kiran-Yoku*《腹證奇覽翼》(The Wings to Extraordinary Views of Abdominal Patterns), it has been traditionally assumed that Inaba was functionally illiterate, and asked his pupils to act as scribes to write down his findings in this work. However, his ability to quote from a wide range of Chinese classics in this work suggests that either he was in fact a humble man of erudition, or that his pupils made substantial additions to the oral teachings of the author.

5. Naniwa 浪華 (also written as 浪速, 難波, or 浪花) is the central district of Ōsaka City.

6. As explained in the text, Kaku Taiei 鶴泰榮 (dates of birth and death unknown) is the mentor of the source of many of the formulae found in this work. However, no information is available concerning his life other than what is written here.

を教ふるに診腹の事を以てせんか。汝も亦た佗を顧みず、夙夜講明し、以て治療を爲せ」と。

[When we met,] my sensei said to me, "I am afraid that not only are you obstinate and foolish, but [your behavior is also] extremely coarse and vulgar. Moreover, you are already well advanced in years. Although I desire to teach you through writing and have you read the books written by the ancients, I fear that you would never become a full-fledged [physician. For this reason,] I shall teach you the art of abdominal examination. You must not divert your attention to other matters. You must train day and night to elucidate [abdominal patterns] in order to perform medical treatment."

Ch: 古有言、病之所根在腹、探以知其壅滯、

Jp: 古へに言有り、「病の根ざす所は腹に在り、探りて以て其の壅滯を知れ」と。

"The ancients had a saying: Diseases reside in the abdomen. Hence, [the physician] must search [the abdomen] to find the [regions of] congestion and stagnation."[7]

Ch: 古謂之診尺、以自鳩尾至臍一尺也、

Jp: 古へのこれを「診尺」と謂ふは、鳩尾より臍に至るまで一尺なるを以てなり。

"The reason why the ancients called this [method] 'cubit examination' is because the distance from *jiū wěi* 鳩尾 (CV-15) to the umbilicus is one cubit."[8]

Ch: 《靈樞》論疾診尺篇曰、黄帝問於歧伯曰、余欲無視色持脉、獨調其尺、以言其病、從外知内、爲之奈何、歧伯曰、審其尺、緩急小大滑澀、肉之堅脆、而病形定矣、

---

7. This philosophy of treatment was shared by other members of the Ancient School (Jp: *kohō-ha* 古方派). Yoshimasu Tōdō 吉益東洞 (1702–1773 CE) had a similar phrase: 腹者有生之本、故百病根於此焉、是以診病必候其腹、外證次之。(The abdomen is the root of life; thus, the hundred diseases take root therein. For this reason, examination of diseases must [involve] examination of the abdomen. The external signs are secondary).

8. The exact length of the cubit (Ch: *chǐ* 尺; Jp: *shaku*) differed depending on the region and era in which it was used; the length generally ranged from 23 to 35 cm.

Jp:『靈樞』「論疾診尺篇」に曰く、「黄帝、歧伯に問ひて曰く、『余、色を視、脉を持ること無く、ひとり其の尺のみを調べ、以て其の病を言ひ、外より内を知らんと欲す。これを爲さんにいかんせん』と。歧伯曰く、『其の尺の緩急・小大・滑澀、肉の堅脆を審らかにすれば、而ち病形定まるなり』」と。

"In the Chapter on *Understanding Sickness by Examination of the Cubit Skin*[9] of *Líng Shū*,[10] it states, 'The Yellow Emperor asked Qí Bó: I wish to examine only the cubit [skin of patients], without looking at their [facial] complexion or feeling their pulses, in order to be able to diagnose their diseases and know the inside [of the patients] by [looking at] the outside [patterns]. What should I do? Qí Bó responded: Examine the cubit to check if the pulse is relaxed or tense, small or great, and slippery or rough. If [the physician] elucidates whether the flesh is hard and brittle, the form of the disease can be decided.'"

Ch:又《内經》曰、尺内兩傍、則季脇也、

Jp:又た『内經』に曰く、「尺内の兩傍、則ち季脇なり」と。

"Furthermore, the [*Huáng Dì*] *Nèi Jīng*[11] states: 'both sides of the cubit [skin] are the free rib [regions].'"[12]

Ch:又按脉動靜、循尺滑澁寒溫之意、視其大小、合之病態、

Jp:又た按ずるに、脉の動靜、尺の滑澁・寒溫の意に循ひ、其の大小を視、之れを合して病態とす。

"I believe that by comprehensively evaluating if the pulse is stirring or tranquil, if the cubit is slippery or rough, cold or warm, great or small, [the physician can elucidate] the pathology [of any disease]."[13]

9. Ch: *Lùn Jí Zhěn Chǐ*《論疾診尺》; Jp: *Ron-Shitsu-Shin-Shaku*, Chapter 18.

10. Jp: *Reisū*; The Magic Pivot.

11. Jp: [*Kōtei-*]*Daikei*; [The Yellow Emperor's] Inner Canon.

12. This is found in Treatise of the Essential Subtleties of the Pulse (Ch: *Sù Wèn, Mài Yāo Jīng Wēi Lùn*《素問·脈要精微論》; Jp: *Somon-Myakuyō-Seibi-Ron*) Plain Questions, Chapter 17. The original text is as follows: "尺内兩傍、則季脅也、尺外以候腎、尺裏以候腹中... The inside of the cubit [skin], on both sides, this is [the region of] the free ribs. The exterior of the cubit serves to examine the kidneys; the interior of the foot-long section serves to examine the abdomen...."

13. As explained in the section for *Dà Huáng Huáng Lián Xiè Xīn Tāng* 大黄黄連瀉心湯, the

Ch:且古人言疾、必言腹心、

Jp:且つ古人、疾を言ふに、必ず腹心を言ふ。

"Moreover, when the ancients spoke of any disease, they invariably spoke of the abdomen as the 'heart' [of the disease]."

Ch:然則診腹之於治療、莫先於斯、令我所知、悉授汝、冀篤志明辨、以救疾病、爲涯之任焉、

Jp:然らば則ち、診腹の治療に於けるは、斯れより先なるは莫し。今、我の知る所を悉く汝に授く。冀くは篤志明辨して、以て疾病を救ひ、生涯の任と爲よ」と。

"If this is true, then there is nothing more important than abdominal examination in treating [patients]. I shall pass on everything that I know to you. It is my hope that you will use your devotion [to medicine] and discernment [in diagnosis] and regard saving [patients from] diseases as your life's work."

Ch:克謹奉教、游歷諸國、每遇病客、沈思苦慮、或從宿儒老醫問之、或與學生小子論之、

Jp:克、謹みて教をうけ、諸國を游歷し、病客に遇ふ每に、沈思苦慮し、或るときは宿儒老醫に從ひてこれを問ひ、或るときは學生小子とともに之れを論ず。

I humbly received his instruction, [and subsequently] traveled around various provinces [as an itinerant physician]. Each time that I encountered an ailing patient, I contemplated deeply and racked my brain [to find the appropriate treatment]. In some cases, I went to inquire of experienced scholars [of medicine] or old physicians concerning treatment, and in other cases I discussed [the cases] with my pupils.

Ch:克謹奉教、游歷諸國、每遇病客、沈思苦慮、或從宿儒老醫問之、或與學生小子論之、壬子歲、游于甲州、登富嶽、而失塗投宿于黑川里之禪院、幸獲知足齋遺書奇方十九、

---

author seemed to consider that the radial-arterial pulse regions form a microcosm of the abdomen, which is itself a microcosm of the entire body.

Jp: みづのえねのとし、甲州に游び、富嶽に登りて、塗を失し、黒川の里の禪院に投宿して、幸ひにして知足齋の遺書『奇方十九』を獲たり。

In the *rén zǐ* year [of the sexagenary cycle, i.e., 1792 CE],[14] I traveled to Kōshū and climbed Mount Fuji.[15] [During the trek,] I lost my way and ended up taking refuge in a Zen [Buddhist] temple, where I was fortunate enough to obtain [a copy of] the testament of Chisokusai,[16] that is, *Kihō-Jiku*《奇方十九》.[17]

Ch: 益精研究皦、而得六十餘方之腹候、痼病篤疾往往而愈、

Jp: ますます精研究皦して、六十餘方の腹候を得、痼病・篤疾往々にして愈ゆ。

[Having obtained the text,] I continued my painstaking research all the more. After elucidating more than sixty different abdominal patterns, [I found that] all manner of long-standing illnesses and critical diseases were often cured [through correct abdominal diagnosis].

Ch: 既傳門人二三子、亦有所發明、能相助以成業、屢請上之梓、然克感往年東都鳳山子之忠告、而未之允也、

Jp: 既にして門人二三子に傳ふ。亦た發明する所有りて、能く相助けて以て業を成し、屢々之れを梓に上さんことと請ふ。然れども克、往年東都鳳山子の忠告に感じて、未だ之れをよしとせざるなり。

I transmitted [the fruits of my studies] to my pupils, [but they] often pleaded with me to publish my findings, which may be useful in assisting [physicians] in clinical practice.

14. *Rén zǐ* 壬子 (Jp: *mizunoene* or *jinshi*) is the forty-ninth year of the traditional sixty-year calendar cycle.

15. Kōshū 甲州 is the abbreviated name of Kai Province (Jp: *Kai-No-Kuni* 甲斐國), the region of Japan that currently comprises Yamanashi Prefecture (Jp: *Yamanashi-Ken* 山梨縣).

16. As explained in the section for *Xiǎo Chái Hú Tāng* 小柴胡湯, Chisokusai 知足齋 is the pen name of Nagata Tokuhon 永田德本.

17. *Kihō-Jiku*《奇方十九》(Nineteen Extraordinary Prescriptions) is an alternate name of *Tokuhon-Ō-Jūku-Hō*《德本翁十九方》(Nineteen Prescriptions of the Venerable Tokuhon), a text that is heavily referenced in this work.

However, still being impressed by the admonishment of Master Hōzan of the eastern capital [i.e., Edo] that I had received many years ago, I refused [at that time].[18]

Ch:乙卯之歲、來游京師、欲以此診術、博施諸海內、

Jp:きのとうの歲、京師に來游し、此の診術を以て、ひろくこれを海内に施さんと欲す。

In the *yǐ mǎo* year [of the sexagenary cycle, i.e., 1785], I traveled to the capital region [i.e., Kyōto], where I desired to widely propagate this method of abdominal examination in Japan.[19]

Ch:然京師四方輻湊之地、其諸君子皆俊才博識、固富文字、又優于言行、如克不才薄行者、不能一歷其眼路、

Jp:然れども京師四方輻湊の地にして、其の諸君子皆、俊才博識にして、固より文字に富み、又た言行に優なり。克が如き不才薄行の者、一も其の眼路にふること能はず。

However, the entire capital region was filled with physicians who were highly talented and erudite; being well read, they were all eloquent and behaved elegantly. They would not take a single look at a person such as I, who was [considered to be] incompetent and had crude behavior.

Ch:適會有一二門生相羽翼、至丁巳之春、療數十病客、雖有間奏其効、或畏攻擊過多、或侮言貌鄙俗、於此克不欲久止、暫待暖和之時、

Jp:たまたま一、二の門生有りて、相羽翼するに會して、ひのとみの春、數十病客を療し、まま其の効を奏すること有りと雖も、或るひは攻擊の過多を畏れ、或るひは言貌の鄙俗を侮る。ここに於いて、克、久しく止むることを欲せず、暫く暖和の時を待つ。

18. There is no available information concerning Hōzan.

19. *Yǐ mǎo* 乙卯 (Jp: *kinotō* or *itsubō*) is the fifty-second year of the traditional sixty-year calendar cycle.

Supported by my pupils, by the spring of the *dīng sì* year [of the sexagenary cycle; i.e., 1797 CE] I had successfully treated several dozens of patients, who all made a recovery.[20] Nevertheless, I [continued to] fear the vicious attacks [of the physicians of Kyōto] and their insults regarding my uncouth speech and vulgar manner. Although I did not wish to cease [treating patients] for a long while, I temporarily waited for an easing [of the situation].

Ch: 而不幸遇疾、羅子半身不遂之患、乃令門生詳診之、攻以數方、累日而覺愉快、

Jp: しかるうち不幸にして疾に遇ひ、半身不遂の患にかかる。すなはち門生をして之れを詳診せしめ、攻るに數方を以てし、累日にして愉快を覺ゆ。

During that period, I had the misfortune of experiencing a disease that left me hemiplegic. I then asked my pupils to examine me. They attacked [the disease] using several formulae, and I made a full recovery after several days.

Ch: 而克居常有嗜酒之癖、病少間、則不堪寂寞欝悶、故態復發、門人親戚雖痛誡之、舊僻遂難改、得而失者數次、

Jp: しかるに克、居常・嗜酒の癖あり。病、少間にして、則ち寂寞欝悶に堪へず。故にさま復た發す。門人・親戚、之れを痛誡すと雖も、舊僻、遂に改め難く、得て失すること數次なりき。

However, I was a habitual drinker of alcohol. Within a short period, I experienced [feelings of] loneliness and oppressive depression that were unbearable. For this reason, [my] previous [condition] recurred. My pupils and family members made strong emotional appeals for me [to stop drinking], but old habits are difficult to break, and I repeated the same cycle a number of times.

Ch: 今春再苦因鋭意誓於鬼神、毀盃碎瓶、益攻以藥劑、累日復故、

20. *Dīng sì* 丁巳 (Jp: *hinotomi* or *teishi*) is the fifty-fourth year of the traditional sixty-year calendar cycle.

Jp:今春再び苦しみ、因りて鋭意、鬼神に誓ひ、盃をやぶり瓶を砕きて、ますます攻むるに藥劑を以てす。累日にして故に復す。

In the spring of this year, I once again experienced [a bout of] suffering. I made a solemn vow to the gods [to cease drinking] and having broken my sake cups and destroyed my bottles [of alcohol], I focused on attacking [my disease] using medicinals all the more. After a number of days, I returned to normal.

Ch:於是乎欲事游歷、廣施其功、開發其所未知、終以身委于溝壑、冀可以長其短綆、而汲其深井、且死于道路、謝于薄行之罪、竊詢諸門生宗輔、

Jp:是に於いて游歷を事とし、廣く其の功を施し、其の未だ知らざる所を開發せんと欲す。終に身を以て溝壑に委ぬるも、以て其の短綆を長じて其の深井を汲む可し、且つ道路に死するも、薄行の罪を謝せんことを冀ひ、竊かに諸れを門生宗輔にとふ。

I thereupon devoted myself to traveling [across Japan] and widely obtained success [in my practice] while desiring to elucidate the points that I did not understand. In order to lengthen my "short rope" to plumb the depths of the well [of medicine, I was willing to do whatever necessary,] even if it meant me finally ending up in a ditch, or even if it meant me dying in the street,[21] I would plead for forgiveness for my careless actions. I secretly inquired of my pupil Sōsuke concerning this.[22]

Ch:宗輔曰、先生性直術精矣、然其言行殆非京師之人、縱令先生留寓于京師、恐不能如素意、有美器而不成其用、實可惜哉、不如如先生之意、而遍傳於天下後世、以博濟篤癃沈痾、爲功之最大矣、

Jp:宗輔曰く、「先生、性直に術くわし。然れども其の言行は殆ど京師の人に非ず。たとひ先生をして京師に留寓せしむるとも、恐らくは素意の如くなること能はざらん。美器有るも其の用を成さ

---

21. This refers to an unbefitting death of a Confucian gentlemen. In the *Zǐ Hǎn* 子罕 (Jp: *Shi-Kan*) chapter of *Lún Yǔ*《論語》(Jp: *Rongo*; The Analects [of Confucius]) Confucius remarked: "且予縱不得大葬，予死於道路乎 And though I may not get a great burial, shall I die upon the road?"

22. There is no available information concerning this person.

ず、實に惜しむべきかな。先生の意の如くにして、遍く天下後世に傳へ、以て博く篤癃沈痾をすくひ、功を爲すの最も大なるには如かず」と。

Sōsuke said [to me:] "Sensei, you are honest [i.e., unpretentious] and well-acquainted with the techniques [for abdominal examination]. However, your speech and behavior are generally unbefitting a person from the capital. Even if you remained in the capital region, you would most likely be unable to freely [treat patients] in accordance with your original intention. [You] can be compared to a beautiful receptacle that remains unused: it is indeed a waste! It would be better to pass on [your knowledge] to younger generations in order [that they may] widely save [persons suffering from] severe and long-standing diseases, and obtain even greater success [than you]."

Ch: 克諾之於是錄此書、以授與焉、

Jp: 克、之れを諾し、是に於いて此の書を錄し、以て授與す。

I agreed to this and subsequently recorded [my knowledge in] this book in order to provide instruction [to physicians concerning abdominal examinations].

寛政己未初夏湖南稻葉克文禮識

Written in the early summer of the first year of the Kansei era, *jǐ wèi* year [of the sexagenary cycle; i.e., 1799] by Konan Inaba Katsu Bunrei.[23]

23. *Jǐ wèi* 己未 (Jp: *tsuchinotohitsuji* or *kibi*) is the fifty-sixth year of the traditional sixty-year calendar cycle.

Introduction

夫れ腹症を按ずるの法、まづ病人を平らかに臥さしめ、志氣を正しうせしめ、さて醫者も亦た平らかに坐し、呼吸をただし、志氣を臍下に收め、あたかも武夫の兵を執りて敵に向かふが如く。大病を怖れず、死生に眩せず、富貴に屈せず、貧賤を侮らず。その病敵を治して、その疾苦を救はんと、心を專一にして、診察すべし。是れ疾醫、病者を診察するの大法なり。

The method to palpate abdominal patterns is to first ask the patient lie supine and make his mind qì right. The physician must then also sit straight and correct his [own] breathing, while focusing his mind qì on his subumbilical region. It is similar to a warrior who takes his sword and faces an enemy. [Such a physician] does not fear any major illnesses. He is not blinded by life or death. He does not yield to riches or nobility. He does not scorn the poor or those of low rank. The physician must perform examinations while keeping his mind focused on the goal of curing the disease and of removing suffering. This is the great method of physicians to examine patients.

凡そ腹症を候ふの法、右のごとく。病者に臨み、まづ右手の掌を徐かに胸心へあて、一息して呼吸を定め靜かにし、こころをしづめて、胸膈の毒をうかがふ。中央より診して左右にをよぶ。而して後、心下へやはらかに指を下して、三指(食指、中指、無名指)の頭にて按ずべし。次に肋骨のはしへ指頭をかかげ入れて、苦滿の有無をうかがひ、次に腹中。次に左右の小腹。次に臍穴。次に左右の臍傍。次に臍下と順々に診察すべし。これ診腹の次第なり。かくのごとくにして後、外證を察し諸患の有無を問ふべし。

The general method to examine abdominal patterns is as follows: While facing the patient, the physician must first slowly and softly stretch out his right palm and place it on the patient's chest. [He will] then take a deep breath to stabilize his breathing and quiet his mind, and then examine the chest and diaphragm for [the presence of] any toxins. Starting from the center, he will then examine the left and right sides. After that, he should softly lower his fingers and palpate the region below the heart using the tips of three fingers (the forefinger, the middle finger, and the ring finger). He should then feel up along the edges of the ribs with his fingertips to examine for the presence or absence of bitter fullness, and after that feel the middle of the abdomen. Next, he should feel the smaller abdomen on the left and right sides. Next is the umbilicus. Next are the left and right sides of the umbilicus. Next is the subumbilical region. This is the order in which the abdominal examination should follow. After having done like this, [the physician] should inspect the external signs of the patient and inquire if the patient is suffering from any type of disease.

Translator's Note Regarding Kampō Medicine

Note: In modern Japan, as with all pharmaceutical products, Kampō drugs are strictly regulated by the MHLW and are generally classified as Schedule II pharmaceuticals (Jp: *dainirui-iyakuhin* 第二類醫藥品). Of the thousands of traditional Chinese/Japanese formulae that have been developed over the centuries, 294 are currently approved to be sold over the counter in a drug store/pharmacy by a pharmacist (Jp: *yakuzaishi* 藥劑師) or registered pharmaceutical distributor (Jp: *tōroku-hanbaisha* 登錄販賣者) licensed by the MHLW. Furthermore, 148 of the aforementioned Kampō drugs may be covered by the National Health Insurance system when prescribed by a physician (Jp: *ishi* 醫師) or dentist (Jp: *shikaishi* 齒科醫師) in accordance with the indications set forth by the MHLW.

桂枝湯之證

The Pattern for Guì Zhī Tāng[24] 桂枝湯

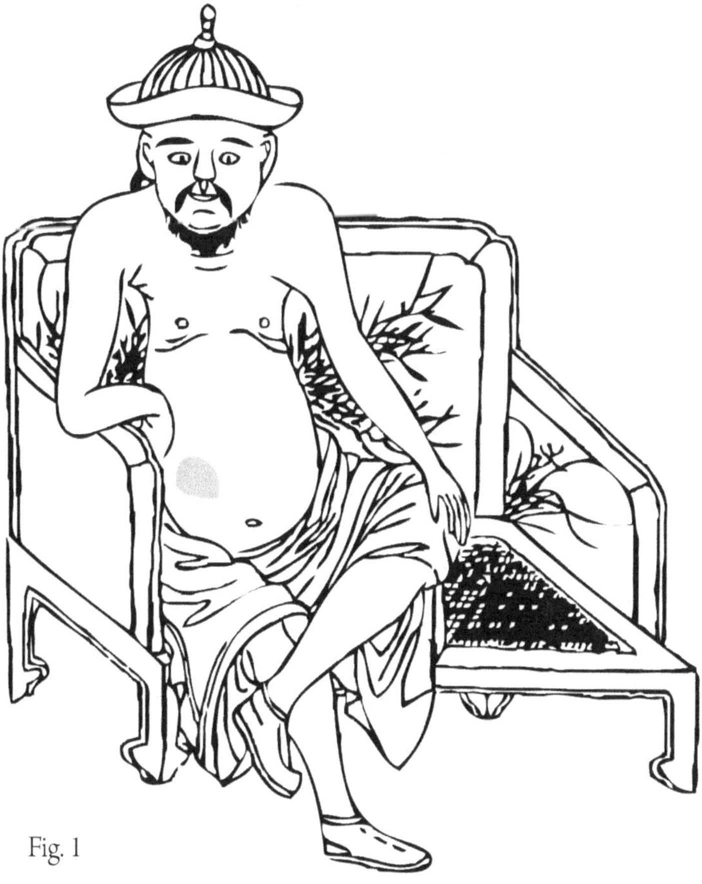

Fig. 1

24. The formula for *Guì Zhī Tāng* 桂枝湯 (Jp: *Keishi-Tō*; cinnamon twig decoction) was originally found in *Shāng Hán Lùn*《傷寒論》(Jp: *Shō-Kan-Ron*; On Cold Damage) and *Jīn Guì Yào Lüè*《金匱要略》(Jp: *Kinki-Yōryaku*; Essential Prescriptions of the Golden Coffer). The extract preparation of the formula is covered by the Japanese National Health Insurance program as a prescription drug, and is also commonly sold in Japanese drug stores as an over-the-counter drug. It is currently indicated by the Japanese Ministry of Health, Labour and Welfare (MHLW; Jp: *Kōsei-Rōdō-Shō* 厚生勞働省) for the following symptoms: initial stages of the common cold in persons with weak physical strength who are experiencing sweating (體力虛弱で、汗が出るものの次の症狀：かぜの初期).

此の證、腹滑にして、底までもこたゆるものなく、圖のごとく、只だ拘攣あり。所謂臟佗病無し。上衝・發熱・頭痛・有汗・惡風する者は、桂枝湯を用ゆる也。拘攣せざる者は、去芍藥湯を用ゆるなり。拘攣劇しき者は、加芍藥湯を用ゆるなり。

In this pattern, the abdomen is slippery and does not spring back,[25] even [when pressed deeply] to the depths [of the abdomen]. As shown in the illustration, the patient presents with only hypertonicity.[26] It is the case of what is called having no other disease in the viscera. When the patient has upward surging [of qì], fever, headache, sweating, or chills, use *Guì Zhī Tāng*.[27,28] When there is no hypertonicity, use [*Guì Zhī*] *Qù Sháo Yào Tāng*.[29] In cases when the hypertonicity is severe, use [*Guì Zhī*] *Jiā Sháo Yào Tāng*.[30]

此の三方を合はせみれば、「上衝」と「拘攣」との二つ。此の症の準據たること知るべし。故に腹證を知らんと欲せば、まづ準據とするところの字義を味はひ考ふべし。「衝」は「突」也、「向」也。毒の頭上へ突き上がるなり。「拘」は物去り手能く之れ

25. Springing back (Ch: *yìng* 應; Modern Jp: *kotaeru* こたえる; Old Jp: *kotayu* こたゆ) is an important concept in this book. The expression literally means "to respond," and refers to the quick rebounding feeling as the hand is released when palpating the abdomen.

26. Hypertonicity (Ch: *jū luán* 拘攣; Jp: *kōren*) is an important concept in this book. It refers to the abnormal stiffness and tension that manifests in inhibited normal bending and stretching of a region. In the case of abdominal hypertonicity, it refers to a cramping sensation or abdominal contracture.

27. For this book, we have decided to only include characters after Japanese names or formulas within the running text. A full list of the Japanese, Chinese, and English names can be found within the appendices.

28. Upward surging (Ch: *shàng chōng* 上衝; Jp: *jōshō*) is an important concept in this book. It refers the qì rising upward, causing a variety of problems such as hot flashes, dizziness, and palpitations.

29. *Guì Zhī Qù Sháo Yào Tāng* 桂枝去芍藥湯 (Jp: *Keishi-Kyo-Shakuyaku-Tō*; cinnamon twig decoction minus peony) is discussed separately in its own section in this book.

30. The details of *Guì Zhī Jiā Sháo Yào Tāng* 桂枝加芍藥湯 (Jp: *Keishi-Ka-Shakuyaku-Tō*; cinnamon twig decoction plus peony) are not explained in this book. This formula was originally found in *Shāng Hán Lùn*. The extract preparation of the formula is covered by the Japanese National Health Insurance program as a prescription drug, and may be sold in Japanese drug stores as an over-the-counter drug. It is currently indicated by the MHLW for: [what is known in Japan as] "strained abdomen," abdominal pain, diarrhea, and constipation in persons with moderate or weak physical strength who have a sense of fullness in the abdominal region. Note: strained abdomen (Jp: *shiburi-bara* 澀り腹) refers to the feeling of incomplete stool evacuation and repeated desire to defecate accompanied by abdominal pain [i.e., tenesmus] (體力中等度以下で、腹部膨滿感のあるものの次の諸症：しぶり腹、腹痛、下痢、便祕。しぶり腹とは、殘便感があり、くり返し腹痛を伴う便意を催すもののことである).

を止むるなり 。また「 擁 」なり 。「 攣 」は「 係攣 」なり 。縄を以て引きずりしばるなり 。然れば拘攣は毒のかかはりひきつるものなり 。

When these three formulae are matched together and compared, it can be known that the two indications for treatment of this pattern are upward surging (Ch: *shàng chōng* 上衝) and hypertonicity (Ch: *jū luán* 拘攣). Therefore, if [the physician] desires to understand abdominal patterns, he must first appreciate and consider the meaning of the words related to the indications for treatment. *Chōng* 衝 [i.e., the character for surging] means "thrusting." It also means "going toward [something]." [It is the case when] a toxin is thrust upward toward the top of the head. *Jū* 拘 [i.e., the first character of the word "hypertonicity"] means "[something] being restrained by the hands as it tries to depart." It also means "being embraced." *Luán* 攣 [i.e., the second character of the word "hypertonicity"] means "tying [something] up," as if tying something tightly with a rope. Thus, [the concept of] hypertonicity [refers to] the toxin pulling [the body] tightly.

これを診する法 、やはらかに指を下して 、腹中をいろひ探ぐるに 、指頭にあたりてかかはり引きつるものあり 。是れすなはち拘攣なり 。夫れ毒 、腹中にあり 、拘攣して上衝す 。是れ即ち桂枝湯の主治する所なり 。衝逆して毒 、心胸を過ぐるを以て 、嘔する氣味ある故 、方中 、生姜あり 。

The method to perform the examination is to softly lower the fingers and touch the middle of the abdomen with the fingertips and search for anything that feels pulled taut. This is hypertonicity. [It is the case] of a toxin existing in the middle of the abdomen, [causing] hypertonicity and upward surging. This is the indication for *Guì Zhī Tāng*. [In this pattern,] the patient presents with a surging counterflow, and a toxin that passes through the heart and chest, which tends to cause retching. Thus, *shēng jiāng* is included in the formula.

又た拘攣・上衝すれば 、攣引急迫も其のうちにこもりある故 、大棗・甘草あり 。是れこの諸藥各主治する所ありといへども 、壹に皆 、桂・芍二味に佐として 、拘攣・上衝の毒を治するものなり 。然れども拘攣のみにて 、上衝なければ 、此の方の證にあらざる故 、上衝をつかまへものにして 、「 上衝の者に桂枝湯を與ふ可し 」と『 傷寒論 』にもいへり 。これを「 方意を明らかにして 、毒の在る所を視る 」といふなり 。

Furthermore, when the patient presents with hypertonicity accompanied with upward surging, hypertonic tautness and distress will eventually reside [in the body]. Thus, *dà zǎo* and *gān cǎo* are included in the formula. Although each of these herbs have their own indications, [in this formula,] they all work as assistant [herbs] to support *guì zhī* and *sháo yào* in treating the hypertonicity and upward surging. However, when the patient presents with only hypertonicity, and no upward surging, this is not the pattern for this formula. Therefore, as it is written in the *Shāng Hán Lùn*, using upward surging as the indication [for treatment], "*Guì Zhī Tāng* may be given to the person with upward flushing."[31] This is known as "elucidating the decision to prescribe medicine by seeing the location of where the toxin exists."

右桂枝湯及び去芍藥、加芍藥の三方、此こに於いてもとむべし。その餘本方より去加の諸方も亦たみな桂・芍二味の證を主として、出入去加したるものなれば、只だ桂・芍二味の意を主として考ふべし。

The previously mentioned three formulae (consisting of *Guì Zhī Tāng* and the variants subtracting or adding *sháo yào*) should be sought after in any of these cases. Not only the standard preparation, but also all of the variant preparations use *guì zhī* and *sháo yào* as the principal flavors [that are matched] to the pattern. Thus, when leaving or entering the formula [i.e., initiating or terminating treatment], or when subtracting from or adding to the formula, [the physician] should only consider the meaning of *guì zhī* and *sháo yào* [when making decisions about treatment].

又た曰く、桂枝加桂枝、桂枝加皁莢、密傳あり、後篇に書す。懇請の人あらば傳ふべし。桂枝去芍藥湯も亦た腹候傳あり。

Furthermore, secret preparations of *Guì Zhī Jiā Guì Zhī* [*Tāng*] and *Guì Zhī Jiā Zào Jiá* [*Tāng*] also exist, which I shall write about in a later volume.[32] If there is any person who

31. As explained in the text, this formula was originally found in *Shāng Hán Lùn*, written by Zhāng Zhòngjǐng 張仲景 (Jp: Chō Chūkei; 150-219 CE) in the Latter *Hàn* (漢) dynasty (25–220 CE). It is the major textual basis for the classical school (Jp: *kohō-ha* 古方派) of Japanese Kampō medicine, which the author of this book and many other famous physicians of the Edo period such as Yoshimasu Tōdō 吉益東洞 belonged to. As a result, most of the formulae found in this book, as well as the majority of the formulae that are commonly used in Japan today, come from *Shāng Hán Lùn* or *Jīn Guì Yào Lüè*, another text written by Zhāng Zhòngjǐng that is heavily referenced in this work.

32. The author does not discuss the details of *Guì Zhī Jiā Guì Zhī Tāng* 桂枝加桂枝湯 (Jp:

makes an earnest request, I shall impart [the knowledge to him]. There is also a text that speaks of an abdominal pattern for *Guì Zhī Qù Sháo Yào Tāng.*

小柴胡湯之證

The Pattern for Xiǎo Chái Hú Tāng[33] 小柴胡湯

胸脇苦滿の毒淺薄なる者の圖也 。之れを按じて知るの傳 、圖の如く 。脇下肋骨の端を指頭にてかかげみるに 、こたゆるものあり 。是れ薄き苦滿の毒なり 。又た心下を按じて少しくこたゆるものなり 。是れ即ち痞鞕なり 。世に「 積聚 」と號するもの此の證多し 。

This is an illustration of a superficial toxin leading to bitter fullness in the chest and rib-sides.[34] It can be felt by palpating as shown in the illustration. When the region under the edges of the rib-sides is pressed with the fingertips, it will spring back. This is weak bitter fullness [caused by a] toxin. Moreover, when the region under the heart is palpated, it will spring back slightly. This is a case of glomus and hardness.[35] What are commonly called "accumulations and gatherings" are often examples of this pattern.

Keishi-Ka-Keishi-Tō; cinnamon twig decoction plus cinnamon twig) and *Guì Zhī Jiā Zào Jiá Tāng* 桂枝加皂莢湯 (Jp: *Keishi-Ka-Sōkyō-Tō*; cinnamon twig decoction plus gleditsia) in this work. At present, both formulae are not covered by the Japanese National Health Insurance program and are not commonly used in Japan.

33. The formula for *Xiǎo Chái Hú Tāng* 小柴胡湯 (Jp: *Shō-Saiko-Tō*, minor bupleurum decoction) was originally found in *Shāng Hán Lùn*. The extract preparation of the formula is covered by the Japanese National Health Insurance program as a prescription drug, and is also commonly sold in Japanese drug stores as an over-the-counter drug. It was, and continues to be, perhaps the most popular traditional Chinese drug prescribed by physicians in Japan. It is currently indicated by the MHLW for: loss of appetite, nausea, gastritis, stomach pain, gastrointestinal weakness, fatigue, and various symptoms of the later stages of the common cold in persons with moderate physical strength who often feel discomfort from the hypochondriac region of the abdomen to the solar plexus, have decreased appetite or a bitter taste in the mouth, and have white tongue fur. (體力中等度で 、ときに脇腹(腹)からみぞおちあたりにかけて苦しく 、食欲不振や口の苦味があり 、舌に白苔がつくものの次の諸症：食欲不振 、はきけ 、胃炎 、胃痛 、胃腸虛弱 、疲勞感 、かぜの後期の諸症狀).

34. Bitter fullness (Ch: *kǔ mǎn* 苦滿; Jp: *kuman*) is an important concept in this book. It refers to a bloated feeling in the chest and hypochondriac region.

35. Glomus and hardness (Ch: *pǐ yìng* 痞鞕; Jp: *hikō*) are important concepts in this book. The two words collectively refer to a feeling of stuffiness associated with local rigidity.

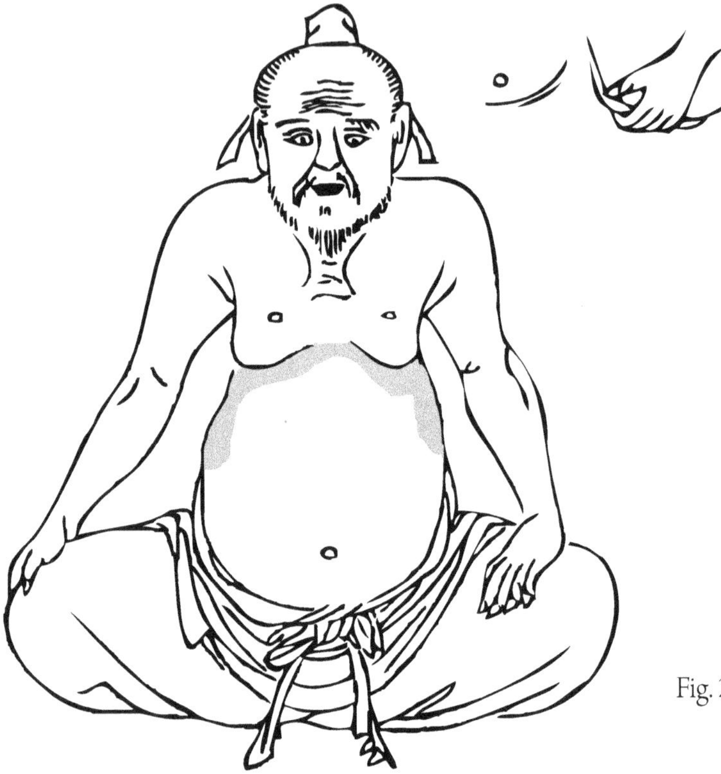

Fig. 2

凡そ腹症を按ずるに、毒の在る所厚深なるものは見易く、淺薄なるものは見難し。然れども又た毒淺薄なるが如くにして、大いに深きものあり。是れ毒腹底に在りて、悉く表に顯はれざるものなり。

When palpating the abdomen, it is easy to see the deep regions where the toxin resides, but difficult to see the superficial regions. However, there are cases in which the toxin appears superficial, yet it is extremely deep. These [cases] are due to a toxin that resides in the depths of the abdomen and does not completely appear on the exterior.[36]

これを攻むるときは、其の毒動いて表に顯はる其の時彌々本劑を投じて止まず。之れを攻むれば、或るひは寒熱往來、或るひは欝々として心煩するもの。是れ方症相對して瞑眩するなり。甚だし

36. The depths of the abdomen (Ch: *fù dǐ* 腹底; Jp: *fukutei*), literally, "the bottom of the abdomen," refer to the deepest part of the abdomen that can be felt when pressing deeply.

きものは、振々戰慄して却つて發熱・汗出・瘧狀の如く覺ゆるもの。是れ病毒去るの時なり。必ず恐惧すべからず。益々本劑を用ひて可なり。

The method to attack [the pattern] is to increasingly administer this formula without ceasing when the toxin moves and appears on the exterior. When attacking [the pattern], in some cases the patient may present with alternating heat [effusion, i.e., fever] and [aversion to] cold,[37] or in some cases, he may present with a depressive vexation of the heart.[38] This is the case of the formula matching the pattern,[39] causing dizziness [in the patient].[40] In severe cases, there is shuddering and even symptoms such as fever, sweating, and malaria-like symptoms. This is the toxin leaving the body. There is no need to fear it. [The physician] may continue to use this formula all the more.

又た其の外、世に所謂疫症、外邪の類、六氣の變に敗れ出でたるものは藥を用ひざる初めより、件の外症など、様々に顯はすもの

37. Alternating heat [effusion, i.e., fever] and [aversion to] cold (Ch: *hán rè wǎng lái* 寒熱往來; Jp: *kan-netsu-ōrai*) refers to chills without fever and fever without chills occurring in alternating succession.

38. Heart vexation (Ch: *xīn fán* 心煩; Jp: *shinhan*) refers to the feeling of restlessness, heat, and oppression in the region of the heart.

39. Formula-pattern matching or formula-pattern correspondence (Ch: *fāng zhèng xiāng duì* 方症相對; Jp: *hō-shō-sōtai*) is an extremely important concept in Kampō medicine that differentiates it from traditional Chinese medical (TCM) theory. In traditional Chinese medical (TCM) diagnostic theory, emphasis was placed on disease identification as the basis for determining treatment (Ch: *biàn bìng lùn zhì* 辨病論治; Jp: *benbyō-ronchi*), often through careful examination of the eight principles (Ch: *bā gāng* 八綱; Jp: *hachi-kō*). Although not all Japanese scholars rejected these theoretical underpinnings of TCM outright, they generally tended to focus on the use of a certain drug to treat a pattern of symptoms. Thus, many Japanese medical texts place little focus on a complex analysis of the pathogenesis of conditions (e.g., disorders of the *zàng-fǔ* organs, external contractions of the six excesses), but rather elucidate which drugs are effective for treating the manifested pathoconditions. Originally propagated by the Ancient School (Jp: *Kohō-Ha* 古方派), the formula-pattern matching system of diagnosis is now common to most schools of Kampō in Japan.

40. Dizziness (Ch: *míng xuàn* 瞑眩; Jp: *menken* or *mengen*) refers to the various symptoms (dizziness, headache, fever, diarrhea, fatigue, rash, etc.) that are experienced by the patient after treatment. The symptoms, which may last up to several days and cause severe discomfort in some cases, were believed to be caused by a pathotoxin leaving the body. In both Japan and China, it was often considered that such symptoms were signs that the treatment was successful. The earliest known use of the word as found in "Charge to Yue, Part I (Ch: *Yuè Mìng Shàng* 說命上; Jp: *Etsu-Mei-Jō*)" of *Shū Jīng* 《書經》 (Jp: *Shokyō*; Book of History) sums up the philosophy of many ancient physicians: "若藥弗瞑眩、厥疾弗瘳" (Unless the medicinal causes distress [i.e., dizziness] in the patient, his disease will not be cured by it).

あり。右の診法を詳らかにして胸脇苦満せば、かまはず此の方を投ずべし。外症に眩して妄りに方を轉ずることなかれ。

Furthermore, some patients present with various types of manifested external signs that were caused by damage [to the body] from before the drug was administered (i.e., damage that is due to what are commonly called epidemic pathoconditions, external evils, or transmutations of the six qì). If, after the above-mentioned method of examination, it is apparent that there is bitter fullness in the chest and rib-sides, this formula may be used without worry. Do not be blinded by the external signs and change the formula carelessly!

又た圖の如く、苦滿ありて心下痞鞕甚だしきものあり。此の時はまず苦滿をさし置きて、痞鞕より攻むべし。人參湯・桂枝人參湯の類、證を詳らかにしてこれを用ゆべし。

Furthermore, as shown in the illustration, there are cases of bitter fullness when severe glomus and hardness are present in the region below the heart. In these cases, [the physician] should first attack the glomus and hardness and leave the bitter fullness for later. After the pattern has been ascertained, [formulae] such as *Rén Shēn Tāng*[41] or *Guì Zhī Rén Shēn Tāng*[42] should be used.

41. *Rén Shēn Tāng* 人參湯 (Jp: *Ninjin-Tō*; ginseng decoction) is also known as *Richū-Gan* 理中丸 (Ch: *Lǐ Zhōng Wán*; center-rectifying pill) in Japan (it may also be found in powder or decoction form), albeit with a slightly different quantity of ingredients. The extract preparation of the formula is covered by the Japanese National Health Insurance program as a prescription drug, and is also commonly sold in Japanese drug stores as an over-the-counter drug. It is currently indicated by the MHLW for: gastrointestinal weakness, diarrhea, vomiting, stomach pain, abdominal pain, and acute or chronic gastritis in persons with weak physical strength who are easily fatigued or have cold extremities (體力虛弱で、疲れやすくて手足などが冷えやすいものの次の諸症：胃腸虛弱、下痢、嘔吐、胃痛、腹痛、急・慢性胃炎).

42. The formula for *Guì Zhī Rén Shēn Tāng* 桂枝人參湯 (Jp: *Keishi-Ninjin-Tō*; cinnamon twig and ginseng decoction) appears several times in this book, but is not discussed separately in its own section. This formula was originally found in *Shāng Hán Lùn*. The extract preparation of the formula is covered by the Japanese National Health Insurance program as a prescription drug, and is also commonly sold in Japanese drug stores as an over-the-counter drug. It is currently indicated by the MHLW for: headache, palpitations, chronic gastroenteritis, gastrointestinal weakness, diarrhea, and other digestive symptoms associated with the common cold in persons with weak physical strength who have poor digestion or experience occasional fever and chills (體力虛弱で、胃腸が弱く、ときに發熱・惡寒を伴うものの次の諸症：頭痛、動悸、慢性胃腸炎、胃腸虛弱、下痢、消化器症狀を伴う感冒).

是れのみに限らず、病人諸症あらば、まづ其の甚だしきものより攻むべし。若し甚だしきものなき時は、上より順に攻むべし、妄りに合方加減して、方法を改易すべからず。必ず功なきのみならず、却つて其の害多かるべし。之れを戒めよ。之れを戒めよ。

This [principle] is not only limited to these cases, but [applies] to any patient presenting any type of pattern [or symptoms]; the severe [symptoms] should be attacked first. If there are no severe [symptoms, the physician] should attack in order starting upward [i.e., the outer symptoms] and move down. He should not carelessly combine formulae, nor add or remove from the formulae, nor change the method [of treatment. Otherwise,] not only will there definitely be no success, but [such actions] will actually bring much harm [to the patient]. Be forewarned! Be forewarned!

凡そ此の症大率心煩あるものなり。即ち柴胡、或るひは人参の心煩なり。兼用は三黄丸、或るひは知足齋の解毒丸等、考へ用ゆ可し。

Generally speaking, patients with this pattern present with heart vexation. It is a type heart vexation that can be treated by *chái hú* or *rén shēn*. Concerning the simultaneous use of other formulae, [the physician] may consider using *Sān Huáng Wán*[43] or Chisokusai's *Gedoku-gan* 解毒丸 formula in combination [with this formula].[44]

43. The details of *Sān Huáng Wán* 三黄丸 (Jp: *San'ō-Gan*; three yellows pill) are discussed in the section concerning *Dāng Guī Sháo Yào Sǎn* 當歸芍藥散 (Jp: *Tōki-Shakuyaku-San*; Chinese angelica and peony powder).

44. Chisokusai 知足齋 is the pen name (Ch: *hào* 號; Jp: *gō*) of Nagata Tokuhon 永田德本 (1513–1630 CE), a famous physician of the late Warring States period and Edo period. *Gedoku-Gan* 解毒丸 (Ch: *Jiě Dú Wán*; toxin-resolving pill) and many of the other original Japanese formulae in this book were originally found in Nagata's most famous work, *Tokuhon-Ō Jūku Hō* 《德本翁十九方》(Nineteen Prescriptions of the Venerable Tokuhon), although the extant text is considered by many scholars to be a forgery. The formula for *Gedoku-Gan* as found in the received text of *Tokuhon-Ō Jūku Hō* is as follows: *dà huáng* (3 *qián*), *huáng lián*, *huáng qín* (2 *qián* each), [*shān*] *zhī zǐ* (1 *qián*). At present, this formula is not covered by the Japanese National Health Insurance program and is not well known in Japan.

小柴胡湯之證（胸肋肪脹）

The Pattern for Xiǎo Chái Hú Tāng 小柴胡湯 (for Distention in the Chest and Ribs)[45]

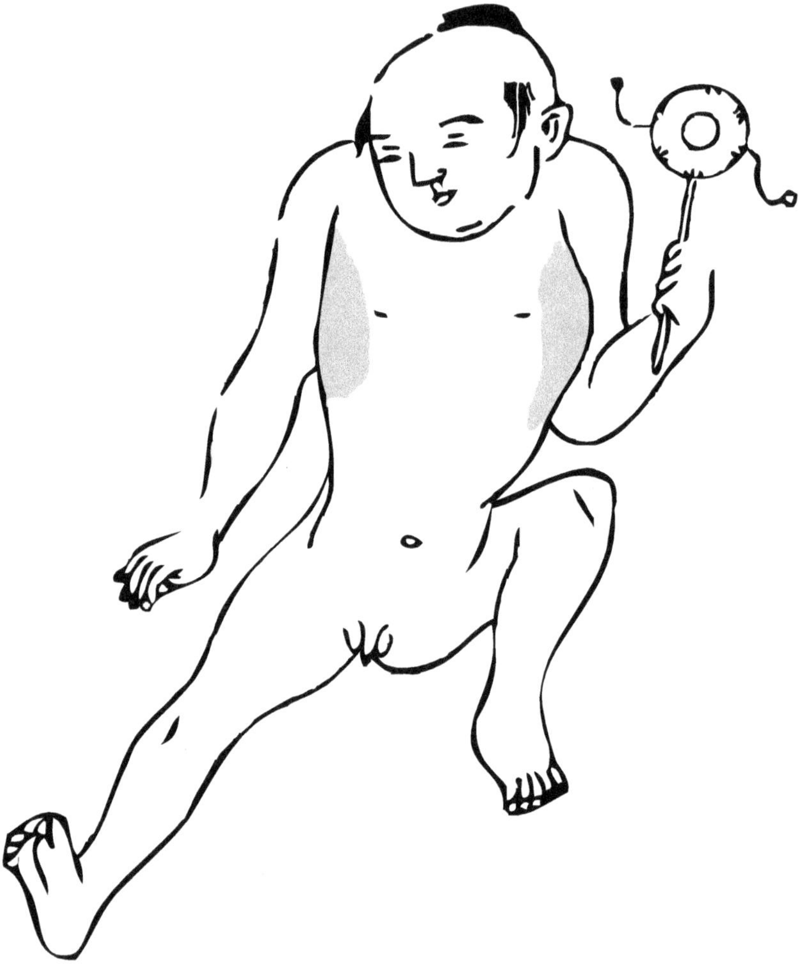

Fig. 3

圖の如く、苦滿・痞鞕見えずして、胸肋ふくれはりたるものなり。俗にこれを蝦蟆腹といふ。小兒に此の症多し。即ち此の方の症なり。外形を以て察すべし。若ししれがたきときは、指頭の横はらを以て肋骨の間をいろひ、をして見るべし。必ず痛むものなり。又た此の症に似て胸高くはり出でたる者あり。是れは大・小陷胸湯の症なり。誤るべからず。

45. This section discusses some of the other applications of *Xiǎo Chái Hú Tāng* 小柴胡湯 not mentioned in the previous section.

As shown in the illustration, some patients do not present with clear cases of bitter fullness or glomus and hardness, yet the chest and ribs are distended. This is popularly called "frog's belly." It is often seen in children, and is [also] a pattern [matched to] this formula. [The pattern] should be observable from the outward appearance [of the patient]. If [the pattern] is difficult to recognize, [the physician] should try to palpate the ribs using the sides of his fingertips to caress the spaces between the ribs; pain will definitely be present. There is also a pattern resembling this one, in which the patient presents with a distended chest and severe bulging. This is the pattern for either *Dà Xiàn Xiōng Tāng* or *Xiǎo Xiàn Xiōng Tāng*.[46] The patterns must not be mistaken!

又た胸肋膨脹して胸高く張り出でたるは、二證相合したる也。此の時は先づ小柴胡湯を用ひて後、時々陷胸丸を以て攻む可し。

There are two corresponding patterns in cases when the chest or ribs are distended and severe bulging is present. In these cases, *Xiǎo Chái Hú Tāng* should be used first, and after that [the symptoms] may be occasionally attacked with [*Dà*] *Xiàn Xiōng Wán*.[47]

若し又た胸肋膨脹結實して、解し難きものは鶴家の滅毒丸、知足齋の玉丹の類、考へ用ゆ可し。

In cases when the patient presents with distension in the chest or ribs and binding fullness that are [both] difficult to resolve, [the physician] may consider using the Kaku family's *Metsudoku-Gan*[48] or Chisokusai's *Gyoku-Tan*.[49]

---

46. *Dà Xiàn Xiōng Tāng* 大陷胸湯 (Jp: *Dai-Kankyō-Tō*; major chest bind decoction) and *Xiǎo Xiàn Xiōng Tāng* 小陷胸湯 (Jp: *Shō-Kankyō-Tō*; minor chest bind decoction) are discussed separately in their own section in this book.

47. In this text, *Dà Xiàn Xiōng Wán* 陷胸丸 (Jp: *Dai-Kankyō-Gan*; major chest bind pill) appears to be the same formula as *Dà Xiàn Xiōng Tāng* 大陷胸湯.

48. The details of *Metsudoku-Gan* 滅毒丸 (Ch: *Miè Dú Wán*; toxin-elimination pill) are not discussed in this work. Kaku Taiei 鶴泰榮 (dates of birth and death unknown) was the teacher of the author, and this formula appears to be a secret shared only with his family members and pupils. Hence, the exact ingredients are unknown.

49. The details of *Gyoku-Tan* 玉丹 (Ch: *Yù Dān*; jade elixir), originally found in *Tokuhon-Ō-Jūku-Hō* 《德本翁十九方》(Nineteen Prescriptions of the Venerable Tokuhon), are also not discussed in this work. According to the received text of *Tokuhon-Ō-Jūku-Hō*, the formula is as follows: *bā dòu*, *shuǐ yín* (5 *fēn* each), *dà huáng* (3 *qián*), *hēi qiān* [i.e., *hēi xī*], *shēng jiāng* (2 *fēn* each). However, as mentioned previously, many scholars are of the opinion that this text is a forgery, thus the veracity of formulae found in the text cannot be confirmed.

大柴胡湯之證

The Pattern for Dà Chái Hú Tāng[50] 大柴胡湯

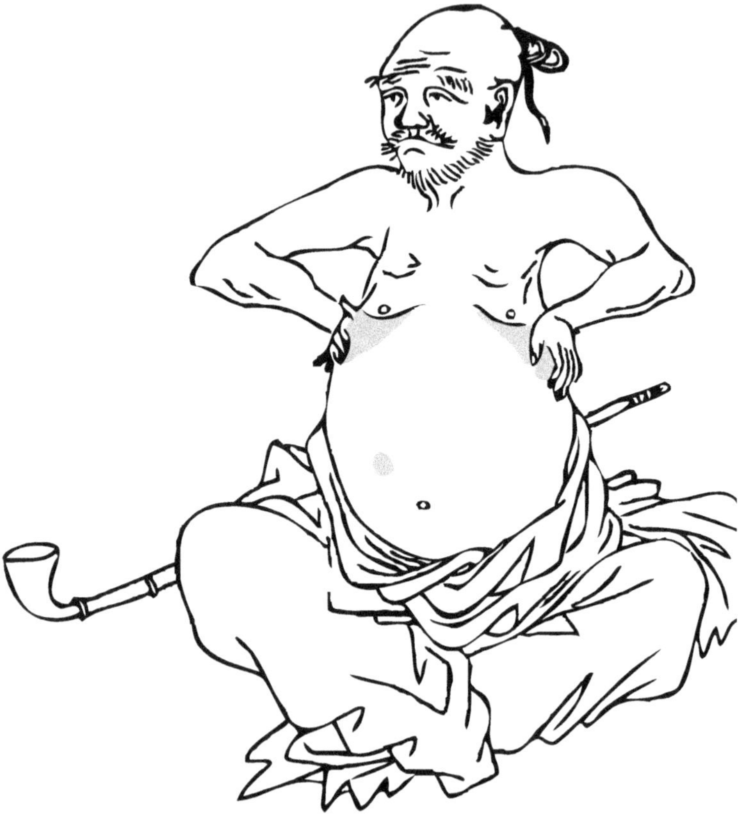

Fig. 4

圖のごとく、胸脇苦滿して、すこしく拘攣あり 。およそ拘攣は塊物とことなり 。指頭にすこしかかはりこたゆるものなり 。又た腹すこしく實滿して心下鞕せず、痞するばかりなり 。よくよく診して考ふべし 。前にいふ小柴胡湯は心下痞鞕ありて實滿なし 。これをもつて分別すべし 。

50. The formula for *Dà Chái Hú Tāng* 大柴胡湯 (Jp: *Dai-Saiko-Tō*; major bupleurum decoction) was originally found in *Shāng Hán Lùn*. The extract preparation of this formula is covered by the Japanese National Health Insurance program as a prescription drug, and is also commonly sold in Japanese drug stores as an over-the-counter drug. It is currently indicated by the MHLW for: gastritis, chronic constipation, stiff shoulders, headache, and constipation associated with hypertension or obesity, neurosis, and obesity in persons with strong physical strength who feel discomfort in the region stretching from the sides of the abdomen to the solar plexus or tend to experience constipation (體力が充實して、脇腹からみぞおちあたりにかけて苦しく、便祕の傾向があるものの次の諸症: 胃炎、常習便祕、高血壓や肥滿に伴う肩こり・頭痛・便祕、神經症、肥滿症).

As shown in the illustration, the patient presents with bitter fullness in the chest and rib-sides, and slight hypertonicity is present. Generally speaking, the hypertonicity is [manifested as] a lump. Some slight tension can be felt, and [the abdomen will] spring back when pressed with the fingertips. The abdomen has slight replete fullness, and the region below the heart has no hardness, but only glomus. [The pattern] should be carefully examined and considered. [In the pattern for] the previously-mentioned *Xiǎo Chái Hú Tāng*, the patient presents with glomus and hardness in the region below the heart with no replete fullness. This should be used to differentiate [the patterns].

およそ『傷寒論』の藥方は其の意精密なるものにして、その方、その證、自然とそなはりて、たがはざること、あざむくべからざるものなり。つつしんで方の主證をあきらかにし、君・佐の意味をかんがへ、これをもちゆるときは、一も病治せざることなかるべし。これ天然自然の方法、三代以上の術たること、うたがひなし。醫者、私智をはなれ、いにしへの法をもちひ、つつしんで其の功あることをしるべし。

Generally speaking, the thinking behind the formulae found in the *Shāng Hán Lùn* is precise; the prescriptions are naturally complete, and include no inaccuracies nor any deceptions. When [the physician] cautiously makes the primary pattern for each formula clear and uses [the formulae] after considering the meaning of the sovereign and the assistants, there should be no disease that cannot be cured. There is no doubt that this natural method has been continuing for over three generations.[51] The physician should leave his own wisdom and use the ancient methods with all due respect. [If he does so,] he will understand [and experience] their efficacy.

51. It is unclear to whose family this passage is referring. It is possible that this refers to the family of the author's teacher, Kaku Taiei 鶴泰榮.

柴胡加芒硝湯之證

The Pattern for Chái Hú Jiā Máng Xiāo Tāng[52] 柴胡加芒硝湯

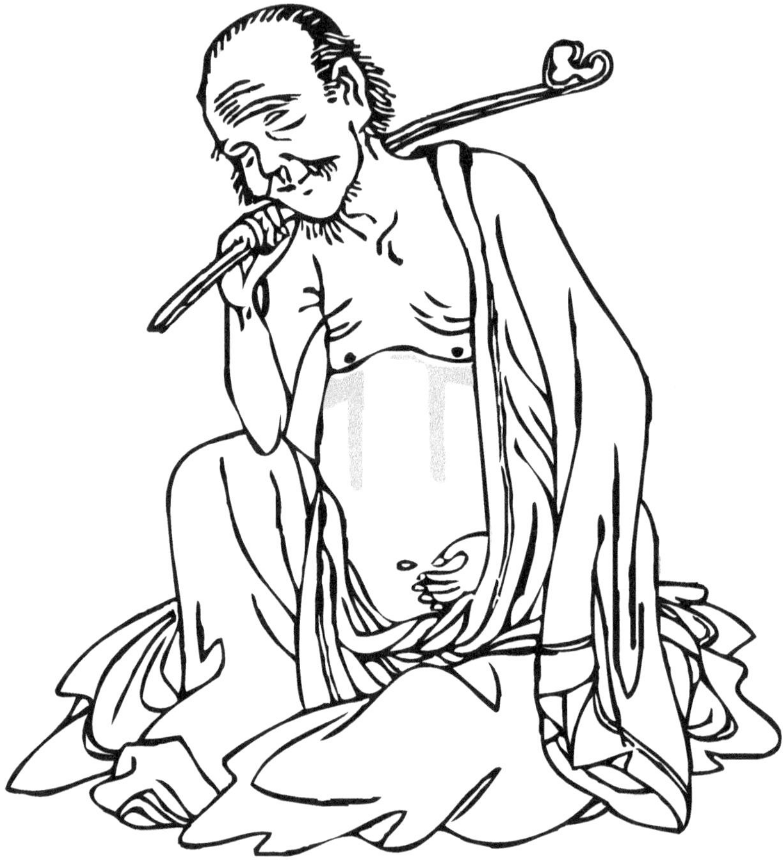

Fig. 5

圖の如く、胸脇苦滿して、二大竹を立てるが如く、之れを按じて堅きものあり。是れ堅塊なり、故に芒硝を加ふ。芒硝は堅き毒を治するものなり。然るに、世の腹診に暗きもの、是れを以て小建中湯の症、或るひは芍藥の拘攣とす。大いに誤りなり。小建中湯の腹症は、拘攣急迫して、數繩をはりたがるが如し。其の說、下に詳らかなり。

52. The formula for *Chái Hú Jiā Máng Xiāo Tāng* 柴胡加芒硝湯 (Jp: *Saiko-Ka-Bōshō-Tō*; bupleurum decoction plus marabilite) was originally found in *Shāng Hán Lùn*. At present, this formula is not covered by the Japanese National Health Insurance program and is not commonly used in Japan.

As shown in the illustration, the patient presents with bitter fullness in the chest and rib-sides, and hardness can be felt when palpated; [upon palpation] it feels as if there are two large bamboo poles that have been placed [in the abdomen]. These are hard lumps. Therefore, *máng xiāo* is included in the formula, as *máng xiāo* treats hard toxins. However, those in the world who are ignorant about abdominal examination take this pattern to be the pattern for *Xiǎo Jiàn Zhōng Tāng* or the pattern for hypertonicity that is treated by *sháo yào*.[53] These are grave errors. In the abdominal pattern for *Xiǎo Jiàn Zhōng Tāng*, there is hypertonicity and distress; it is similar to the feeling of [the abdomen] being pulled taut by several ropes. The explanation [of the pattern] will be made clear below.

此の證、芒硝の酸味を嫌ひて藥を服しかぬるものあり。故にかくの如き者に至つては、大率本方に鶴家の鶴丸を兼用すること、毎夜、一戔にして功あり。考ふべし。按ずるに、『傷寒論』中、大・小柴胡、其の餘去加の方、凡そ七方あり。柴胡加龍骨牡蠣湯は別に說ありて、ここに說かず。

This pattern despises the sour flavor of *máng xiāo*, making it impossible for [the patient] to take this drug. Therefore, in cases such as this, the simultaneous use of this formula with one *qián*[54] of the Kaku family's *Kaku-Gan*[55] 鶴丸 every night is generally effective, and should be considered [by the physician for use]. I believe that the *Shāng Hán Lùn* contains approximately seven different formulae related to *chái hú*, including *Dà Chái Hú Tāng*, *Xiǎo Chái Hú Tāng*, and the other variants adding or removing [ingredients]. *Chái Hú Jiā Lóng Gú Mǔ Lì Tāng* is discussed separately [in the present work]. Therefore, I will not discuss it here.[56]

---

53. The formula for *Xiǎo Jiàn Zhōng Tāng* (Jp: *Shō-Kenchū-Tō*; minor center-fortifying decoction) is discussed separately in its own section in this book.

54. *Qián* (Ch: *qián* 錢; Jp: *sen*, although more popularly referred to as *monme* 匁) is a traditional Chinese measurement of weight used throughout East Asia. Although the exact weight differs depending on the region and period in which it was used, in the case of Japan, the Weights and Measures Act of 1893 prescribed 1 *qián* to be calculated as 3.75 grams. Moreover, in this work, the author uniformly uses the character 戔, but because it is a simplified version of 錢, I have translated each instance of the word as "*qián*."

55. *Kaku-Gan* 鶴丸 (Ch: *Hè Wán*; Kaku's pill) is discussed separately in its own section in this book.

56. Perhaps due to the oversight of the author, the formula for *Chái Hú Jiā Lóng Gú Mǔ Lì Tāng* 柴胡加龍骨牡蠣湯 (Jp: *Saiko-Ka-Ryūkotsu-Borei-Tō*; bupleurum decoction plus dragon bone and oyster shell) is not discussed again in the present work. This formula was originally found in *Shāng Hán Lùn*. The extract preparation of the formula is covered by the Japanese National Health Insurance program as a prescription drug, and is also commonly sold in Japanese drug stores as an over-the-counter drug. It is currently indicated by the MHLW for: associated

その外、ここに圖せざる三柴胡も同じく皆、胸脇苦滿を以て主とす。故にこれを略す。乃ち、渴して嘔せざるものは、柴胡去半夏括蔞湯。又た上衝して少しく拘攣あるものは、柴胡桂枝湯。又た渴して嘔せず、痞鞕なく腹中動ある者は、柴胡桂枝乾姜湯の證也。

In addition to [the above formulae], there are three other formulae using *chái hú* that I have not illustrated. In all cases, [the presence of] bitter fullness in the chest and rib-sides is the primary indication for the pattern. Therefore, I will omit [the explanations for] these [patterns]. Moreover, when the patient presents with thirst but no vomiting, it is [the pattern for] *Chái Hú Qù Bàn Xià [Jiā] Guā Lóu Tāng*.[57] Furthermore, if the patient presents with upward surging and slight hypertonicity, it is [the pattern for] *Chái Hú Guì Zhī Tāng*.[58] Also, if the patient presents with thirst that is not accompanied with vomiting and has neither glomus nor hardness, but experiences stirring in the middle of the abdomen, it is the pattern for *Chái Hú Guì Zhī Gān Jiāng Tāng*.[59]

---

symptoms of hypertension (i.e., palpitations, anxiety, insomnia), neurosis, menopausal neurosis, pediatric nocturnal crying episodes, and constipation in persons with moderate or strong physical strength who have mental anxiety, palpitations, insomnia, or constipation (體力中等度以上で、精神不安があって、動悸、不眠、便祕などを伴う次の諸症: 高血壓の隨伴症狀[動悸、不安、不眠]、神經症、更年期神經症、小兒夜泣き、便祕).

57. The formula for *Chái Hú Qù Bàn Xià Guā Jiā Lóu Tāng* 柴胡去半夏加栝蔞湯 (Jp; *Saiko-Kyo-Hange-Karō-Tō*; bupleurum decoction minus pinellia plus trichosanthes root) was originally found in *Jīn Guì Yào Lüè*. At present, this formula is not covered by the Japanese National Health Insurance program and is not commonly used in Japan.

58. The formula for *Chái Hú Guì Zhī Tāng* 柴胡桂枝湯 (Jp: *Saiko-Keishi-Tō*; bupleurum and cinnamon twig decoction) was originally found in *Jīn Guì Yào Lüè*. The extract preparation of the formula is covered by the Japanese National Health Insurance program as a prescription drug, and is also commonly sold in Japanese drug stores as an over-the-counter drug. It is currently indicated by the MHLW for: gastroenteritis and other symptoms associated with the middle and later stages of the common cold in persons with moderate or slightly weak physical strength who sometimes experience symptoms such as mild fever, chills, headache, or nausea that is often accompanied by abdominal pain. (體力中等度又はやや虛弱で、多くは腹痛を伴い、ときに微熱・寒氣・頭痛・はきけなどがあるものの次の諸症：胃腸炎、かぜの中期から後期の症狀).

59. The formula for *Chái Hú Guì Zhī Gān Jiāng Tāng* 柴胡桂枝乾薑湯 (Jp: *Saiko-Keishi-Kankyō-Tō*; bupleurum, cinnamon twig, and dried ginger decoction) was originally found in the *Shāng Hán Lùn*. The extract preparation of the formula is covered by the Japanese National Health Insurance program as a prescription drug, and is also commonly sold in Japanese drug stores as an over-the-counter drug. It is currently indicated by the MHLW for: menopause, [what is known in Japan as] "blood path disease," insomnia, neurosis, palpitations, shortness of breath, symptoms associated with the late stages of the common cold, and bronchitis in persons with moderate physical strength who have cold extremities, anemia, neurologic hypersensitivity, palpitations, shortness of breath, and occasionally experience night sweats, head sweating, or dry mouth. Note: Blood path disease (Jp: *chi-no-michi-shō* 血の道症) refers to neuropsychiatric and

余、諸州を經歷し、衆病人を療するに、十に六、七人までは、柴胡の證多し。醫者、よく腹證を熟知せば、これを用ひて功あることを知るべし。

Through my experiences traveling throughout various provinces and treating a multitude of patients, I have found that as many as six or seven out of ten patients present with a pattern for *chái hú*. If the physician becomes [more] deeply acquainted with abdominal patterns, he will be able to use these [formulae correctly] and come to understand their effectiveness.

吳茱萸湯之證

The Pattern for Wú Zhū Yú Tāng[60] 吳茱萸湯

圖の如き、即ち吳茱萸湯の證なり。余、此の證を得ざること久し。苦心刻意して、近ごろ漸く審らかにすることを得たり。門人、東民と共に論ず。東民も亦た苦心すること多年。時に此の證を患ふる者、兩三人に遇へり。因つて共に單思して、始めて此の證を理會することを得たり。柴胡を用ひて治せざるもの、間この證あり。何となれば、胸脇苦滿して嘔巳まざる者なればなり。然れども、胸脇苦滿して嘔するものは、柴胡を用ひて愈ゆ柴胡の證にして、唯だ胸滿するもの、是れ吳茱萸湯の證なり。

---

physical symptoms such as anxiety and irritation that occur [in women] due to hormonal fluctuations associated with menstruation, pregnancy, childbirth, postpartum period, menopause, etc. (體力中等度以下で、冷え症、貧血氣味、神經過敏で、動悸、息切れ、ときにねあせ、頭部の發汗、口の乾きがあるものの次のの諸症：更年期障害、血の道症、不眠症、神經症、動悸、息切れ、かぜの後期の症狀、氣管支炎。血の道症とは、月經、姙娠、出產、產後、更年期など女性のホルモンの變動に伴って現れる精神不安やいらだちなどの精神神經症狀および身體症狀のことである).

60. The formula for *Wú Zhū Yú Tāng* 吳茱萸湯 (Jp: *Goshuyu-Tō*; evodia decoction) was originally found in *Jīn Guì Yào Lüè* and *Shāng Hán Lùn*. The extract preparation of the formula is covered by the Japanese National Health Insurance program as a prescription drug, and is also commonly sold in Japanese drug stores as an over-the-counter drug. It is currently indicated by the MHLW for: headache, nausea and vomiting accompanied by headache, and hiccups in persons with moderate or weak physical strength who have cold extremities, stiff shoulders, and an occasional sense of fullness in the solar plexus (體力中等度以下で、手足が冷えて肩がこり、ときにみぞおちが膨滿するものの次の諸症：頭痛、頭痛に伴うはきけ・嘔吐、しゃっくり).

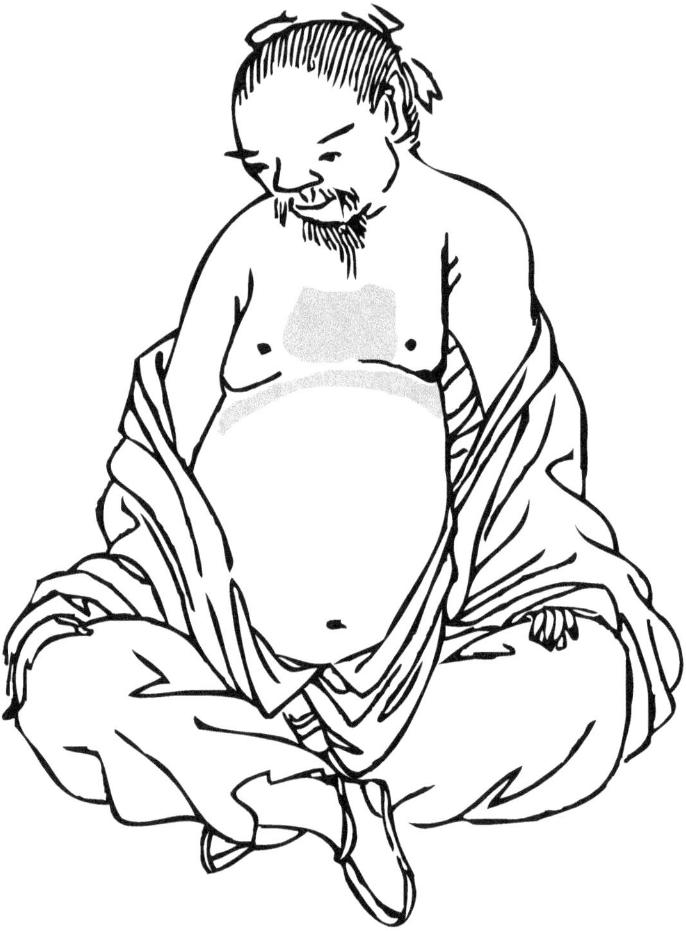

Fig. 6

As shown in the illustration, this is the pattern for *Wú Zhū Yú Tāng*. I was long unable to grasp this pattern. It was only after great pain and considerable effort that I was recently able to elucidate it. I had much discussion about it with Tōmin, my pupil.[61] Tōmin had also spent many years of hard work in [trying to solve] the problem. It just so happened that we encountered two or three patients who were suffering from this pattern. We therefore consulted with each other [concerning the cases], and it was only then that we were able to understand this pattern: some patients who do not respond to [initial] treatment with *chái hú* actually have this pattern. The reason why [we initially administered *chái hú*] was because these patients presented with bitter fullness in the chest and rib-sides, as well as ceaseless retching. However, when a patient presents with bitter fullness in the chest and rib-sides and retching that are cured after treatment with *chái*

61. There are no available records concerning the details of the pupils of the author, including Tōmin 東民.

hú [then this patient] has [one of] the patterns for *chái hú*, whereas in a case in which the patient presents with only fullness in the chest, it is actually an example of the pattern for *Wú Zhū Yú Tāng*.

其の胸滿するに、二證あり。あらはれて胸滿するあり、其のあらはれざる者、これを按ずるに實中に一點の空所なし。是れ即ち此方の證なり。

[Thus,] there are two types of patterns in which fullness in the chest is present: [the first is the case in which] the patient presents with apparent fullness in the chest, and [the second is the case in which the patient] presents with fullness in the chest that is not apparent; repletion and no empty spaces [can be felt] on palpation [in such a pattern]. This [case] is the pattern for this formula.

其の餘、猶をあまたあり。食せんとして嘔する者あり、手足厥冷・煩燥・吐利して死せんと欲するものあり、乾嘔・喘沫・頭痛するものあり。又た嘔して胸滿するものあり、この四證要するに、胸脇苦滿・心下痞鞕して嘔するを準據とすべし。柴胡の症、大略かくのごとし。しかれども、痞鞕に至つては、吳茱萸の證を大いなりとす。

There are also many other types of cases besides these. [For example,] there are cases when the patient vomits when trying to eat. There are also cases of reversal cold in the extremities, vexation, agitation, vomiting, and diarrhea in which the patient is near death.[62] There are also cases when the patient presents with dry retching, drool foaming at the mouth, and headache. There are also cases in which the patient presents with retching and fullness in the chest. In summary, the indications for these four patterns are: bitter fullness in the chest and rib-side, glomus and hardness in the region below the heart, and retching. Roughly speaking, in the patterns for *chái hú* [the symptoms are] the same as these. However, in the pattern for *Wú Zhū Yú Tāng*, [the degree of] glomus and hardness is much greater.

62. Reversal cold in the extremities (Ch: *shǒu zú jué lěng* 手足厥冷; Jp: *shusoku-ketsurei*) refers to pronounced cold in the extremities up to the knees and elbows or beyond, also the same as cold extremities.

人参芎軍桃花湯之證

The Pattern for Ninjin-Kyū-Gun-Tōka-Tō[63] 人参芎軍桃花湯

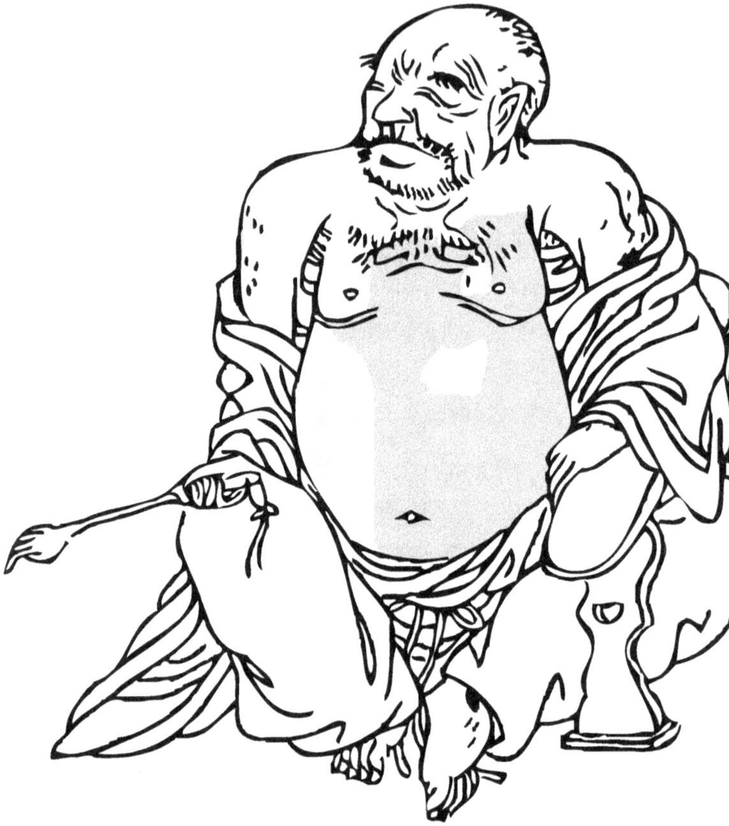

Fig. 7

圖の如く、腹張滿、心下痞鞕、食下らず、一身悉く浮腫、兩便利せず。百藥、効なきもの。此の腹證、張滿はなはだしきゆへ、腹底の毒、診察しがたし。此の時、浮水を去つて而して后、舊毒を知つて、方證相對の藥劑を以つて毒をせむるにあらざれば、治しがたし。

As shown in the illustration, [the patient presents with] abdominal distension and fullness, glomus and hardness in the region below the heart, puffy swelling in the entire

63. This formula for *Ninjin-Kyū-Gun-Tōka-Tō* 人參芎軍桃花湯 (Ch: *Rén Shēn Xiōng Jūn Táo Huā Tāng*; ginseng, chuanxiong, rhubarb, and peach blossom decoction) is not found in any known Chinese or Japanese text: it appears to be an invention of the author or perhaps one of his teachers. At present, this formula is not covered by the Japanese National Health Insurance program and is not well known in Japan.

body, and inhibited urination and defecation.[64] The hundred medicinals are ineffective [in treating the pattern]. Because the [abdominal] distension and fullness is severe in this pattern, the toxin residing in the bottom of the abdomen is difficult to examine. [Therefore, the symptoms are] difficult to treat unless the water causing the puffy swelling is first eliminated, so that the physician may understand the [nature of the] old [i.e., long-standing] toxin and attack [the pattern] using a medicinal selected according to formula-pattern matching theory.

而れども、又た始めより、本劑きはむることあり。一もみな、腹診の審らかなればなり。ここに云ふ人參芎軍桃花湯は、張滿、心下痞鞕して、これを按じて腹中雷鳴す。此れ大いに白桃花湯の證なり。

However, in some cases, initial treatment using this formula is successful. In all such cases, it is because the abdominal pattern was made clear during examination. In [the pattern for] *Rén Shēn Xiōng Jūn Táo Huā Tāng* mentioned here, the patient presents with distension and fullness, and glomus and hardness in the region below the heart. Upon palpation, a thunderous rumbling [can be heard] in the abdomen. This is exactly the pattern for *Bái Táo Huā Tāng*.[65]

余、諸州を遊歴して、浮腫脹滿のものは治療數多にして、これを覺ふ。この證、或るひは鼓脹、あるひは中風半身不隨。みな難治として、衆醫、手をそかぬ。その毒、積年あつまり、一時に發するものなり。

I learned this during my travels across various provinces as I treated a great number of patients who presented with puffy swelling, distention, and fullness. Some patients who have this pattern may present with drum distention, but other patients may present with hemiplegia associated with wind strike. [These cases are] all difficult to cure, and a multitude of physicians are unable to successfully treat them. [In such cases,] the toxin has accumulated [in the patients] for many years, and [finally] emerges at once.

64. Inhibited urination (Ch: *xiǎo biàn bù lì* 小便不利; Jp: *shōben-furi*) is an important concept in this book. It refers to difficult discharge of urine, usually scanty in amount, the same as dysuria.

65. There are several formulae with similar names to *Bái Táo Huā Tāng* 白桃花湯 (Jp: *Hakutōka-Tō*; white peach blossom decoction), thus it is unclear to which the author is referring. However, based on the symptoms described in this section, this formula appears to refer to *Kaku-Ka Kanzui-Tōka-Tō* 鶴家甘遂桃花 (Ch: *Hè Jiā Gān Suì Táo Huā Tāng*; the Kaku family's kansui and peach blossom decoction), which is discussed separately in its own section in this work.

故に浮水を去つて、つつしんで腹底の舊毒を考ふるに、凡そ大承氣湯、あるひは桃軍圓、あるひは癥痼圓、あるひは大黄牡丹皮湯。この四方、過半大劑を以て長く攻むるにあらざれば、治しがたし。

Therefore, in order to eliminate the water causing the puffy swelling, the physician should carefully consider the long-standing toxin residing in the depths of the abdomen; generally speaking, *Dà Chéng Qì Tāng, Tō-Gun-En, Chōko-En,* or *Dà Huáng Mǔ Dān Pí Tāng*[66] [should be] used [to treat patients with the pattern]. In the majority of cases, [the toxin] will be difficult to treat unless it is attacked with a major formula such as one these four formulae for a long period of time.

『内經』に曰く、「重きものは因つて之を減じ、故に凡そ積年の患へ、豈に一藥にして愈ゆべけんや。漸く減じてこれを去るべし」と云々。克、衆病人を療して合するに、此のこと是れなり。都べて陳寒痼冷のもの、みなかくのごとし。

In the [*Huáng Dì*] *Nèi Jīng,* it says, "...after [the disease] has become heavy, eliminate it. Therefore, how can any suffering that has accumulated over many years be cured if only one medicinal is used?"[67] As I have treated a multitude of patients and matched [their patterns, I have found] this to be so; it is also the same in all cases of old [i.e., long-standing] cold or intractable cold [in the body].

66. *Dà Chéng Qì Tāng* 大承氣湯 (Jp: *Dai-Jōki-Tō*; major qì-infusing decoction), *Tō-Gun-En* 桃軍圓 (Ch: *Táo Jūn Yuán*; peach kernel and rhubarb pill), *Chōko-En* 癥痼圓 (Ch: *Zhēng Gū Yuán*; intractable concretion pill), and *Dà Huáng Mǔ Dān Pí Tāng* 大黄牡丹皮湯 (Jp: *Daiō-Botanpi-Tō*; rhubarb and moutan decoction) are all discussed separately in their own sections in this book.

67. The original quote as found in the "Great Treatise on the Correspondences and Manifestations of Yīn and Yáng (Ch: *Yīn Yáng Yìng Xiàng Dà Lùn* 《陰陽應像大論》(Chapter 5); Jp: *In-Yō-Ō-Shō-Tairon*)" of *Sù Wèn* 《素問》 is slightly different: "故曰、病之始起也、可刺而已、其盛、可待衰而已。故因其輕而揚之、因其重而減之、因其衰而彰之" (When a disease begins to emerge, one can pierce and [the disease] ends. When it abounds, one must wait until it weakens and [the disease] ends. Thus, after it has become light, scatter it. After it has become heavy, reduce it. After it has become weak, let it shine [again]). Furthermore, some ancient commentaries are of the opinion that *jiǎn* 減 (to reduce) is a mistake, and should be read as *xiè* 瀉 (to drain) or *dàng* 蕩 (to dissipate). Therefore, this would read as: [The drug] should be gradually reduced until [the disease] is eliminated.

又た云はく、凡そ死證のものを考ふるに、予知るもの三あり。一に云はく、臍穴張り出で、英の如し。二に云はく、足裏、一面に滿ち腫るること甚だしきもの。三に云はく、尸惡臭、下痢するもの。この三つのもの、一つもあれば、かならず死す。

Moreover, when considering death patterns, there are three that I know of. In the first [pattern], the umbilicus is distended and protuberant, resembling a bloom. In the second [pattern], there is severe swelling spreading across the soles of the feet. In the third [pattern, the patient presents with] dysentery, producing a cadaverous malign odor. If [the patient] has even one of these [patterns], he will surely die.

又た云はく、あるひは此の三、四の方中、一方の證有つて、自若としてうごかざるものあり。あるひはこの一、二の證ありて、傍ら佗證一、二、若しくは二、四かぬるものあり。その治方、まづその大なるものを攻むることあり。あるひはまづ、その小なるものを除きさりて後、大なるものを攻むることあり。又た、たがひにその證をあらはすときは、たがひにその毒を攻むることあり。

Furthermore, in some cases [when one] of these three or four formulae [is used], there might be one pattern (corresponding to the formula) that remains unmoved [i.e., uncured]. In some cases, the patient may present with one or two [primary] patterns and have one or two side [i.e., concurrent] patterns, or even from two to four other [concurrent] patterns. [In such cases,] the method to treat [the disease] is to first attack the major [pattern]. In some cases, the minor [pattern] must be first eliminated, and then the major [pattern] may be attacked. In other cases, when multiple patterns are manifested, the toxins must be attacked together [simultaneously].[68]

此等の數件いやしくも診腹につまびらかなる者にあらざれば、機にのぞみ變に應ずることあたはず。豈に一時筆頭のつくすべきことならんや。したしく口授を受けて、刻意苦慮するにあらざれば、その奥に入ることあたはず。

---

68. The author and many other classical practitioners of Japanese-style abdominal examination seem to have believed that diseases are generally caused by a single specific toxin, which manifests itself in the body as a unique abdominal pattern that can be matched to a single medicinal formula. However, as stated in the text, it was thought possible for multiple patterns (caused by multiple toxins) to coexist with the main pattern in a patient. Such concurrent patterns are normally known as *jiān zhèng* 兼證 (Jp: *kenshō*), but in this work, they are referred to as "side (Jp: *katawara* 傍ら[旁ら]) patterns."

Unless the person [treating the disease] is well versed in abdominal examination, he will be unable to adapt and respond according to the circumstances. How can I fully express [everything concerning abdominal patterns] at one time [in this book] through the tip of a brush? Unless one intimately receives oral instruction and makes considerable effort to understand through racking his brain, he will be unable to penetrate the depths [of abdominal examination].

桃軍圓之證二圖

The Pattern for Tō-Gun-En[69] 桃軍圓 (Two Illustrations)

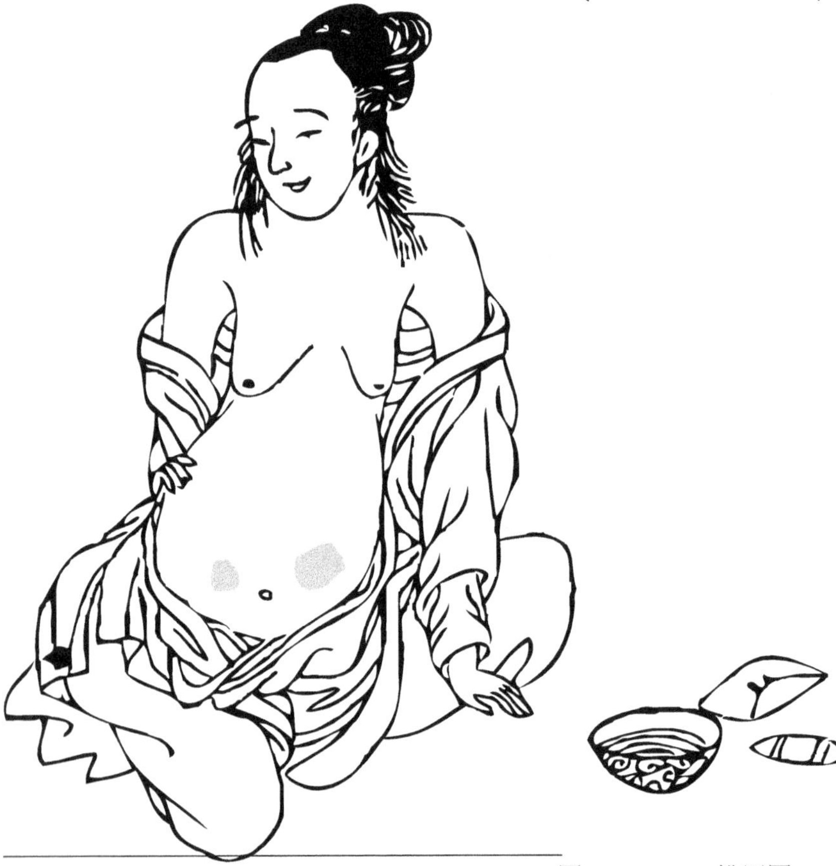

Fig. 8

69. As with the other formulae in this book that end in *-en* (圓), *Tō-Gun-En* 桃軍圓 (Ch: *Táo Jūn Yuán*; peach kernel and rhubarb pill) is one of the "secret" preparations that the author obtained during his travels or learned from his teachers. Naturally, they were never commonly used in Japan. At present, this formula is not covered by the Japanese National Health Insurance program and is not well known in Japan. Although similar to *Táo Hé Chéng Qì Tāng* 桃核承氣湯 (discussed separately in this book), *Tō-Gun-En* 桃軍圓 contains different quantities of ingredients and the addition of *qiáo mài* 蕎麥.

圖の如く、形ありて、これを按して痛むもの、即ちこの證なり。世にいはゆる「男女積聚」なるもの、あるひは勞瘵欝證と號するものにも、間この證あり。是れ血證なるが故にあるひは吐血・衂血・下血・痔疾・脫肛・淋瀝・經水不調等の患へあるものなり。

As shown in the illustration, in cases when [the patient] presents with a form as shown in the illustration, and there is pain when [the abdomen is] pressed, it is this pattern. What are commonly known as "accumulations and gatherings in male and female [patients]" or what are called consumption or depression patterns are also examples of this pattern.[70] This is a blood pattern; therefore, in some cases, the patient may suffer from blood ejection,[71] spontaneous external bleeding,[72] descent of blood, hemorrhoidal disease, prolapse of the rectum, dribbling [blood], or menstrual flow irregularities.

しかりといへども、其の毒敗れざるものは、さまでに患ふることなきもあり。しかれども、この腹症あるもの、桃軍圓を永久に用ひば、諸患發することなし。

Nevertheless, [even] in cases in which the toxin is not vanquished, the patient may not [necessarily] suffer so much [from these symptoms]. However, if a patient who has this abdominal pattern permanently uses *Tō-Gun-En* 桃軍圓, [the above-mentioned] various symptoms will never develop.

---

70. The term "accumulations and gatherings (Ch: *jī jù* 積聚; Jp: *shakuju*)," also known as "aggregation-accumulation" or "abdominal masses," is a general term referring to mass formation in the chest and abdomen. It is similar to the term "concretions and conglomerations (*zhēng jiǎ* 癥瘕; Jp: *chōka*)." Strictly speaking, the pathology of *jī jù* 積聚 and *zhēng jiǎ* 癥瘕 differ; in *Zhōng Zàng Jīng* 《中藏經》 (Jp: *Chūzō-Kyō*; Central Treasury Canon), attributed to Huá Tuó 華佗 (c. 145–208 CE), it is explained that "積者系於臟也、聚者系於腑也、癥者系於氣也、瘕者系於血也 (accumulations are tied to the viscera, gatherings are tied to the bowels, concretions are tied to qì, and conglomerations are tied to blood)."

However, in this work, and in many other classical works, the terms do not seem to be clearly differentiated and are used together (especially in describing diseases in female patients). In *Zhū Bìng Yuán Hòu Lùn* 《諸病源候論》 (Jp: *Shobyō-Genkō-Ron*; The Origin and Indicators of Disease), published by Cháo Yuánfāng 巢元方 (dates of birth and death unknown) in 610 CE, it is stated that "...瘀久不消，則變成積聚癥瘕也 (...when blood stasis is enduring and does not disperse, accumulations, gatherings, concretions, and conglomerations develop)."

71. Blood ejection (Ch: *tù xuè* 吐血; Jp: *toketsu*) refers to spitting of blood (i.e., expulsion of blood with saliva.

72. Spontaneous external bleeding (Ch: *nǜ xuè* 衂血 [although normally written as 衄血]; Jp: *jikuketsu*) refers to epistaxis (i.e., non-traumatic external bleeding, including bleeding from the ear, nose, gum, and tongue, and subcutaneous hemorrhage).

The Second Illustration of the Pattern for Tō-Gun-En 桃軍圓

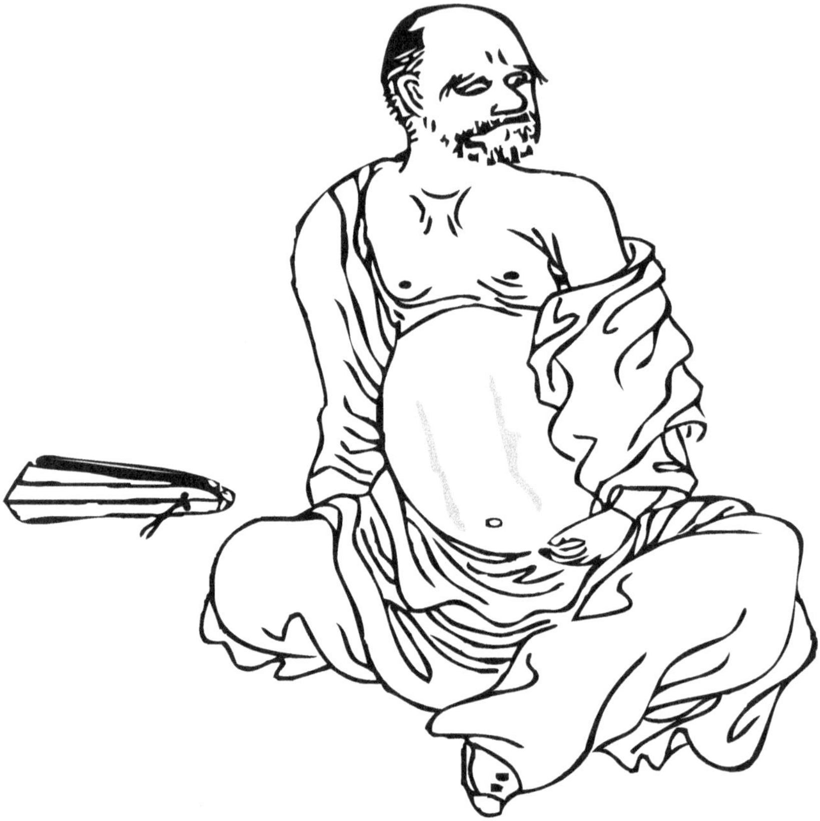

Fig. 9

又た一證、此の圖の如く、紐を結びたがるが如きもの、これを按してすなはち痛む。亦た桃軍丸の證なり。始めに云ふ腹症と異なり、其の腹やはらかにして知れがたし。心を沈めて探り求むべし。凡そ此の證、毒の肯綮(肯綮は骨肉の相著くところなり、『莊子』に出づ)にあたりたるときは、大いに下血することあり。驚くべからず。

Another pattern [matching *Tō-Gun-En* is shown here]. As seen in this illustration, it appears similar to strings that are tied [in the abdomen]. When [these regions are] pressed, pain is present. [This is] also the pattern for *Tō-Gun-Gan* 桃軍丸. *Tō-Gun-Gan* is the same as *Tō-Gun-En*. *Gan* 丸 (Ch: *wán*) and *en* 圓 (Ch: *yuán*) both mean "pill," although the use of *gan/wán* 丸 is more common. Differing from the first abdominal pattern mentioned, the abdomen is soft and difficult to discern. [The physician] should quiet his heart and search [for the pattern]. In many cases of this pattern, there is a great descent of blood when the toxin reaches the membranous ligatures (the areas where bones and flesh attach to each other, as described in **Zhuāng Zǐ**《莊子》). There is no need to be frightened.[73]

然りといへども、世醫、これらの證に至りては、腹症を審らかにせざるゆへに、治を取ることあたはず。終身の患へを抱かしめ、又は治せずして夭死に及ばしむ。豈に哀しからずや。

However, because the physicians of the world do not elucidate these abdominal patterns, they are unable to cure [the patients]. They make the patients suffer from their afflictions for their entire lives, or cause the patients to die prematurely from lack of [effective] treatment. Is this not sad?

又た曰く、古今の醫書、大率臍より以下を「小腹」と名づく。吾が門、臍傍より上腹の左右、少しばかりの所を以て小腹とす。蓋し古今の醫書と合はずといへども、醫はもとより事實にして、動かざるところあるを主とする者なれば、すなはち毒のある所を以てその名を定む。

Ancient and contemporary medical texts have generally regarded the smaller abdomen to be the region inferior to the umbilicus. In my school, the regions somewhat to the upper left and right sides of the umbilicus are defined as the smaller abdomen. Although this does not match what is commonly written in ancient or contemporary medical texts, if the physician [focuses on] facts and [selects] the [abdominal] regions that remain unmoved to be the primary [indications of the pattern], the name of the pattern [will become clear] based on where the toxin is actually located.[74]

---

73. The expression "membranous ligatures (Ch: *kěn qǐng* 肯綮; Jp: *kōkei*)" was originally found in the "Nourishing the Lord of Life Chapter (Ch: *Yǎng Shēng Zhǔ* 養生主; Jp: *Yō-Seishu*)" of *Zhuāng Zǐ*《莊子》(Jp: *Sōji* or *Sōshi*), an ancient Chinese Daoist philosophical text from the late Warring States period (3rd century BCE). In context, this expression was used to describe the technique of a certain dexterous butcher cutting up an ox. The original text and translation by the eminent Sinologist James Legge (1815–1897 CE) is as follows: "依乎天理、批大郤、導大窾、因其固然、技經肯綮之未嘗、而況大軱乎" (Observing the natural lines, [my knife] slips through the great crevices and slides through the great cavities, taking advantage of the facilities thus presented. My art avoids the membranous ligatures, and much more the great bones).

74. In traditional abdominal examination, *shào fù* 少腹 (Jp: *shōfuku*; lesser abdomen) and *xiǎo fù* 小腹 (Jp: *shōfuku*; smaller abdomen) were generally differentiated, but the author does not differentiate the two. This may be because the present work was intended to be a clinical reference book for physicians to quickly find cures for patients, rather than a treatise on the theoretical framework of elucidating abdominal patterns.

凡そ此の方の證、世に甚だ多きものにして、余、数百人を治して後、其の効をいふものなれば、容るること有るべからず。且つ我が師、鶴先生は、東洞翁を慕ひたる者なれども、其の門に入らずして、自ら天機の力を以て腹診をきはめられしものなれば、其の精妙なる所に至つては、世俗の論の及ぶ所にあらず。

An extremely high number of patients in the world present with the pattern matching this formula. I speak on the efficacy [of the medicinal] after having [successfully] treated hundreds of patients; therefore, [I] cannot accept [contrary opinions]. Furthermore, although my teacher, Kaku-Sensei, admired the venerable [Yoshimasu] Tōdō, he did not enter his school, and he perfected [the art of] abdominal examination on his own using his own natural skills.[75] Therefore, the treatises of common [physicians] in the world are unable to match [his level of depth] concerning the subtleties of [abdominal examination].

括蔞薤白白酒湯之圖

Illustration of the Pattern for Guā Lóu Xiè Bái Bái Jiǔ Tāng[76,77]

栝蔞薤白白酒湯

圖の如く、胸膈痞塞、喘息、咳唾、及び氣急促迫、胸背痛のもの。克案ずるに、舊年喘息を患ふるもの、此の證多し。或るひは、勞咳と號して、百藥効なきもの、譬へば大小青龍湯、あるひは麻黄甘草湯、あるひは葛根湯等の證に似て効なきもの。

As shown in the illustration, the patient presents with glomus blockage in the chest and diaphragm, panting, coughing and spitting, distressed rapid breathing, and pain in the

75. Kaku Taiei 鶴泰榮 was a renowned physician of the Edo period, although little is known of his life outside of what is written in the present work and *Fukushō-Kiran-Yoku*《腹證奇覽翼》(The Wings to Extraordinary Views of Abdominal Patterns), written by Wakuda Yoshitora 和久田叔虎 (1768-1824), who studied under the author.

76. *Guā lóu* 栝蔞: The original text used the character 括 (a mistake for the standard character 栝); I have changed all instances of the character in the translation to 栝 for clarity.

77. The formula for *Guā Lóu Xiè Bái Bái Jiǔ Tāng* 栝蔞薤白白酒湯 (Jp: *Karo-Gaihaku-Hakushu-Tō*; trichosanthes, Chinese chive, and white liquor decoction) was originally found in *Jīn Guì Yào Lüè*. The extract preparation of the formula is approved by the MHLW to be sold in Japanese drug stores as an over-the-counter drug, although it is largely unknown, as it was newly approved in 2012. It is currently indicated by the MHLW for: pain in the chest and solar plexus that resonates to the back, and an oppressive feeling in the chest. This drug may be used regardless of physical strength (背部にひびく胸部・みぞおちの痛み、胸部の壓迫感、體力に關わらず、使用できる).

chest and back. I am of the opinion that many patients who suffer from long-standing panting have this pattern. In some cases, [the pattern] may be called "taxation cough," but [conventional treatments using] the hundred medicinals are ineffective to treat it. The pattern may appear similar to the patterns for *Xiǎo Qīng Lóng Tāng,*[78] *Má Huáng Gān Cǎo Tāng,*[79] or *Gé Gēn Tāng,*[80] etc. However, these formulae are ineffective.

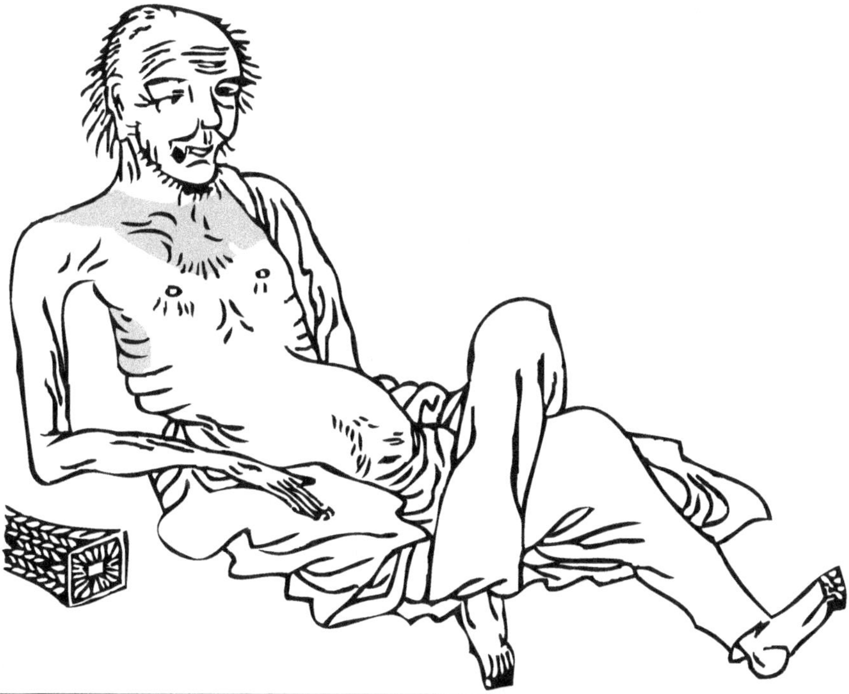

Fig. 10

78. The details of *Xiǎo Qīng Lóng Tāng* 小青龍湯 (Jp: *Shō-Seiryū-Tō*; minor green-blue dragon decoction) are not discussed in this work. The formula was originally found in *Jīn Guì Yào Lüè* and *Shāng Hán Lùn*. The extract preparation of the formula is covered by the Japanese National Health Insurance program as a prescription drug, and is also commonly sold in Japanese drug stores as an over-the-counter drug marketed as a treatment for hay fever and allergies. It is currently indicated by the MHLW for: bronchitis, bronchial asthma, rhinitis, allergic rhinitis, edema, common cold, and hay fever in persons with moderate or slightly weak physical strength who have symptoms such as cough accompanied by thin watery phlegm or a runny nose (體力中等度又はやや虚弱で、うすい水様のたんを伴うせきや鼻水が出るものの次の諸症:氣管支炎、氣管支ぜんそく、鼻炎、アレルギー性鼻炎、むくみ、感冒、花粉症).

79. The details of *Má Huáng Gān Cǎo Tāng* 麻黃甘草湯 (Jp: *Maō-Kanzō-Tō*; ephedra and licorice decoction) are not discussed in this work. The formula was originally found in *Shāng Hán Zǒng Bìng Lùn* 《傷寒總病論》(Jp: *Shōkan-Sōbyō-Ron*; On Cold Damage and General Diseases), written by Páng Ānshí 龐安時 (ca. 1043–1100 CE). At present, this formula is not covered by the Japanese National Health Insurance program and is not commonly used in Japan.

80. The formula for *Gé Gēn Tāng* 葛根湯 (Jp: *Kakkon-Tō*; pueraria decoction) is discussed separately in its own section in this work.

此の證、許多あり。然れども又た此の證に似て、茯苓杏仁甘草湯の證、ままあり。謹んで診察あやまるべからず。その別心下悸甚だしく、小便不利。これ茯苓杏仁甘草湯の正證なり。心下悸の有無を以て分別すべし。

[This is because] in many [such cases, patients actually have] this pattern [matching *Guā Lóu Xiè Bái Bái Jiǔ Tāng*]. However, another pattern that resembles this is the pattern for *Fú Líng Xìng Rén Gān Cǎo Tāng*.[81] [The physician] must carefully perform the examination so as to not mistake [the patterns. When the patient presents with] severe palpitations in the region below the heart and inhibited urination, it is the pattern for *Fú Líng Xìng Rén Gān Cǎo Tāng*. The patterns should be differentiated by the presence or absence of palpitations in the region below the heart.

磁石丸之證

The Pattern for Jishaku-Gan[82] 磁石丸

圖の如く、手足羸瘦して腹脹滿、所謂鼓脹、顏色黃青白のもの。證に髓ひて本劑を與へ、每夜此の丸、あるひは二錢、或るひは三錢、もしくは小兒あるひは五分、毒の淺深厚薄に從つて、藥の分量多少、謹んで考ふべし。

As shown in the illustration, the patient presents with marked emaciation of the extremities, abdominal distention and fullness (what is known as "drum distention,") and a yellow, green-blue, or white complexion. This formula should be given [to the patient] in

81. The formula for *Fú Líng Xìng Rén Gān Cǎo Tāng* 茯苓杏仁甘草湯 (Jp: *Bukuryō-Kyōnin-Kanzō-Tō*; poria, apricot kernel, and licorice decoction) was originally found in *Jīn Guì Yào Lüè*. The extract preparation of the formula is approved by the MHLW to be sold in Japanese drug stores as an over-the-counter drug. It is currently indicated by the MHLW for: shortness of breath, chest pain, bronchial asthma, cough, and palpitations in persons with moderate or weak physical strength who have the feeling of a knot in the chest (體力中等度以下で、胸につかえがあるものの次の諸症: 息切れ、胸の痛み、氣管支ぜんそく、せき、動悸).

82. As explained in the text, the formula for *Jishaku-Gan* 磁石丸 (Ch: *Cí Shí Wán*; loadstone pill) original formula was taken from *Tokuhon-Ō-Jūku-Hō*《德本翁十九方》(Nineteen Prescriptions of the Venerable Tokuhon). At present, this formula is not covered by the Japanese National Health Insurance program and is not well known in Japan. Kojima Shōen 小島蕉園 (1771–1826 CE), a samurai of the Edo period, claimed in his collection of essays that the copy of *Tokuhon-Ō-Jūku-Hō* that the author saw was a forgery written by a Buddhist monk who did not want to reveal the secrets of the book. Thus, it is unclear if the formulae taken from that book are genuine Tokuhon originals. Moreover, the quantities of the ingredients used in this work are slightly different from those found in the version of extant version of *Tokuhon-Ō-Jūku-Hō*.

accordance with the pattern: in some cases two, and in some cases 3 *qián* of the pill be should given. In the cases of children, 5 *fēn* should be given.[83] The quantity of the drug should be given in accordance with depth and thickness of the toxin.

此の方、もと甲斐の徳本翁十九方中の名方なり。世に知るものなし。余、遊歴の中、故あつて此れを得る。尤もその効あること、神變微妙。學ぶ者、用ひて以て妙をしるべし。其の方法の密なるが如きは、後篇に出だす。然れども吾が門に入つて懇請する人あらば、詳らかに之れを傳へん。其の佗、詳らかならざるものは之れに傚へ。

This formula is a famous formula originally [obtained] from *Tokuhon-Ō-Jūku-Hō*《徳本翁十九方》(Nineteen Prescriptions of the Venerable Tokuhon) written by Tokuhon of Kai Province.[84] [However,] there are none in the world that know [the details of the formula]. During my travels, I was able to obtain it due to certain circumstances. Its miraculous effects are indeed subtle and wondrous. Those who study [abdominal patterns] should use [the formula] in order to understand its wondrousness. I will explain its secret methods of use in a later volume. However, if there is

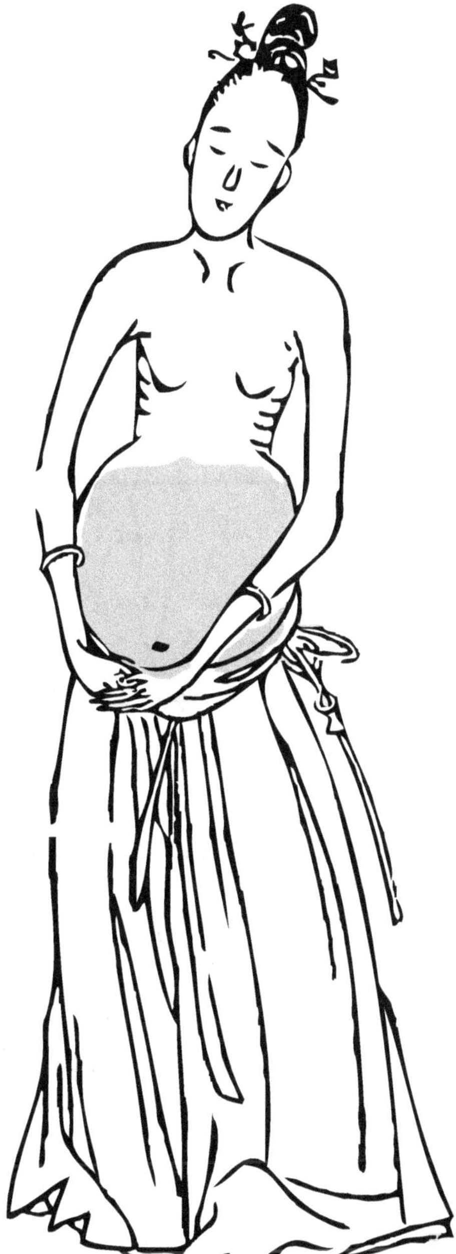

Fig. 11

83. *Fēn* (Ch: *fēn* 分; Jp: *fun*) is a traditional unit of weight that was used in East Asia. The exact weight differed depending on the region and period in which it was used, but it was calculated as one-tenth of a *qián*, or approximately 0.375g in Japan during the Meiji period.

84. Kai Province (Jp: *Kai-No-Kuni* 甲斐國) was the region of Japan that currently comprises Yamanashi Prefecture (Jp: *Yamanashi-Ken* 山梨縣).

anyone who enters my school and earnestly requests [to learn the uses], I will pass on the details to that person. For other cases that are unclear, refer to this.

橘皮大黄朴硝湯之證

The Pattern for Jú Pí Dà Huáng Máng Xiāo Tāng[85] 橘皮大黄芒硝湯

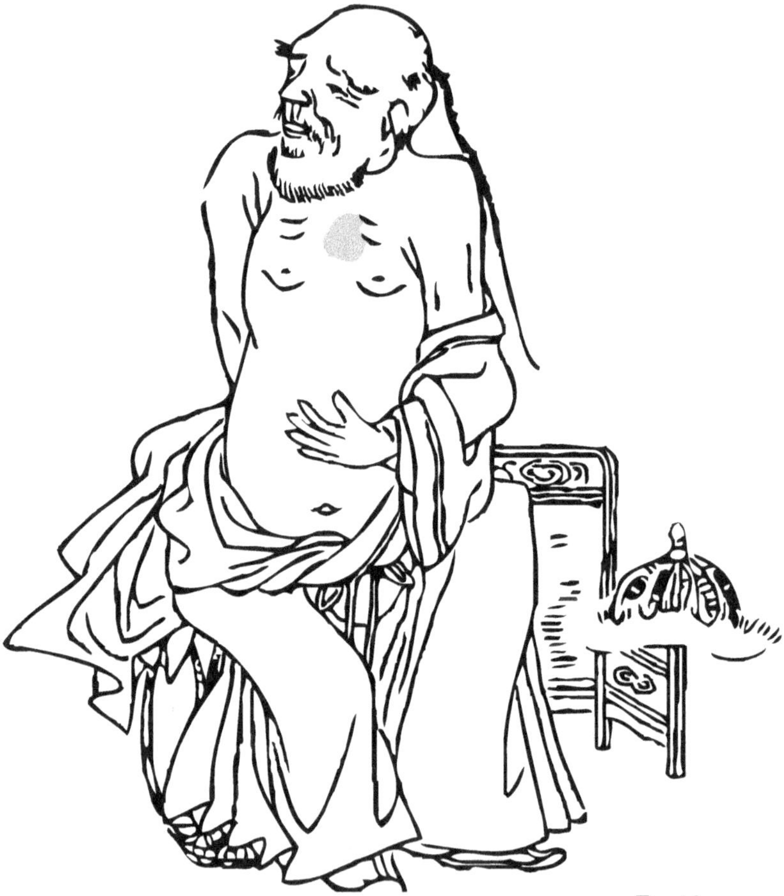

Fig. 12

圖の如く、心胸の間、宿食あつて結するもの。『論』に曰く、「鱠食の心胸の間に在りて化せず、吐復た出でざるは、速やかに之れを下し、久成の癥病を除く」。

85. The formula for *Jú Pí Dà Huáng Máng Xiāo Tāng* 橘皮大黄芒硝湯 (Jp: *Kippi-Daiō-Bōshō-Tō*; tangerine peel, rhubarb, and mirabilite decoction) was originally found in *Jīn Guì Yào Lüè*, although the formula itself was not named. At present, this formula is not covered by the Japanese National Health Insurance program and is not well known in Japan.

As shown in the illustration, the patient presents with abiding food that is bound in the heart and chest. The text [of *Jīn Guì Yào Lüè*] states that "when [the patient] eats sliced raw fish that remains in the heart and chest and is not transformed, it should be quickly precipitated in order to eliminate enduring conglomeration disease."[86]

克、案ずるに敢へて宿食・鱠食にかぎるべからず。心胸のあいだ、これを按じて凸にして堅し。按じて病者痛みを覺ふ。これ舊毒あるを以てなり。此の方の以てまつたく治す。餘藥の及ぶべからざるなり。

In my opinion, this does not mean that "abiding food" should be limited to only sliced raw fish. When the region between the heart and chest is palpated, a hard bulge can be felt. [Moreover,] the patient feels pain upon palpation. This is due to the presence of a long-standing toxin. This formula can completely cure [the pattern in cases when] other medicinals cannot reach [the toxin].

六君子湯之證

The Pattern for Liù Jūn Zǐ Tāng[87] 六君子湯

86. The Japanese text in this book uses the term *zhēng bìng* 癥病 (Jp: *chōbyō*; concretion disease), but the original Chinese text of *Jīn Guì Yào Lüè* uses the expression *jiǎ bìng* 瘕病 (Jp: *kabyō*; conglomeration disease). The original text as found in the "Contraindications Regarding Fowl, Beasts, and Insects Chapter (Ch: *Qín Shòu Yú Chóng Jìn Jì Bìng Zhì* 禽獸魚蟲禁忌并治; Jp: *Kin-Jū-Chō-Kinki-Heichi*)" of *Jīn Guì Yào Lüè* is as follows: "鱠食之、在心胸間不化、吐復不出、速下除之、久成瘕病."

87. The formula for *Liù Jūn Zǐ Tāng* 六君子湯 (Jp: *Rikkunshi-Tō*; six gentlemen decoction) was originally found in *Yī Xué Zhèng Zhuàn*《醫學正傳》(Jp: *Igaku-Seiden*; The Orthodox Tradition of Medicine), written by Yú Tuán 虞摶 (Jp: Gu Tan; 1438-1517 CE) and published in 1515. However, it seems to have become famous in Japan through *Wàn Bìng Huí Chūn*《萬病回春》(Jp: *Manbyō-Kaishun*; Return-of-Spring for All Diseases), compiled by Gōng Tíngxián 龔廷賢 (Jp: Kyō Teiken; 1522-1619 CE) and published in 1587. Dài Màn Gōng 戴曼公 (Jp: Tai Mankō; 1596-1671), a student of Gōng, moved to Japan and helped to popularize the text, which became a "best-seller" during the Edo period, and one of the core texts of the Later School of Kampō medicine (Jp: Gosei-Ha 後世派). The extract preparation of the formula is covered by the Japanese National Health Insurance program as a prescription drug, and is also commonly sold in Japanese drug stores as an over-the-counter drug. It is one of the most popular Chinese formulae in Japan, and is currently indicated by the MHLW for: gastritis, gastrointestinal weakness, gastroptosis, indigestion, loss of appetite, stomach pain, and vomiting in persons with moderate or weak physical strength who have poor digestion, decreased appetite, feeling of a knot in the solar plexus, fatigue, or cold extremities associated with anemia (体力中等度以下で、胃腸が弱く、食欲がなく、みぞおちがつかえ、疲れやすく、貧血性で手

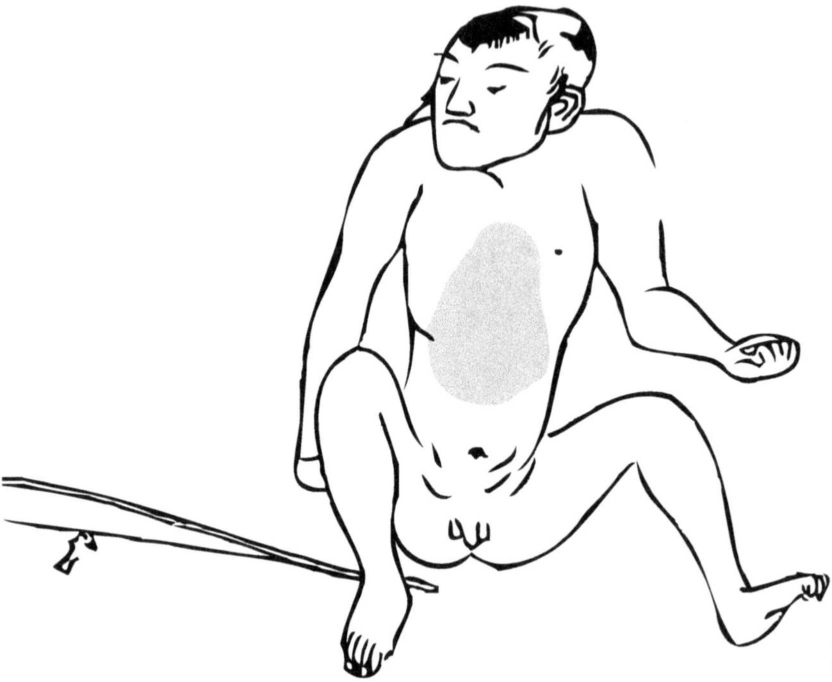

Fig. 13

圖の如く、中脘より上、腹力ありて、下脘腹力なし。苓姜朮甘湯の腹證に似たり。臍下脱して力なく、小便不利、あるひは氣急促迫、その人氣短く。

As shown in the illustration, [the patient] has strength in the region above the center stomach duct, but there is no abdominal strength in the region below the center stomach duct. [This pattern] resembles the abdominal pattern for *Líng Jiāng Zhú Gān Tāng*;[88] The region below the umbilicus has no strength, and urination is inhibited.

足が冷えやすいものの次の諸症：胃炎、胃腸虚弱、胃下垂、消化不良、食欲不振、胃痛、嘔吐).

88. The details of *Líng Jiāng Zhú Gān Tāng* 苓薑朮甘湯 (Jp: *Ryō-Kyō-Jutsu-Kan-Tō*; poria, ginger, white atractylodes, and licorice decoction) are not discussed in this work. The formula was originally found in *Shāng Hán Lùn*. The extract preparation of the formula is covered by the Japanese National Health Insurance program as a prescription drug, and is also commonly sold in Japanese drug stores as an over-the-counter drug. It is currently indicated by the MHLW for: low back pain, cold sensation in the lower back, nocturnal enuresis, and neuralgia in persons with moderate or weak physical strength who have a cold sensation and pain in the lower limbs below the waist and polyuria (體力中等度以下で、腰から下肢に冷えと痛みがあって、尿量が多いものの次の諸症：腰痛、腰の冷え、夜尿症、神經痛).

あるひはことにふれておどろく 。あるひは歩行してよく倒るる 。尤も小兒にこの證多し 。世に癇症と號するもの 、此の證 、間々あり 。その餘 、某々の病 、その憂を問はず 、この腹に合するもの 、六君子湯を用ひて治せざるものなし 。學者 、用ひて以て効を知るべし 。

In some cases the patient presents with both hasty and distressed rapid breathing and shortness of breath. In other cases, the patient experiences fright. In some cases, the patient collapses while walking. This pattern is quite common in children. [The condition] that is commonly called epilepsy fits this pattern. Regardless of the affliction or disease [that the patient presents with], there is no [condition] matching this abdominal [pattern] that cannot be cured by using *Liù Jūn Zǐ Tāng*. As the student [of abdominal patterns] uses [this formula], he will come to understand its efficacy.

大柴胡湯・甘草乾姜湯

[A Comparison of the Patterns for] Dà Chái Hú Tāng 大柴胡湯 and Gān Cǎo Gān Jiāng Tāng[89] 甘草乾薑湯

圖の如く 、二方相合するもの 。前の圖にいふ大柴胡湯 、胸脇苦滿 、腹實滿 、二方の證に比すれば 、大柴胡湯の毒もつとも深し 。甘草乾姜湯の毒 、胸中にあつて淺しといへども 、まづさきに上より順に治療をなし 、後 、大柴胡湯を用ゆべし 。大柴胡湯は說前につぶさにあり 。

As shown in the illustration, there are two formulae that match [the pattern]. Similar to the previous illustration for *Dà Chái Hú Tāng*, the patient presents with bitter fullness in the chest and rib-sides and replete fullness in the abdomen. Upon comparison of the two patterns, the toxin is located deeper in [the pattern for] *Dà Chái Hú Tāng*. Although the toxin [in the pattern for] *Gān Cǎo Gān Jiāng Tāng* is located more superficially inside

89. The formula for *Gān Cǎo Gān Jiāng Tāng* 甘草乾薑湯 (Jp: *Kanzō-Kankyō-Tō*; licorice and dried ginger decoction) was originally found in *Shāng Hán Lùn*. The extract preparation of the formula is approved by the MHLW to be sold in Japanese drug stores as an over-the-counter drug. It is currently indicated by the MHLW for: frequent urination, urinary incontinence, hypersalivation, rhinitis, hiccups, and dizziness in persons with weak physical strength who have cold extremities and thin saliva that collects in the mouth (體力虛弱で 、手足が冷え 、薄い唾液が口に溜まるものの次の諸症：頻尿 、尿もれ 、唾液分泌過多 、鼻炎 、しゃっくり 、めまい).

the chest, treatment should first focus on the superficial [symptoms] and then *Dà Chái Hú Tāng* may be later used [to attack the root]. I have already explained the details concerning *Dà Chái Hú Tāng* [in an earlier section].

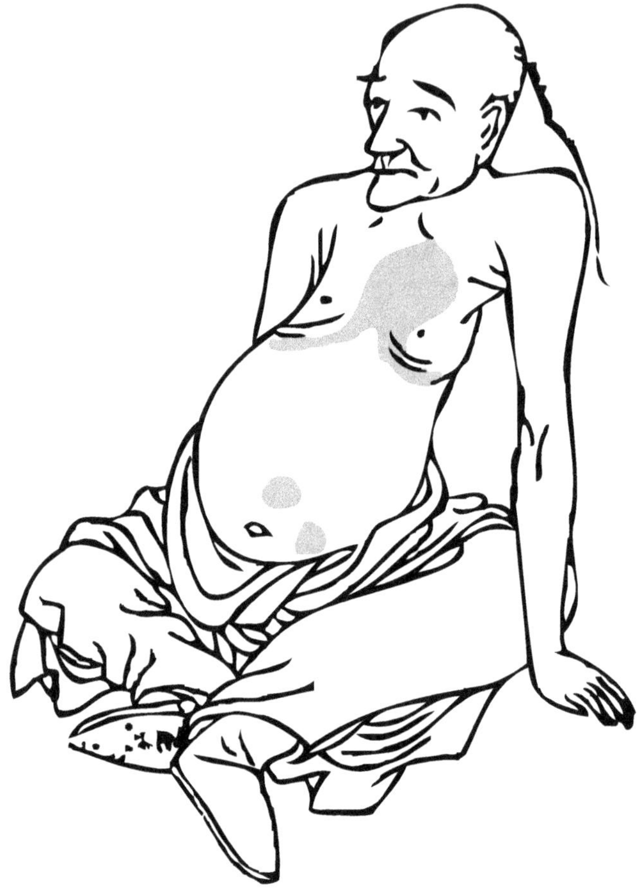

Fig. 14

甘草乾姜湯 、胸中煩燥急迫 、時に涎痰を吐するもの 、これなり 。小便不利 、世俗にいふ「 よばりたれ 」といふもの 、此の證多し 。八味丸の證もまたかんがふべし 。

[In the pattern for] *Gān Cǎo Gān Jiāng Tāng*, the patient presents with vexation, agitation, and distress in the chest, and ejects phlegm-drool. Many patients who have this pattern present with inhibited urination; they are colloquially referred to as "bedwetters." [In such cases,] *Bā Wèi Wán* may also be considered.[90]

90. The formula for *Bā Wèi Wán* 八味丸 (Jp: *Hachimi-Gan*; eight-ingredient pill) is discussed separately in its own section in this book.

大黄甘遂湯之證

The Pattern for Dà Huáng Gān Suì Tāng[91] 大黄甘遂湯

圖の如く、腹實滿して青筋一、二寸ばかりのもの、横に幾筋も染めなせしがごとくあらはれ、腹の色うす赤くして光りあり。又た一證、前のごとく腹張りて縦に煙を畫きし如き青筋、いくすぢも生ず。倶にみな、此の方の證にして、すなはちいはゆる「敦状」の如きもの、これなり。「敦」は都・内の切、音は對。黍稷を盛るの器なり。

As shown in the illustration, the patient presents with replete fullness in the abdomen, and several horizontal green-blue vessels [i.e., veins] approximately one or two *cun* in size are visible on the abdomen, [which appears] as if it were dyed. The abdomen is light red in color and has a bright luster. There is another pattern that is similar to the above-mentioned pattern in which the patient presents with a tense abdomen visible vertical blue vessels on the abdomen. Both [of these patterns] correspond to this formula. That is, any pattern [in which the abdomen] appears similar to a "*duì* vessel" is an example of this pattern.[92] The *fanqie* pronunciation for the character *duì* (敦) is composed of *dū* 都 and *nèi* (内); the pronunciation is the same as the character *duì* 對.[93] [A *duì* vessel] was a vessel to serve broomcorn millet and non-glutinous broomcorn millet.

91. The formula for *Dà Huáng Gān Suì Tāng* 大黄甘遂湯 (Jp: *Daiō-Kanzui-Tō*; rhubarb and kansui decoction) was originally found in *Jīn Guì Yào Lüè*. At present, this formula is not covered by the Japanese National Health Insurance program and is not well known in Japan.

92. As explained in the text, a *duì* vessel was a type of bronze food container that was used as a ritual vessel in the late *Zhōu* Ch: *Zhōu* 周; Jp: *Shū*; c. 1046–256 BCE) and the Warring States (Ch: *Zhàn Guó* 戰國; Jp: *Sengoku*; c. 475–221 BCE) periods of ancient China. *Duì* vessels were typically spherical in shape, possessing a half-domed bowl on bottom with a similarly shaped container fitting on top. The containers themselves possessed highly intricate detailing, varying in geometric and curvilinear designs distributed in symmetrical registers, which the author believed resembled the patterns created by visible abdominal vessels.

93. In traditional Chinese lexicography, *fanqie* (Ch: *fǎn qiè* 反切; Jp: *hansetsu*) was a method to indicate the pronunciation of a monosyllabic character by using two other characters (one with the same initial consonant as the desired syllable and one with the same rest of the syllable). The method was introduced in the 3rd century CE and used in dictionaries and commentaries on the Chinese classics until the modern period. As seen from this example, the system does not always work perfectly when reading the characters using modern Mandarin pronunciation. Although very few Japanese had a chance to study spoken Chinese during the Edo period, most learned persons had at least some knowledge of *fanqie*, as literacy was taught through study of the Chinese Confucian classics and their respective commentaries, similar to the education systems of China and Korea.

その圖、三才圖會及び唐土訓蒙圖彙・器用の部にのす。有虞氏の兩敦、これなり。蓋し敦の器爲るや、その腹面、張りて波を畫き、烟を畫きたるごとき模様あり。これその形のすこしく似たるを以て、たとへたるのみにて、直に圖と同じからず。

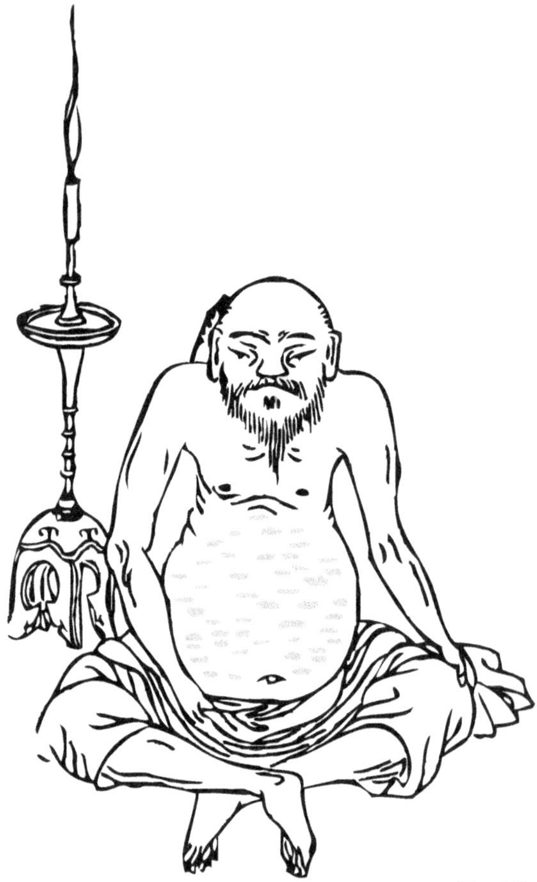

Fig. 15

Illustrations [of this vessel] can be found in the [*Wakan*]-*Sansai-Zue*[94] and in the section concerning vessels in the *Morokoshi-Kinmō-Zui*.[95] The two *duì* vessels of Yǒu Yúshì are examples of this.[96] *Duì* vessels are decorated with patterns that appear similar to waves or streams of rising smoke spread along the body of the vessels. Because the designs of the vessels appear somewhat similar to this pattern, I have only used this as an example for comparison, but it does not mean that the designs [on the abdomen] necessarily appear exactly the same as the illustration.

---

94. The title of this work can refer to either: *Sān Cái Tú Huì* 《三才圖會》, an illustrated Chinese encyclopedia compiled by Wáng Qí 王圻 and published in 1609, or *Wakan-Sansai-Zue* 《和漢三才圖會》([Sino-Japanese] Illustrated Compendium of the Three Talents), an illustrated Japanese encyclopedia inspired by *Sān Cái Tú Huì*, which was compiled by the physician Terajima Ryōan 寺島良安 (1654–ca. 1720) over a period of 30 years. In context, the author seems to be referring to the latter work. Consisting of 105 volumes in 81 books, *Wakan-Sansai-Zue* covers a variety of subjects, and was quite popular during the Edo period. It is still used as a reference work for the history of Kampō medicine.

95. *Morokoshi-Kinmō-Zui* 《唐土訓蒙圖彙》(Illustrated Encyclopedia of China), published in 1719, was also a best-selling Japanese encyclopedia of Chinese knowledge compiled by the physician Hirazumi Sen'an 平住專安 (unknown–1734 CE).

96. Yǒu Yúshì 有虞氏 (c.2300–c.2200 BCE) is an alternate name of Emperor Shùn 舜 (Jp: Shun), a legendary leader of ancient China, who was glorified for his virtue by Confucian philosophers.

此の證、大率難治なり。然れども、此の方を用ゆるときは、右の青筋盡く下りて功を奏することもつとも著し。克、しばしば此の方を用ゆ。凡そ死症なり。此の症まづ本劑を二、三劑施し、腹滿少しく減ずれば、直ちに後服をとどむ。琥珀湯を投じて以て調和して後、本劑を施す。しばしば此くの如くにして、救ふことを得べし。

This pattern is generally difficult to cure. However, this formula has the most notable success in causing the above-mentioned blue lines to descend completely. I have often used this formula. [This pattern] is generally a death pattern. [When the patient presents with] this pattern, [this] base formula should be administered two or three times, and when the abdominal fullness has been slightly reduced, administration of the formula should be immediately stopped. *Kohaku-tō* should be administered to harmonize [the body], and then this formula may be administered [again].[97] If repeatedly administered in this way, [the physician] should be able to save [the patient].

琥珀湯の方：琥珀（一戔半）・反鼻（五分）・商陸（一戔、生に非ざれば効無し）・豬苓（八分）・桂枝（一戔、上衝無き者は、桂を去りて、丁子を加ふ。若し有悸者ならば、茯苓を加ふ）。水二盞を以て一盞を取る。

The formula for *Kohaku-Tō* [is as follows]: *hǔ pò* (1 and 1/2 *qián*), *fǎn bí* (5 *fēn*), *shāng lù* (1 *qián*; there will be no effect if it is not fresh), *zhū líng* (8 *fēn*), *guì zhī* (1 *qián*; in cases in which there is no upward surging, *guì zhī* should be removed, and *dīng zǐ* should be added. If the patient has palpitations, then *fú líng* should be added). Boil [the ingredients] in two cups of water to make one cup [of the decoction].

97. Although there are various formulae in China with the name *Hǔ Pò Sǎn* 琥珀散 (Jp: *Kohaku-San*; amber powder), *Kohaku-Tō* 琥珀湯 (Ch: *Hǔ Pò Tāng*; amber decoction) seems to be a Japanese original formula that was copied from *Meika-Hōsen*《名家方選》(Selected Formulae of Distinguished Masters; compiled by Yamada Genrin 山田元倫 (also known as Wake Koreyuki 和氣惟享; 1760–1824 CE) in 1781 CE. However, as with most of the formulae in this book, the quantities of ingredients slightly differ from the original. At present, the formula is not covered by the Japanese National Health Insurance program and is not well known in Japan.

大承氣湯之證二圖

Two Illustrations of Dà Chéng Qì Tāng[98] 大承氣湯

前は腹堅滿、後は毒堅滿

The first illustration shows abdominal hard fullness, and the second shows hard fullness [caused by a] toxin.

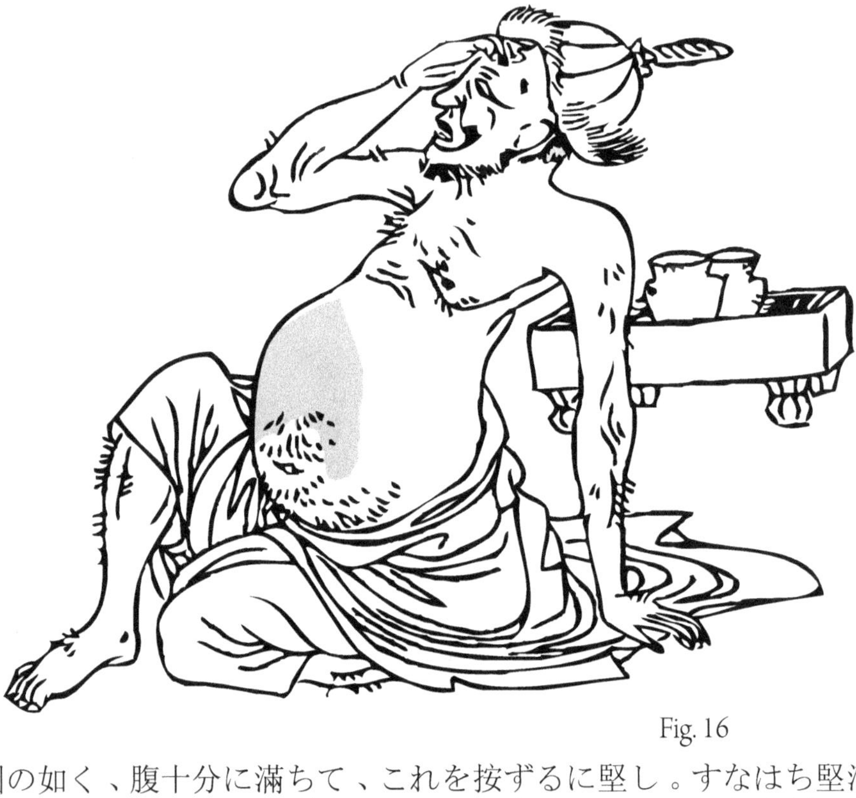

Fig. 16

圖の如く、腹十分に滿ちて、これを按ずるに堅し。すなはち堅滿なり。所謂「傷寒・疫利」の類にこの症多し。このとき大劑にして、急速にこれを攻むるときは、臭穢の毒物下り盡きて後、治すべきなり。

98. The formula for *Dà Chéng Qì Tāng* 大承氣湯 (Jp: *Dai-Jōki-Tō*; major qì-infusing decoction) was originally found in *Shāng Hán Lùn*. At present, this formula is not covered by the Japanese National Health Insurance program, although it is rather well known among Kampō specialists and is commonly sold in Japanese drug stores as an over-the-counter drug. It is currently indicated by the Tsumura ツムラ, the largest Kampō drug maker in Japan, for: chronic constipation, acute constipation, hypertension, neuralgia, and food poisoning in persons who have the feeling of a knot in the abdominal region, have constipation, or are obese and experience constipation (腹部がかたくつかえて、便祕するもの、あるいは肥滿體質で便祕するもの。常習便祕、急性便祕、高血壓、神經症、食當たり).

As shown in the illustration, the abdomen is completely full and feels hard upon palpation. It is [a case of] hard fullness. This pattern is common in patients who have what is known as "cold damage" or "epidemic dysentery." When [the toxin] is rapidly attacked using a major formula, the pattern will be cured after completely causing the foul-smelling toxic agent to descend.[99]

The Second Illustration of the Pattern for Dà Chéng Qì Tāng 大承氣湯

又た一證。此の圖のごとく、敢へて腹堅滿なるにてもなく、腹の中央に長く堅きものあり。これを按ずるに敢へて痛まず。これすなはち堅塊なり。あるひは身體羸痩して、堅塊あるものあり。世にいはゆる中風・脹滿、あるひは勞瘵等にこの證多し。

[Here is] another pattern [matching the formula]. As seen in this illustration, the patient may not necessarily present with hard fullness in the abdomen, but there is a long hard region in the center of the abdomen. When palpated, pain may not necessarily be present. This is a hard lump. In some cases, the body [of the patient] is markedly emaciated, and a hard lump is present. Many patients who present with [diseases] such as what is commonly known in the world as "wind strike" or "distention and fullness," or patients who present with consumption actually have this pattern.

謹んで藥品をあらため、數百劑を以て攻むること、或るひは半年、一年より、二年、三年に及ぶものあり。凡そ此の症もしくは燥屎あるものなり。燥屎あるものは、臍下必ず磊砢として、あた

---

99. At present, the *dà huáng* 大黃-based formulae covered by the Japanese National Health Insurance program as drugs for the treatment of abdominal inflation and fullness associated with a fecal block (i.e., constipation) are: *Xiǎo Chéng Qì Tāng* 小承氣湯 (Jp: *Shō-Jōki-Tō*; minor qì-infusing decoction), *Tiáo Wèi Chéng Qì Tāng* 調胃承氣湯 (stomach-regulating qì-infusing decoction), and *Táo Hé Chéng Qì Tāng* 桃核承氣湯 (peach kernel qì-infusing decoction). Of these formulae, *Tiáo Wèi Chéng Qì Tāng* and *Táo Hé Chéng Qì Tāng* are discussed in separate sections in this book. Because *Xiǎo Chéng Qì Tāng* is not discussed in this work, I will present the details here: the formula was originally found in *Jīn Guì Yào Lüè* and *Shāng Hán Lùn*. The extract preparation of the formula is approved by the MHLW to be sold in Japanese drug stores as an over-the-counter drug. It is currently indicated by the MHLW for: constipation in persons with comparatively strong physical strength who have abdominal bloating and fullness and occasionally experience fever (比較的體力があり、腹部が張って膨滿し、ときに發熱するものの次の症狀：便祕).

かも衆石を包みて、上より按ずるがごとし。肌膚枯燥して、ばさばさとしたるものなり。あるひは時々下痢臭穢、あるひは結糞・兔屎の如きものを下す。總て何病ひを問はず、腹底中央深くをすに、底へこたへて、其のかたち長きものあるは、みな大承氣湯の證なり。

When the medicinals used are carefully changed [after much consideration] and [the pattern] is attacked using [one of the] hundred medicinals, in some cases, [treatment] may last a half year, or in some cases up to one, two, or three years. In this pattern, the patient generally has dry stools. When palpating the subumbilical region of patients who have dry stools, it feels similar to touching many rocks that are loose. [These patients present with] skin that is desiccated and feels flaky. In some cases, the patient presents with foul-smelling diarrhea, and in other cases, the stools are dry and bound or appear similar to the passing of stools which are like rabbit droppings. Regardless of the disease [that was diagnosed], any pattern in which the center region of the abdomen springs

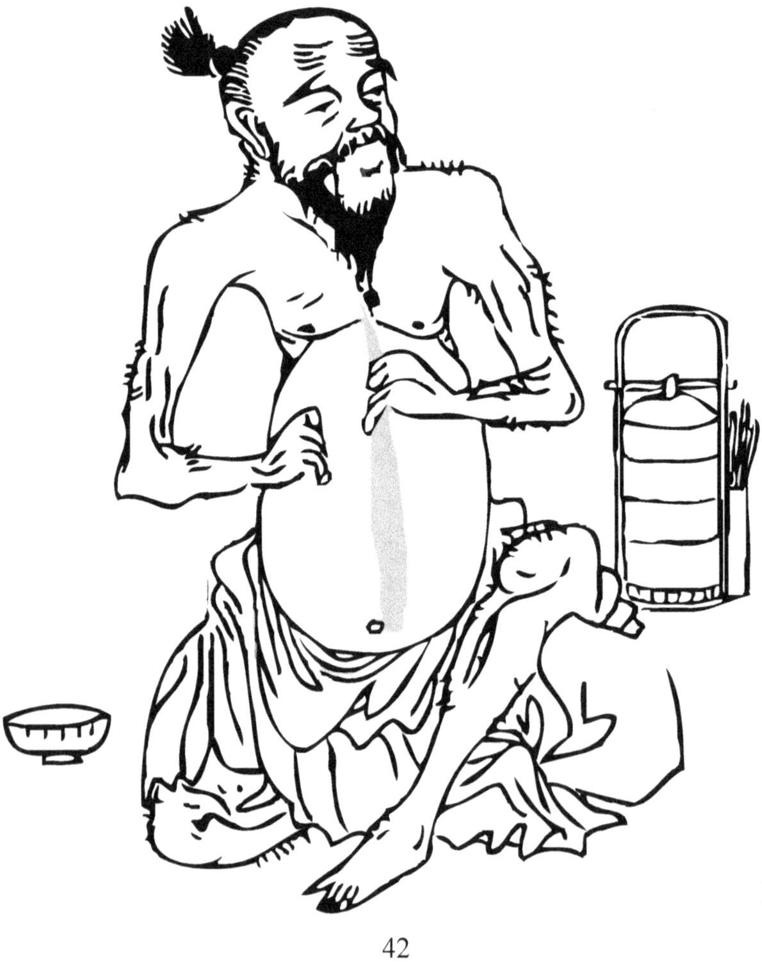

Fig. 17

back when pressed deeply to the depths of the abdomen, and the appearance [of the affected region] is long, this is the pattern for *Dà Chéng Qì Tāng*.

さて、またこの證を攻むるときは、まま脇に引いて掣痛するものあり。このとき本方を止めて、十棗湯をもちひ、掣痛治して後、本方に復りてこれを攻むべし。これ兼用の法なり。あるひはこの時に臨んで、知足齋の直行丸考ふべし。

Furthermore, when the pattern is attacked, some patients experience pulling pain in the rib-sides. In these cases, [administration of] this formula should be terminated, and *Shí Zǎo Tāng* should be used instead.[100] After the pulling pain has been cured, [the physician] may return to this formula and continue to attack [the toxin]. In some cases, when faced with this situation, Chisokusai's *Chokkō-Gan* may be considered for use.[101]

小建中湯之證

The Pattern for Xiǎo Jiàn Zhōng Tāng[102] 小建中湯

圖の如く、腹皮拘急して、縱横數繩を引つぱりたるが如く、これを按ずるにたゆまず。たとへば弓弦を押すがごとし。世にいはゆ

100. *Shí Zǎo Tāng* 十棗湯 (Jp: *Jissō-Tō*; ten jujubes decoction) is discussed separately in its own section in this book. This is the method for simultaneous use [of the formulae].

101. *Chokkō-Gan* 直行丸 (Ch: *zhí xíng wán*; direct-moving pill) was originally found in *Tokuhon-Ō-Jūku-Hō*. As with all of the "secret" formulae of Chisokusai 知足齋 (i.e., Nagata Tokuhon 永田德本), this formula is not covered by the Japanese National Health Insurance program and is not well known in Japan. The formula as found in the received text of *Tokuhon-Ō-Jūku-Hō* is as follows: *dà jǐ, dà huáng* (1 *qián* each), *yuán huā, gān suì, qiān niú zǐ* (5 *fēn* each).

102. The formula for *Xiǎo Jiàn Zhōng Tāng* 小建中湯 (Jp: *Shō-Kenchū-Tō*; minor center-fortifying decoction) was originally found in *Jīn Guì Yào Lüè* and *Shāng Hán Lùn*. The extract preparation of the formula is covered by the Japanese National Health Insurance program as a prescription drug, and is also commonly sold in Japanese drug stores as an over-the-counter drug. It is currently indicated by the MHLW for: pediatric weak physical constitution, fatigue, chronic gastroenteritis, abdominal pain, nervousness, and pediatric nocturnal enuresis in persons with weak physical strength who feel easily fatigued and have abdominal pain, poor complexion, occasional palpitations, feeling of hot flashes in the extremities, sensitivity to cold, night sweats, nosebleeds, frequent urination, or polyuria (體力虚弱で、疲勞しやすく腹痛があり、血色がすぐれず、ときに動悸、手足のほてり、冷え、ねあせ、鼻血、頻尿および多尿などを伴うものの次の諸症: 小兒虚弱體質、疲勞倦怠、慢性胃腸炎、腹痛、神經質、小兒夜尿症、夜泣き).

る労瘵癇症。あるひは欝證と號するもの、この證多し。醫者、文辭に眩せず、腹症によつて方を處するときは、百發百中、失するといふことなし。

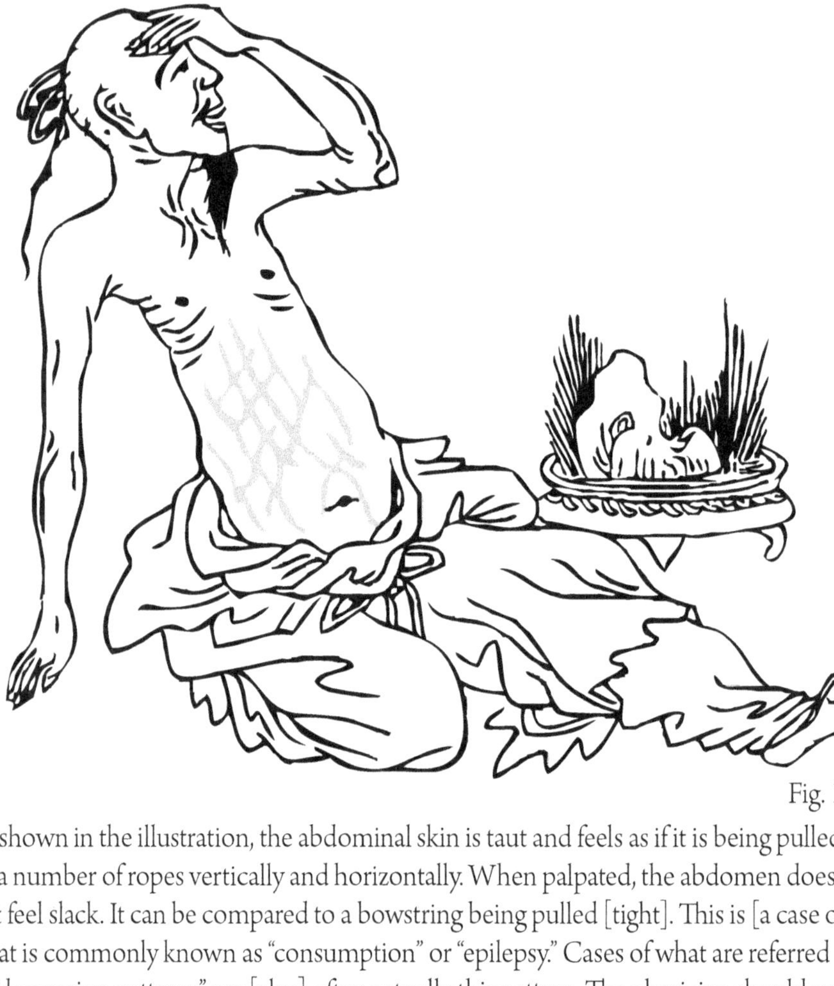

Fig. 18

As shown in the illustration, the abdominal skin is taut and feels as if it is being pulled by a number of ropes vertically and horizontally. When palpated, the abdomen does not feel slack. It can be compared to a bowstring being pulled [tight]. This is [a case of] what is commonly known as "consumption" or "epilepsy." Cases of what are referred to as "depression patterns" are [also] often actually this pattern. The physician should not be blinded by terminology [i.e., the name of the disease]. If he prescribes formulae according to the abdominal patterns [rather than based on the name of the disease], then [the treatments] will be effective in 100 out of 100 cases.

桂姜棗草黄辛附湯之證

The Pattern for Guì Jiāng Zǎo Cǎo Huáng Xīn Fù Tāng[103] 桂薑棗草黄辛附湯

附枳朮湯證及び堅塊・結塊・血塊解せざるの論

The pattern for Fù Zhǐ Zhú Tāng[104] 附枳朮湯 and hard lumps, binding lumps, and blood clots that are not resolved

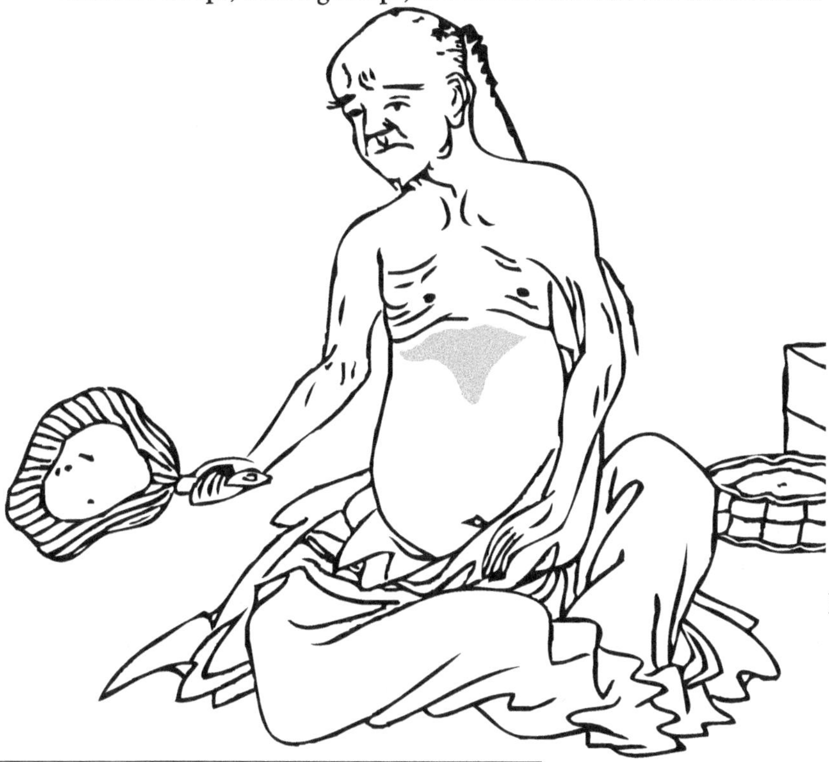

Fig. 19

103. The formula for *Guì Jiāng Zǎo Cǎo Huáng Xīn Fù Tāng* 桂薑棗草黃辛附湯 (Jp: *Kei-Kyō-Sō-Sō-Ō-Shin-Bu-Tō*; cinnamon twig, ginger, jujube, licorice, ephedra, asarum, and aconite decoction) was originally found in *Jīn Guì Yào Lüè*. The extract preparation of the formula is approved by the MHLW to be sold in Japanese drug stores as an over-the-counter drug. It is currently indicated by the MHLW for: the common cold, bronchitis, joint inflammation and pain, watery nasal discharge associated with rhinitis, neuralgia, back pain, and cold extremities in persons with moderate or weak physical strength who complain of chills (體力中等度以下で、さむけを訴えるものの次の諸症：感冒、氣管支炎、關節のはれや痛み、水様性鼻汁を伴う鼻炎、神經痛、腰痛、冷え症).

104. *Fù Zhǐ Zhú Tāng* 附枳朮湯 (Jp: *Bu-Ki-Jutsu-Tō*; aconite, unripe bitter orange, and [white] atractylodes decoction) seems to be an original combination of the formula for *Zhǐ Zhú Tāng* 枳朮湯 (*Ki-Jutsu-Tō*; unripe bitter orange and [white] atractylodes decoction), originally found in *Jīn Guì Yào Lüè*, with the addition of *fù zǐ* 附子. At present, both formulae are not covered by the Japanese National Health Insurance program and are not commonly used in Japan.

圖の如く、心下に毒ありて、其の形、圓なり。所謂盤の如く、邊り旋杯の如きもの、これなり。これを按ずるに、堅くして大承氣湯の堅塊に似たり。然れども、大承氣湯の堅塊は其の形長きを以てこれを別かつ。又た圖の如く、心下堅大なるものに、枳朮湯の證あり。

As shown in the illustration, the patient presents with a toxin in the region below the heart; [the affected region] has a round shape. Patterns in which [the region affected by the toxin] appears to be in the shape of a platter or a rotating cup are examples of this pattern. Upon palpation, [the affected region] feels hard, and the hard lumps are similar to [those seen in the pattern for] *Dà Chéng Qì Tāng*. However, [the pattern for] *Dà Chéng Qì Tāng* can be differentiated by the long shape of the hard lump. Furthermore, as shown in the illustration, when the region below the heart is hard and enlarged, it is the pattern for *Zhǐ Zhú Tāng*.

是れ其の外證に依つてこれを別つべし。此の方の證は、上衝喘急、或るひは自汗、或るひは惡寒、或るひは身痛むもの、是れなり。枳朮湯の證は小便不利なるもの是れなり。

These [patterns] can be differentiated by the external signs that the patient presents with; in the pattern for this formula, the patient presents with signs of upward surging and rapid panting. In some cases, he may experience spontaneous sweating.[105] In some cases, he may have an aversion to cold.[106] In some cases, he may have generalized pain. These are [all the signs of] this pattern. Patterns in which the patient presents with inhibited urination are [examples of] the pattern for *Zhǐ Zhú Tāng*.

余、諸州を游歷して、衆病人を療するに、ままこの二方の證あり。これを用ゆるに、枳朮湯に於いてはしばしば効を得れども、此の方に於いては効を得ることなし。依つて之れを疑ふこと久し。曩に吉益修夫に謁して問ふていはく、「克、古醫の術を慕ひ、諸國を周流して、陳痾を療するに、十に八、九は治を奏せざるものなし。其の一、二に於いて方證相對すといえへども、如何ともすべからざるものあり。之れを如何」と。

105. Spontaneous sweating (Ch: *zì hàn* 自汗; Jp: *jikan*) refers to excessive sweating during the daytime with no apparent cause such as physical exertion, hot weather, thick clothing, or medication.

106. *Wù hán* 惡寒 (Jp: *okan*) is generally translated as "aversion to cold," in Japan, this term commonly refers to any type of chills.

I have experienced these two patterns during my travels around various provinces treating a multitude of patients. Although I have often obtained effective results from using *Zhĭ Zhú Tāng*, this formula was ineffective [in treating such cases]. For this reason, I long had questions about it. I once visited Yoshimasu Shūfu[107] and asked him [about this problem,] saying, "I have great admiration for the techniques of the ancient physicians. I have traveled around the various provinces, [and used the ancient techniques] when treating [all] long-standing diseases; out of every ten cases, I have been able to obtain success in eight or nine. In the one or two cases [that cannot be cured], I try to match the formulae to the patterns, but I am helpless to treat them. What should I do?"

修夫答へて曰く、「昔、吾が翁もまたその事あり。全く大承氣湯の證具はりて、數月これを攻むるといへども、稍や微攻あるのみにして、塊物解せず。翁、依つて考ふるに、旁ら眞武湯の證あり。是を以て、眞武湯の方内に附子を倍して、これを與へ、効を得たり」と。

Shūfu responded, "My father experienced the same situation as you in the past. [The patient] presented with all [of the signs matching] the pattern for *Dà Chéng Qì Tāng*, so he attacked [the disease] for several months, but [the treatment] was only mildly successful, and the lump was not resolved. For this reason, my father thought that [the patient] had the comorbid pattern for *Zhēn Wŭ Tāng*.[108] He therefore doubled the amount of *fù zĭ* (included in the formula for *Zhēn Wŭ Tāng*), and when the formula was administered [to the patient], he obtained a successful result."

又た土州の醫小松久吾なる者の父某が曰く、「堅塊・血塊解せざるもの、附子を用ひて効を得たり」と。此れ等の事ども、思ひ合せて考ふるに、桂姜棗草黄辛附湯の方論に云はく、「心下堅大、盤の如し。邊り、旋杯の如し」と。

---

107. Yoshimasu Nangai 吉益南涯 (1750–1813 CE) was the oldest son of Yoshimasu Tōdō 吉益東洞, and a renown physician himself. As his courtesy name (Ch: *zì* 字; Jp: *azana*) was Shūfu 修夫, he is referred to as Yoshimasu Shūfu in this work. Nangai broke with his father's theory of "myriad diseases arising from one toxin" (Jp: *manbyō-ichidoku-setsu* 萬病一毒說; Ch: *wàn bìng yī dú shuō*) and established a new pathogenetic theory based on imbalances in qì, blood, and water [i.e., bodily fluids] (Jp: *ki-ketsu-sui-ron* 氣血水論; Ch: *qì xuè shuĭ lùn*). This concept has since become one of the foundations underpinning Japanese Kampō medical theory.

108. The formula for *Zhēn Wŭ Tāng* 眞武湯 (Jp: *Shinbu-Tō*; true warrior decoction) is discussed in its own section in this book.

Furthermore, a certain esteemed father, [i.e., teacher] of a physician in Doshū[109] named Komatsu Kyūgo once said, "I have been successful in using *fù zǐ* to treat patients who present with unresolved hard lumps or blood lumps."[110] [If we] consider these facts together, [the condition is exactly as it] is written in the section concerning *Guì Jiāng Zǎo Cǎo Huáng Xīn Fù Tāng* [in *Shāng Hán Lùn*]: "There is great hardness in the region below the heart that appears to be in the shape of a platter, and the sides are similar to rotating cups."[111]

東洞翁云はく、「此の方證、備はざる也。桂枝去芍藥湯と麻黄附子細辛湯と二方の證合するものなり。其の分量、桂枝・生姜・大棗（各々六分）・附子（三分）・麻黄・細辛・甘草（各四分）。水二盞四分を以て煮て六分を取る」と。これによつてこれをみれば、大きさ盤の如く、邊り旋杯の如きものは、是れ塊物なり。

The venerable old [Yoshimasu] Tōdō [once] said, "This formula-pattern is incomplete. The two formulae of *Guì Zhī Qù Sháo Yào Tāng* and *Má Huáng Fù Zǐ Xì Xīn Tāng* should be used simulataneously.[112] The quantity of the ingredients are as follows: *guì zhī, shēng jiāng, dà zǎo* (six *fēn* each), *fù zǐ* (three *fēn*), *má huáng, xì xīn, gān cǎo* (four *fēn* each). Boil the ingredients in two cups and four *fēn* of water to make six *fēn* [of the decoction]." When looked at in this way, "[the hardness in the region below the heart] that is the same size as a platter and sides that are similar to rotating cups" are actually lumps.

109. Doshū 土州 is the abbreviated name of Tosa Province (Jp: *Tosa-No-Kuni* 土佐國), which comprises present-day Kōchi Prefecture (Jp: *Kōchi-Ken* 高知縣) on Shikoku 四國 Island.

110. There appear to be no available records concerning this person or other related persons.

111. This quote is from *Jīn Guì Yào Lüè*, Chapter 14 "On Identification of Pulse, Symptom Complex, and Treatment of Water Qì Diseases (Ch: *Shuǐ Qì Bìng Mài Zhèng Bìng Zhì* 水氣病脈證并治; Jp: *Suiki-Byō-Myaku-Shō-Hei-Chi*)," although the phrase was actually used concerning *Zhǐ Zhú Tāng* 枳朮湯 rather than *Guì Jiāng Zǎo Cǎo Huáng Xīn Fù Tāng* 桂薑棗草黄辛附湯. The original text is as follows: "心下堅、大如盤、邊如旋盤、水飲所作、枳朮湯主之" (When there is great hardness in the region below the heart that appears to be in the shape of a platter, and the sides are similar to rotating cups, [it is a condition] due to water-rheum, which is governed by *Zhǐ Zhú Tāng*).

112. The formula for *Má Huáng Fù Zǐ Xì Xīn Tāng* 麻黄附子細辛湯 (Jp: *Maō-Bushi-Saishin-Tō*; ephedra, aconite, and asarum decoction) was originally found in *Shāng Hán Lùn*. The extract preparation of the formula is covered by the Japanese National Health Insurance program as a prescription drug, and is also commonly sold in Japanese drug stores as an over-the-counter drug. It is currently indicated by the MHLW for: allergic rhinitis, bronchitis, bronchial asthma, and neuralgia in persons with weak physical strength who have cold extremities and occasional chills (體力虚弱で、手足に冷えがあり、ときに惡寒があるものの次の諸症：感冒、アレルギー性鼻炎、氣管支炎、氣管支ぜんそく、神經痛).

凡そ附子の分量多き方劑には、煎方・水量、佗方に比するに尤も多し。然るに此の方、附子の分量少くして、水煎の分量尤も多し。是れ蓋し傳寫の誤りならんと、心に疑ふこと數年。後、東都に遊ぶの日、一病人をみるに正に此の症なり。因つて附子を五倍して與ふるに、盤の如き堅塊、速やかに解けたり。此こに於いて多年の畜疑、一時にとけたり。後、この證に値ふごとに、數しば試みてしばしば功あり。

The quantity of water used to decoct formulae that include a large amount of *fù zǐ* is generally greater in comparison with other formulae. However, the amount of *fù zǐ* in this formula is small, and the quantity of water used to make the decoction is the largest. For many years, I had doubts in my heart that this might be a copyist error in the text. One day, when I was traveling in the eastern capital [i.e., Edo], I examined a patient who fit this pattern exactly.[113] When I increased the quantity of *fù zǐ* five fold and administered [the formula to the patient], the hard lump resembling a platter rapidly resolved. Thus, my doubts that had lingered for many years disappeared in an instant. After that, each of the numerous times that I have encountered this pattern, I have tried using [this formula] and have often able to achieve success.

又た案ずるに、世間に年來難治と稱するもの、或るひは大承氣湯、或るひは桃核承氣湯、あるひは大黄牡丹皮湯、あるひは芎歸膠艾湯、或るひは豬苓湯、あるひは枳朮湯及び此の方の類。其の餘、何等の證を問はず、塊物或るひは急結、或るひは結實堅滿の類。大黄・芒硝を以て動くものあり。枳實を以て動くものあり。附子を以て動くものあり。輕粉・水銀を以て動くものあり。凡そ方證相對して數月これを攻むるといへども、自若として動かざるものは、みな是れ所謂沈寒、涸冷、美疢、痼毒なり。

I believe that what are commonly referred to as long-standing intractable diseases are in some cases [the pattern for] *Dà Chéng Qì Tāng, Táo Hé Chéng Qì Tāng, Dà Huáng Mǔ Dān Pí Tāng, Xiōng Guī Jiāo Ài Tāng, Zhū Líng Tāng, Zhǐ Zhú Tāng,* or other formulae such as this formula.[114] In other cases, regardless of [the name of the] pattern [that was

113. The eastern capital refers to Edo 江戸, which is present-day Tōkyō Metropolis (Jp: *Tōkyō-To* 東京都). From the establishment of the headquarters of the Tokugawa shogunate 德川幕府 (1603-1868 CE) in Edo, the city became the de facto capital and center of political power, although Kyōto 京都, where the emperor continued to reside, remained the official capital of the country.

114. The formulae for *Xiōng Guī Jiāo Ài Tāng* 芎歸膠艾湯 (Jp: *Kyū-Ki-Kyō-Gai-Tō*; Chinese

diagnosed], the patient may present with a lump, tense bind, binding fullness, or hard fullness. In some cases, [the toxin] is moved by *dà huáng* or *máng xiāo*. In some cases, [the toxin] is moved by *zhǐ shí*. In some cases, [the toxin] is moved by *fù zǐ*. In some cases, [the toxin] is moved by *qīng fěn* or *shuǐ yín*. In general, cases in which [the toxin] remains unmoved after being attacked for several months in accordance with formula-pattern matching theory, are examples of what is known as sinking cold, desiccated cold, feverish eruption, or a disease toxin.[115]

是こに於いて、一概して大黄朴硝の主治と極むべからず。詳らかに診察して、附子の證あらば附子を以て攻むべし。若し夫れしからざるものは、或るひは水銀・輕粉・礬石の類、毒を鎔化し下すものに非ずんば、治すべからず。於是乎、東洞家の七寶・礬黄、知足齋の瀉心・玉丹。鶴家の滅毒丸、龜井家の三花神祐丸、村瀨家の雲龍散の類。

In these cases, [the physician] must not make the generalization that *dà huáng* or *máng xiāo* are always indicated [for these patterns. The physician] should perform a detailed examination, and if the patient presents with the pattern for *fù zǐ*, then *fù zǐ* should be used to attack the pattern. In other cases, if ingredients such as *shuǐ yín*, *qīng fěn*, or *fán shí* are not used to melt and precipitate the [long-standing] toxin, [the pattern] will not be cured. In these cases, drugs such as the following [should be administered]: the Tōdō

angelica, ass hide glue, and mugwort decoction) and *Zhū Líng Tāng* 豬苓湯 (Jp: *Chorei-Tō*, polyporus decoction) are discussed together and separately in a different section in this work.

115. Following the translation by James Legge, *měi chèn* 美疢 (Jp: *bichin*) has been translated here as "feverish eruption," although the meaning of the term is somewhat unclear. The *Shuō Wén Jiě Zì*《說文解字》(Jp: *Setsumon-Kaiji*; Etymological Explanation of both Simple and Complex Characters) glosses *chèn* 疢 as a febrile disease (original text: 疢、熱病也), whereas the *Guǎng Yùn*《廣韻》(Jp: *Kōin*; Extended Rhymes) explains it as a type of disease that is commonly written using the character of *zhěn* 疹, i.e., a disease characterized by papules (original text: 疢, 病也。俗作疹). The term *měi chèn* 美疢 was originally used in the *Chūn Qiū Zuǒ Shì Zhuàn*《春秋左氏傳》(Jp: *Shunjū-Sashi-Den*; Commentary of Zuǒ of the Spring and Autumn Annals). It appears to have referred to a disease caused by eating delicious food. The original text and translation by James Legge are as follows: "…季之愛我、疾疢也。孟孫之惡我、藥石也。美疢不如惡石。夫石猶生我、疢之美、其毒滋多..." (…the love of *Jì Sūn* produced in me a feverish eruption. The hatred of *Mèng Sūn* was like a medicinal stone [i.e., *bian* stone] to me. The good eruption was not so beneficial as the painful stone, which brought me to life again, while the eruption increased its venom more and more...).

family's *Shichihō-Gan* or *Ban-Ō-Gan,*[116] Chisokusai's *Shashin-En*[117] or *Gyoku-Tan,* the Kaku family's *Metsudoku-Gan* 滅毒丸, the Kamei family's[118] *Sanka-Shin'yū-Gan,*[119] or the Murase family's *Unryū-San* 雲龍散.[120]

其の餘、水銀・輕粉等の組み入れたる方劑、其の證を詳らかにしてこれを用ゆべし。然りといへども、結實・堅塊となりたるものは皆、多年の舊毒、荏苒して凝結したるものなれば、年月の功を積まざれば、治を奏することあるべからず。是こに於いて病家、其の功遲きに疑ひを起こすときは、治術を盡くすことあたはず。能々教へ諭して後、藥を與ふべし。醫を業とするもの、此の場を考へて、口實とせずんばあるべからず。

In other cases, formulae that contain a mix of *shuǐ yín* and *qīng fěn* should be used after elucidating the pattern. However, because all cases of binding fullness and hard lumps are due to long-standing toxins that have naturally congealed over a period of many years, unless the treatment is [also] continued for a long period, said treatment will be ineffective. Thus, when the patient has doubts [concerning the treatment] on account of

---

116. The details of the formulae for *Shichihō-Gan* 七寶丸 (Ch: *Qī Bǎo Wán*; seven-jewel decoction) and *Ban-Ō-Gan* 礬黃丸 (Ch: *Fán Huáng Wán*; alum and rhubarb pill) are discussed in the final section of the book.

117. The formula for *Shashin-En* 瀉心圓 as found in the received text of *Tokuhon-Ō-Jūku-Hō* 《德本翁十九方》 (Nineteen Prescriptions of the Venerable Tokuhon) is as follows: *dà huáng* (4 *qián*), *fán shí* (2 *qián*), *qīng fěn*, *bā dòu* (5 *fēn* each). At present, this formula is not covered by the Japanese National Health Insurance program and is not commonly used in Japan.

118. The Kamei family refers to the school of Kamei Nanmei 龜井南冥 (1743–1814), a famous Confucian scholar and physician from Chikuzen Province (Jp: *Chikuzen-No-Kuni* 筑前國), which is now part of Fukuoka Prefecture (Jp: *Fukuoka-Ken* 福岡縣) in Kyūshū 九州. He studied briefly under Yoshimasu Tōdō in 1762, but quickly left after feeling dissatisfied with the methods of the Tōdō school. Differing from the Ancient School (Jp: *Kohō-Ha* 古方派), which almost totally relied on *Shāng Hán Lùn* and *Jīn Guì Yào Lüè*, he borrowed newer formulas and ideas from medical books of later Chinese dynasties such as the *Sòng* (宋) and *Míng* (明) dynasties.

119. The formula for *Sanka-Shin'yū-Gan* 三花神祐丸 (Ch: *Sān Huā Shén Yòu Wán*; three flowers spirit protection pill) is unclear. However, there is a Chinese formula of the same name (usually written as 三花神佑丸) found in *Yī Fāng Kǎo* 《醫方考》 (Jp: *Ihō-kō*; Medical Remedies Researched), which was published by Wú Kūn 吳崑 in 1584. It is unknown if Kamei borrowed this formula and the author was confused about the source or if it is an original formula by Kamei. The formula as found in *Yī Fāng Kǎo* is as follows: *gān suì* (one-half *liǎng*), *dà jǐ* (one-half *liǎng*), *yuán huā*, (one-half *liǎng*), *qiān niú* (2 *liǎng*), *dà huáng* (1 *liǎng*), *qīng fěn* (1 *qián*).

120. The details of *Unryū-San* 雲龍散 and the identity of the Murase 村瀬 family are unclear.

the belated [signs of] efficacy [of the medicinals], he will be unable to be continue the treatment to completion. [The physician] should therefore carefully instruct [the patient about this fact] and then administer the medicinals. Anyone who engages in the practice of medicine must consider [what to say] in these cases and not make excuses [to the patient].

腹證奇覽上册終

End of Volume I of Fukushō-Kiran
《腹證奇覽》
(Extraordinary Views of Abdominal Patterns)[121]

121. This work includes four volumes in total. The first two volumes were published together, and the final two were published two years later.

大陥胸湯之證 (幷大陥胸丸之證)

The Pattern for Dà Xiàn Xiōng Tāng[118] 大陥胸湯 (Including Dà Xiàn Xiōng Wán 大陥胸丸)

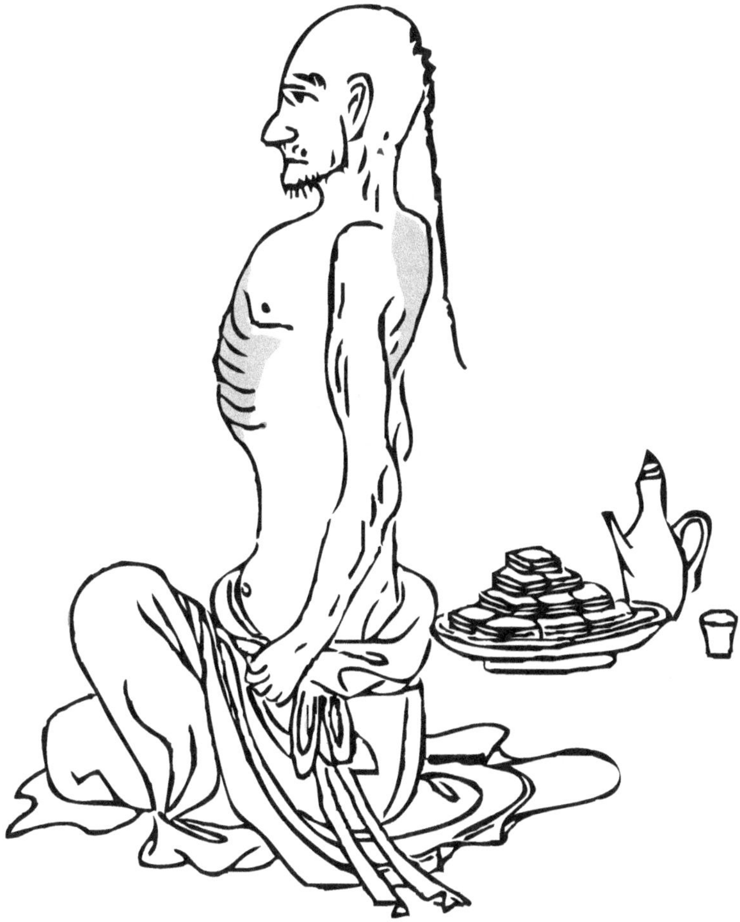

Fig. 20

圖の如く、胸高く張り出でて、これを按すに堅し。世にいはゆる膈噎・反胃の類、この證多し。あるひは心痛、久年治せざるもの、此の證あり。其の餘病名を問はず、この證あるときは、みな此の方を用ゆべし。然れども、この方を用ゆるの傳、たとへば小腹急結して、桃黄丸の證あるものの如きに、圖のごとく、胸間に

118. The formulae for *Dà Xiàn Xiōng Tāng* 大陥胸湯 (Jp: *Dai-Kankyō-Tō*; major chest bind decoction) and *Dà Xiàn Xiōng Wán* 大陥胸丸 (Jp: *Dai-Kankyō-Gan*; major chest bind pill) were originally found in *Shāng Hán Lùn*. At present, both formulae are not covered by the Japanese National Health Insurance program and are not commonly used in Japan.

毒ありて、凸きものは、まづ此の方を用ひ、胸毒を去りて後、急結をせむべし。

As shown in the illustration, the chest is highly distended and protruding, and feels hard when pressed. Patients who present with conditions such as what are commonly known as "dysphagia-occlusion" or "stomach reflux" often have this pattern. In some cases, when the patient has long-standing intractable heart pain, it is actually this pattern. In other cases, this formula should be used when the patient presents with this pattern, regardless of the name of the disease. However, according to the traditional method to use this formula, when the patient presents with a tense and bound smaller abdomen and has a toxin in the chest that causes a bulge, as shown in the illustration (similar to the pattern for *Tō-Kō-Gan*),[119] this formula should be used first. After eliminating the chest toxin, the tense bind may then be attacked.

結毒着項背之圖

Illustration of Toxin Bind Affixed to the Nape and Back[120]

又た大陥胸湯を用ゆるの法は、まづ小陥胸湯をあたふること、日々に二、三服にして、夜大陥胸丸一戔を用ひ、時々大陥胸湯を以てせむべし。餘證にして胸毒あるものも、また之れに傚へ。又た一證此の圖のごとく、胸腹より背脊にいたるまで、その毒凝結して、痛みはなはだしく、手も近づくべからざるものあり。これ毒の厚深にして、劇しきものなり。右の法の如く、大陥胸丸を以てこれを攻むべし。

The method to use *Dà Xiàn Xiōng Tāng* is to first administer two or three daily doses of *Xiǎo Xiàn Xiōng Tāng* [to the patient], give one *qián* of *Dà Xiàn Xiōng Wán* at night, and

119. The details concerning *Tō-Kō-Gan* (Ch: *Táo Huáng Wán* 桃黄丸; peach kernel and rhubarb pill) are unclear. It has been suggested that this refers to the pill form of *Táo Hé Chéng Qì Tāng* 桃核承氣湯.

120. This section explains the difference in clinical indications of *Dà Xiàn Xiōng Tāng* 大陷胸湯 and *Dà Xiàn Xiōng Wán* 大陷胸丸. Both are indicated for chest bind (Ch: *jié xiōng* 結胸; Jp: *kekkyō*), a diseased state attributable to accumulation of pathogens in the chest and abdomen, often manifested by local rigidity, fullness, and tenderness (also the same as chest constriction). However, because *Dà Xiàn Xiōng Wán* contains the additions of *xìng rén* and *tíng lì*, it is indicated in *Shāng Hán Lùn* for cases of concurrent chest bind and stiffness of the neck (Ch: *xiàng jiàng* 項強; Jp: *kōkyō*; i.e., muscular contraction and rigidity of the neck and the upper back with impaired movement).

occasionally attack [the toxin] with *Dà Xiàn Xiōng Tāng*. Follow this [guide] for [treating] other patterns in which the patient presents with a chest toxin. Furthermore, as shown in this illustration for the pattern, in some cases, the toxin congeals and spreads from the chest and abdomen to the back and spine, causing severe pain and stiffness, so much so that pain is exacerbated by the slightest pressure of palpation. The toxin is thick and deep, causing severe [symptoms. In such cases,] *Dà Xiàn Xiōng Wán* should be used in accordance with the above-mentioned method.

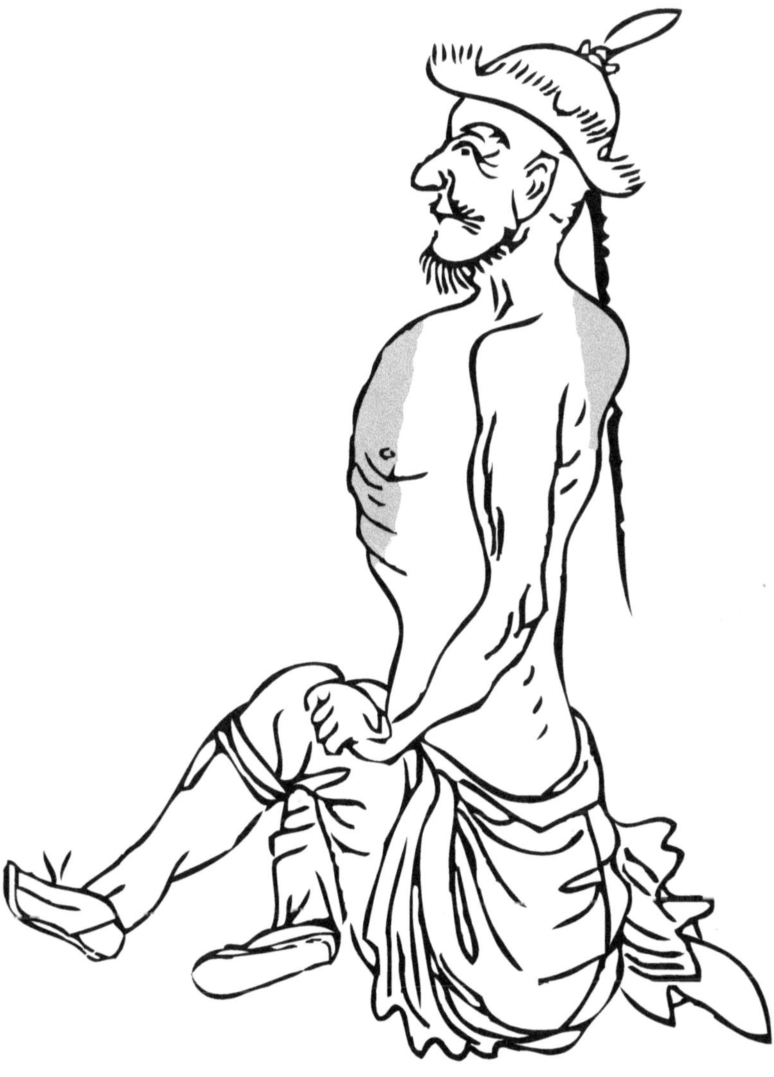

Fig. 21

小陷胸湯之證

The Pattern for Xiǎo Xiàn Xiōng Tāng[121] 小陷胸湯

圖の如く、胸に毒ありて胸高く、時々胸痛し、あるひは心煩し、あるひは胸たとへんかたなく惡く、所謂心痛嘈雜などといふもの、この證多し。まづ小陷胸湯をあたへ、時々大陷胸湯を以て、これを攻むべし。あるひは知足齋の直行丸、可なり。

As shown in the illustration, the patient presents with a toxin in the chest: The chest is highly [distended] and occasional chest pain is present.[122] In some cases, the patient presents with heart vexation, and in other cases, there is an incomparably bad [feeling] in the chest. Patients who have conditions known as "heart pain" or "clamoring [stomach]" often have this pattern. [In such cases,] *Xiǎo Xiàn Xiōng Tāng* should be administered first, and then *Dà Xiàn Xiōng Tāng* may be occasionally [used] to attack [the pattern]. Chisokusai's *Chokkō-Gan* may also be used.

又た圖の如く、頸のめぐりに毒あり。凝結して痛み、あるひは痰喘、あるひは項背強急するもの、何病ひによらず、みな南呂丸の治すところなり。これまた直行丸大いによろし。考へ用ゆべし。たとへば本劑小陷胸湯の證ありて、傍ら南呂丸の證あるときは、

121. The formula for *Xiǎo Xiàn Xiōng Tāng* 小陷胸湯 (Jp: *Shō-Kankyō-Tō*; minor chest bind decoction) was originally found in *Shāng Hán Lùn*. At present, this formula is not covered by the Japanese National Health Insurance program and is not commonly used in Japan. However, a combination of this formula mixed with *Xiǎo Chái Hú Tang* 小柴胡湯 called *Chái Xiàn Tāng* 柴陷湯 (Jp: *Sai-Kan-Tō*; Bupleurum Chest Bind Decoction) is covered by the Japanese National Health Insurance program as a prescription drug, and is also commonly sold in Japanese drug stores as an over-the-counter drug. It is currently indicated by the MHLW for: cough, chest pain, and bronchitis in persons with moderate or strong physical strength who occasionally feel discomfort in the region stretching from the sides of the abdomen to the solar plexus and have decreased appetite accompanied by a bitter taste in the mouth, white tongue fur, severe cough accompanied by phlegm that is difficult to expel, or occasional chest pain (體力中等度以上で、ときに脇腹(腹)からみぞおちあたりにかけて苦しく、食欲不振で口が苦く、舌に白苔がつき、強いせきが出てたんが切れにくく、ときに胸痛があるものの次の諸症：せき、胸痛、氣管支炎).

122. Chest pain (Ch: *xiōng tòng* 胸痛; Jp: *kyōtsū*) refers to pain in the middle or lateral part of the chest. It can be seen in cases of diseases of lung, heart, chest and diaphragm, such as chest impediment with heart pain, lung abscess, lung heat disease, thoracic retention of fluid, pneumothorax, whooping cough, lung cancer, and traumatic chest injury.

毎夜南呂丸を兼用すべし。大陥胸湯を用ゆるときは、南呂丸の兼用を止むべし。

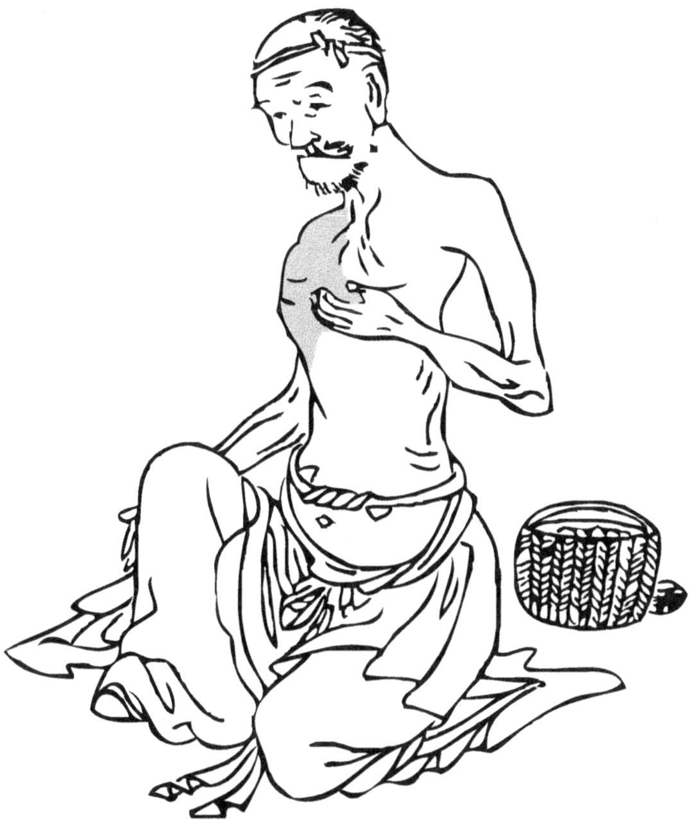

Fig. 22

Furthermore, as shown in the illustration, there is a toxin in the neck region. Any case in which [the toxin] has congealed, causing pain and in some cases phlegm panting or stiffness of the nape and back, should be treated with *Nanryo-Gan,*[123] regardless of [the name of] the disease [that the patient may present with]. *Chokkō-Gan* is also highly effective [for this pattern], and may be considered for use. For example, when the patient has

123. The formula for *Nanryo-Gan* 南呂丸 (Ch: *Nán Lǚ Wán*; nán lǚ pill) was originally found in *Tōdō-Sensei-Kajuku-Hō* 《東洞先生家塾方》 (Ch: *Dōng Dòng Xiān Shēng Jiā Shú Fāng*; Master Tōdō's Family Formulary). The name of the formula is taken from the tenth note (Ch: *nán lǚ* 南呂; Jp: *nanryo*) of the ancient Chinese twelve-note chromatic scale (Ch: *shí èr lǜ* 十二律; Jp: *jūni-ritsu*): several formulae of Yoshimasu Tōdō were named after notes in the scale. The formula as found in *Tōdō-Sensei-Kajuku-Hō* is as follows: *huáng qín* (4 *liǎng*), *gān suì*, *qīng méng shì*, (2 *qián* each), *dà huáng* (8 *qián*). This formula was adapted from the Chinese formula *Gǔn Tán Wán* 滾痰丸 (Jp: *Kontan-Gan*; phlegm-rolling pill) by substituting *gān suì* for *chén xiāng*. At present, both drugs are not covered by the Japanese National Health Insurance program and are not commonly used in Japan.

the pattern for the base formula of *Xiǎo Xiàn Xiōng Tāng* and the comorbid pattern for *Nanryo-Gan, Nanryo-Gan* should be concurrently administered each night. When *Dà Xiàn Xiōng Tāng* is used, the concurrent use of *Nanryo-Gan* should be discontinued.

あるひは桃黄丸の證ありて、傍ら南呂丸の證あるがごときもまた本劑をやめて南呂丸を用ゆべし。凡て大黄芒硝本劑にあるときは、兼用あることなし。やむことを得ざるときは、本劑をやめて用ゆべし。凡そいづれの方によらず、本劑に大黄芒硝あらば、此の例を以て考ふべし。

Furthermore, when the patient has the pattern for *Tō-Kō-Gan* and appears to [also] have the concurrent pattern for *Nanryo-Gan,* this medicinal should be discontinued and *Nanryo-Gan* should be used. The concurrent use of a base formula containing *dà huáng* or *máng xiāo* should be avoided in all cases. When the use [of these ingredients] is unavoidable, this formula should be discontinued. When concurrently using any formula that contains *dà huáng* or *máng xiāo* with this formula, [the physician] should consider this example [as a reference].

芍藥甘草湯之證

The Pattern for Sháo Yào Gān Cǎo Tāng[124] 芍藥甘草湯

圖の如く、腹底ひつぱるものあり、又たかかはるものあり。指頭をもつて輕く按してこれを知る。かかはるものは拘攣なり。ひつぱるもの、急迫なり。芍藥、拘攣を治し、甘草、急迫を治す。あるひは腰脚にひきつり、あるひは手足にひきつりて、いたむものに、この證多し。

As shown in the illustration, the patient feels as if the depths of the abdomen are being pulled taut, as if being tied [with ropes]. It can be felt when lightly pressing [the abdo-

124. The formula for *Sháo Yào Gān Cǎo Tāng* 芍藥甘草湯 (Jp: *Shakuyaku-Kanzō-Tō*; peony and licorice decoction) was originally found in *Shāng Hán Lùn*. The extract preparation of the formula is covered by the Japanese National Health Insurance program as a prescription drug, and is also commonly sold in Japanese drug stores as an over-the-counter drug. It is currently indicated by the MHLW for: cramps, muscle spasm, abdominal pain, and low back pain in persons who have pain associated with sudden muscle spasm. This drug may be used regardless of physical strength (體力に關わらず使用でき、筋肉の急激なけいれんを伴う痛みのあるものの次の諸症：こむらがえり、筋肉のけいれん、腹痛、腰痛).

men] with the fingertips. The feeling of being tied up is hypertonicity. The tautness is distress. *Sháo yào* cures the hypertonicity, and *gān cǎo* cures the distress. Most cases in which the patient presents with cramping in the lumbus and legs or cramping in the extremities are actually examples of this pattern.

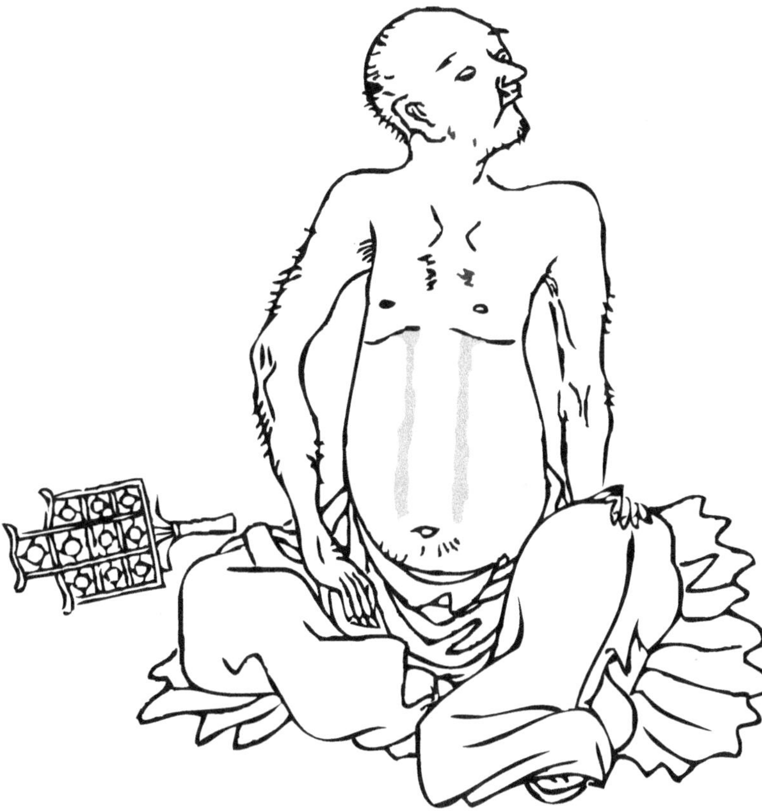

Fig. 23

又たあるひは世に云ふ「積聚」なるものにも此の症多し。なに病をとはず、拘攣急迫するものは此方を用ゆべし。「積聚」と號するものには、鶴丸、あるひは三黄丸・解毒丸の類をつまびらかにして兼用すべし。腰脚手足ひきつりいたむものには、平水丸、あるひは礬黄丸の類、證にしたがひて兼用すべし。然れども、腰脚手足ひきつるものにはまま十棗湯の證あり。十棗湯は掣痛の準據とし、礬黄丸は惡腫を準據とす。いづれも病名に眩せず、その證をつまびらかにして誤失することなかれ。

Moreover, what are commonly called "accumulations and gatherings" are also often seen in this pattern. Regardless of [the name of] the disease [that the patient has], if the patient presents with hypertonicity and distress, this formula should be used. For cases of the so-called "accumulations and gatherings," formulae such as *Kaku-Gan, Sān Huáng Wán*, or *Gedoku-Gan* may be considered for concurrent use after the pattern has been [correctly] elucidated. When cramping is present in the lumbus, legs, or extremities, formulae such as *Píng Shuǐ Wán* or *Ban-Ō-Gan* may be used concurrently in accordance with the pattern.[125] However, in cases when there is cramping in the lumbus, legs, and extremities, it is the pattern for *Shí Zǎo Tāng*.[126] The indication for use of *Shí Zǎo Tāng* is the presence of a pulling pain, and the indication for use of *Ban-Ō-Gan* is the presence of malign swelling. Do not be blinded by the name of the disease! [Correctly] elucidate the [abdominal] pattern and do not make mistakes [in treating patients]!

葛根湯之證

The Pattern for Gé Gēn Tāng[127] 葛根湯

項背強急劇しき者之圖

Illustration of Severe Stiffness of the Nape and Back

125. The formula for *Píng Shuǐ Wán* 平水丸 (Jp: *Heisui-Gan*; water-calming pill) was originally found in *Bèi Jí Qiān Jīn Yào Fāng* 《備急千金要方》(Jp: *Bikyū-Senkin-Yōhō*; Essential Prescriptions Worth a Thousand in Gold For Every Emergency), published by the eminent Chinese physician Sūn Sīmiǎo 孫思邈 (Jp: Son Shibaku; ca. 581–682) in the middle of the seventh century. In Japan, it was also known by the name *Suihin-Gan* 蕤賓丸 (the name of which was taken from *ruí bīn* 蕤賓 (Jp: *suihin*), the seventh note of the Chinese twelve-note musical scale [Ch: *shí èr lǜ* 十二律]), as found in *Tōdō-Sensei-Kajuku-Hō* 《東洞先生家塾方》(Master Tōdō's Family Formulary), albeit with slightly differing quantities of ingredients. The formula found in *Bèi Jí Qiān Jīn Yào Fāng* is as follows: *shāng lù* (4 *liǎng*), *gān suì* (1 *liǎng*), *máng xiāo*, *wú zhū yú*, *yuán huā* (2 *liǎng* each). At present, this formula is not covered by the Japanese National Health Insurance program and is not commonly used in Japan.

126. *Shí Zǎo Tāng* 十棗湯 (Jp: *Jissō-Tō*; ten jujubes decoction) is discussed separately in its own section in this work.

127. The formula for *Gé Gēn Tāng* 葛根湯 (Jp: *Kakkon-Tō*; pueraria decoction) was originally found in *Jīn Guì Yào Lüè* and *Shāng Hán Lùn*. The extract preparation of the formula is covered by the Japanese National Health Insurance program as a prescription drug, and is perhaps the most well-known Chinese drug sold in Japanese drug stores as an over-the-counter drug. Although *Gé Gēn Tāng* is commonly marketed as a remedy for the common cold, it is currently indicated by the MHLW for: initial stages of the common cold (in cases when sweating has not yet occurred), head cold, rhinitis, headache, stiff shoulders, muscle pain, and hand and shoulder pain in persons with moderate physical strength (體力中等度以上のものの次の諸症：感冒の初期「汗をかいていないもの」、鼻かぜ、鼻炎、頭痛、肩こり、筋肉痛、手や肩の痛み).

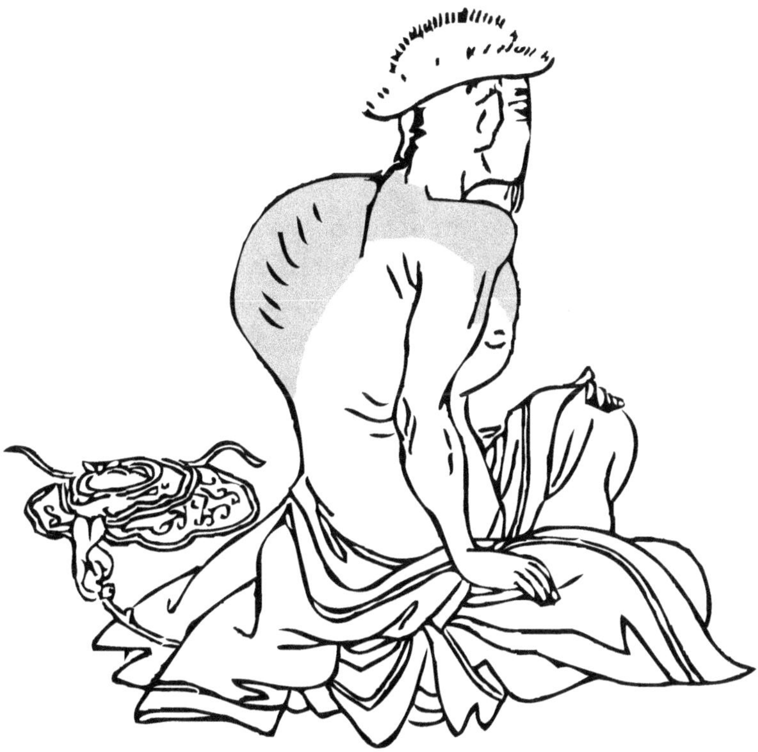

Fig. 24

圖の如きもの、所謂「龜背」。俗に「背蟲」といふもの、これ葛根湯の證の劇しきものなり。此の證、世に間々ありといへども、醫者難治の者として敢へて療せず。病家も亦た不具の生質なりとして、生涯を終らしむ。惜しい哉。男女ともに此の患へにかかるもの、人に接はりて其の形の醜きを愧ぢざるものなし。豈に哀しからずや。

As shown in the illustration, it is a case of what is known as "turtle's back." The pattern for *Gé Gēn Tāng* is a severe version of what is colloquially referred to as "insect back" [i.e., hunchback]. Although this pattern is common in the world, physicians regard it as an intractable [condition] and therefore do not attempt to treat it. Patients [with this pattern] are regarded as being predisposed to being crippled, and are thus forced to live their entire lives [as cripples]. It is indeed regrettable! Both men and women are afflicted [by this pattern], and there are no [patients] who remain unashamed of their ugly appearance when coming into contact with others. Is this not sad?

是れ生質なる者といへども、元是れ病毒のなす所なり。即ち先天の毒、劇しきものなり。凡そ天地の間、萬物各々淺深・厚薄あるものなり。其の淺薄なるものは、庸人も是れをなす。其の深厚に至りては、人、皆及ばざるものとして爲さず。いはゆる自暴自棄なり。

Although these patients are said to have a predisposition [to the condition, the pattern] is actually caused by a pathotoxin. [This pathotoxin] is, in fact, a severe congenital toxin. Of the myriad things [i.e., toxins] that exist between heaven and earth, some are shallow (superficial), some are deep, some are thick, and some are thin. Common people attempt to perform [treatment] in cases of shallow or thin [toxins. However,] people all regard deep or thick [toxins] as being too difficult [to treat] and do not perform [treatment]. This is what is known as "abandoning oneself to despair."

余、これを憂へて、古醫道にいり、治療をなすに、其の厚深なるものを救はんと欲す。圖の如くにして、龜背と號するものは、一身に毒凝結して、項背強急するものなり。凡そ堅塊・血塊の類。これを按じて痛む者あり、痛まざるものあり。之れを按じて痛まざるものは、毒の大いなるものなり。此の證亦た毒大いなるが故に、項背強急することを覺へず。

Being anxious about this, I entered into the way of ancient physicians and perform [ancient] treatments with the desire of curing [patients who have] thick or deep [toxins]. As shown in the illustration, those who are said to have "turtle's back" [actually] have a toxin in the body that has congealed, causing stiffness of the nape and back.[128] [In such cases,] hard lumps or blood lumps are generally [present. Upon palpation,] some patients may [feel] pain, but others may have no pain. Patients who [feel] no pain upon palpation have a large toxin. Because the toxin is large in this pattern, [the patient] is unable to notice the stiffness of the nape and back.

是れを治するの法。葛根湯本劑の分量、二倍若しくは三倍にして、水二盞を以て煮て六分を取つて、之れを服すること。日々三貼。毎夜、南呂丸二戔目を兼用し、時々大陷胸丸、或るひは先天滅毒丸、或ひは凝腐除圓、或ひは直行丸の類を兼用し、其の毒を

128. Stiffness of the nape and back (Ch: *xiàng bèi qiáng jí* 項背強急; *kōhai-kyōkyū*) is an important concept in this book. The expression refers to contracture (i.e., muscular spasm and rigidity) of the nape and back.

吐下し去るときは、其の形、漸々に減じて終に常人となる。然れども、その毒凝結して大いなるが故に、服薬すること一年あるひは一年半、甚だしきは二、三年にも及ばざれば、全く治することあたはず。

The method to treat this [pattern] is as follows: The quantity of *Gé Gēn Tāng* used should be doubled or tripled. Boil in two cups of water to make six *fēn* of the decoction, and administer to the patient. Three doses [of the powder] should be administered each day. Each night, two *qián* of *Nanryo-Gan* should be simultaneously administered, and *Dà Xiàn Xiōng Wán*, *(Senten-)Metsudoku-Gan*, *Gyō-Fu-Jo-En*,[129] or *Chokkō-Gan* may also be administered on occasion. As the toxin is eliminated through vomiting or precipitation, the physical form [of the toxin] will be gradually reduced in size, and [the patient] will finally become a normal [healthy] person. However, because the toxin has congealed and become large, unless administration of the drug is continued for as long as one or one and one-half years, or in severe cases [up to] two or three years, [the physician] will be unable to be completely cure [the patient].

余、往年甲州薤崎縣令の請ひに因つて、田中に客遊せし日、同州加志加澤の邑、喜平次なる者の男、年十九。この證をうれへ、これに加ふるに、兩脚攣急して、歩行することあたはざるものを療するに、すなはちこの方法を以て、これを攻むること二月餘にして、歩行することを得。半歳餘にして、龜背の形漸減ず。

Some years ago, I traveled to the Nirazai area in Kōshū at the request of the local governor. One day, when I was staying in [a house located among] the rice fields, [I met] the 19-year old son of a man named Kiheiji, who lived in the vicinity of Kashi and Kasawa villages of Kōshū.[130] He was suffering from this pattern, but also presented with hypertonicity in both legs and was unable to walk. I used this method to treat the patient, and after more than two months of attacking [the toxin], he was able to walk again. After a little more than half a year, the turtle's back gradually decreased in appearance.

時に余、まさに東都に往かんとす。故に多く丸・散・湯・圓を作りて殘し置き去る。余、東都にいたりて、京橋南紺街に僑居す。

129. The details of *Gyō-Fu-Jo-En* 凝腐除圓 are unclear; the formula appears to have never been popularly used in Japan.

130. Kōshū 甲州 is the abbreviated name of Kai Province (Jp: *Kai-No-Kuni* 甲斐國), the region of Japan that currently comprises Yamanashi Prefecture (Jp: *Yamanashi-Ken* 山梨縣).

喜平次また書を以て請ふて曰く、「先生の治療を得て、吾が男の龜背日々に減ず。今遺すところの服藥、みな盡きたり。願はくは又た藥を賜へ」と。余、諾して本劑及び丸圓を作り與ふること、又た半歳ばかり。前後一年餘にして、まつたく治して常人となる。後、門人關宗俊が療するところの病者、またこの證なり。其の齢四十ばかり、また此の方を用ひて三月ならずして全く治す。

At the time, I was planning to go to the eastern capital, [i.e., Edo]. I therefore made many pills, powders, and decoctions, and left them [for the patient]. I arrived in the eastern capital and was temporarily living in the Nankan area of Kyōbashi [in Edo] when Kiheiji sent me another letter saying, "My son took the medicine that you gave us, and his turtle's back has been improving day by day. [However,] he has just used up all of the medicinals that you left for him. I humbly beg you to send us more medicinals." I agreed to his request and prepared this formula and pills, which were administered [to the patient] for approximately half a year. After approximately one year, [the patient] was completely cured, and became a normal healthy person. Seki Sōshun, one of my pupils, also treated a patient who presented with this pattern.[131] The patient was approximately 47 years of age, and was completely cured within less than three months [after] start of treatment.

黄連湯之證

The Pattern for Huáng Lián Tāng[132] 黄連湯

圖の如く、上脘中脘の邊、塊物に似たるものあつて、時々いたみ、心下敢へて痞鞕せず。食臭をきいて、嘔氣を欲するもの。或るひは曰ふ、心煩、心下痞鞕、嘔吐を欲し、上衝のもの。

131. Seki Sōshun 關宗俊 also acted as a scribe for the author, who has traditionally been considered to be at least partially illiterate. Seki wrote down an earlier work on abdominal patterns *Fukushō-To-I*《腹證圖彙》(Illustrated Compendium of Abdominal Patterns) as dictated by the author. No records concerning the details of the life of Seki are available.

132. The formula for *Huáng Lián Tāng* 黄連湯 (Jp: *Ōren-Tō*; coptis decoction) was originally found in *Shāng Hán Lùn*. The extract preparation of the formula is covered by the Japanese National Health Insurance program as a prescription drug, and is also commonly sold in Japanese drug stores as an over-the-counter drug. It is currently indicated by the MHLW for: stomach pain, acute gastritis, hangover, and stomatitis in persons with moderate physical strength who have a sense of stagnation and heavy feeling in the stomach, decreased appetite, or occasional nausea or vomiting (體力中等度で、胃部の停滯感や重壓感、食欲不振があり、ときにはきけや嘔吐のあるものの次の諸症：胃痛、急性胃炎、二日酔、口内炎).

As shown in the illustration, the patient presents with something resembling a lump in the upper and center stomach duct regions. Pain is sometimes present [in the abdomen], but there is no glomus and hardness in the region below the heart. Food malodor can be smelled, and the patient feels like retching. One [physician] said that patients who present with heart vexation, have glomus and hardness in the region below the heart, experience retching or vomiting, and have upward surging [are also indicated for this pattern].

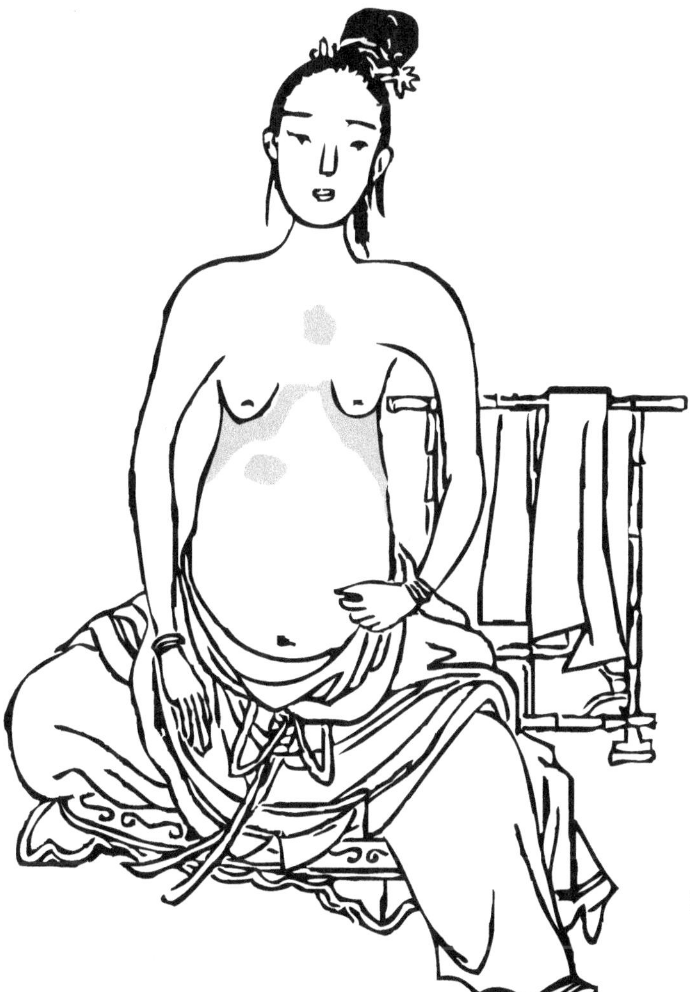

Fig. 25

『論』に云はく、「胸中熱有り、胃中邪氣有り、腹中痛んで嘔吐せんと欲する者」。克、案ずるに、「心中熱有り」、心煩と思ふ可し。「胃中邪氣有り」、心下實痞と思ふ可し。

It is stated in the [*Shāng Hán*] *Lùn* that "patients who have heat in the chest, evil qì in the stomach, abdominal pain, and a desire to retch or vomit [are indicated for *Huáng Lián Tāng*]."[133] I believe that what is meant by "heat in the heart [i.e., chest]" refers to heart vexation, and what is meant by "evil qì in the stomach" refers to replete glomus in the region below the heart.

甘遂半夏湯之證

The Pattern for Gān Suì Bàn Xià Tāng[134] 甘遂半夏湯

圖の如く、心下の毒鞕滿して、或るひは便閉、或るひは下痢すと雖も、鞕滿やまず。食すと雖も、心下より下らず、或るひは心下痛み、或るひは氣急促迫、或るひは脚弱歩行を憂ふ。譬へば桂枝人參湯、或るひは朮防己去石膏加茯苓芒硝湯、或るひは枳朮湯、或るひは桂姜草棗黃辛附湯、或るひは調胃承氣湯等の證に似て、諸藥如何ともすべからざる者、此の方、謹んで考ふ可し。

As shown in the illustration, a toxin causes hard fullness in the region below the heart, although in some cases, the patient might present with a fecal block in some cases or diarrhea in others.[135] However, [in all cases,] the hard fullness does not cease. Although the patient may eat, [the food] does not descend past the region below the heart. In some cases, pain is present in the region below the heart. In some cases, [the patient presents with] hasty and distressed rapid breathing. Furthermore, in some cases, the patient suffers from weak legs and poor gait. The pattern may appear similar to other patterns such

133. The original text is found in *Shāng Hán Lùn*, Line 173 in the Tàiyáng chapter: On Identification of Pulse, Symptom Complex, and Treatment of Tàiyáng [Diseases] (Ch: *Biàn Tài Yáng Mài Zhèng Bìng Zhì Xià* 辨太陽脈證并治下; Jp: *Ben-Taiyō-Myakushō-Hei-Chi-Ka*) is as follows: "傷寒胸中有熱、胃中有邪氣、腹中痛、欲嘔吐者、黃連湯主之。"

134. The formula for *Gān Suì Bàn Xià Tāng* 甘遂半夏湯 (Jp: *Kanzui-Hange-Tō*; kansui and pinellia decoction) was originally found in *Shāng Hán Lùn*. At present, this formula is not covered by the Japanese National Health Insurance program and is not commonly used in Japan.

135. Fecal block (Ch: *biàn bì* 便閉; Jp: *benpei*), also known as constipation (Ch: *biàn mì* 便祕; Jp: *benpi*), is an important concept in this book. It refers to the inability to defecate, prolonged course of defecation, or difficulty in defecation. Apart from intestinal diseases, constipation also can be seen in anal diseases, muscular flaccidity, hemiplegia due to wind stroke, pressure of lumps outside the intestines, febrile disease, excessive taking of antidiarrheal or medicinals, or abdominal operation and general weakness.

as the patterns for *Guì Zhī Rén Shēn Tāng*, *Jutsu-Bōi-Kyo-Sekkō-Ka-Bukuryō-Bōshō-Tō*,[136] *Zhǐ Zhú Tāng*, *Guì Jiāng Zǎo Cǎo Huáng Xīn Fù Tāng*, or *Tiáo Wèi Chéng Qì Tāng*.[137] In cases when a variety of drugs are ineffective, [the physician] may carefully consider the use of this formula.

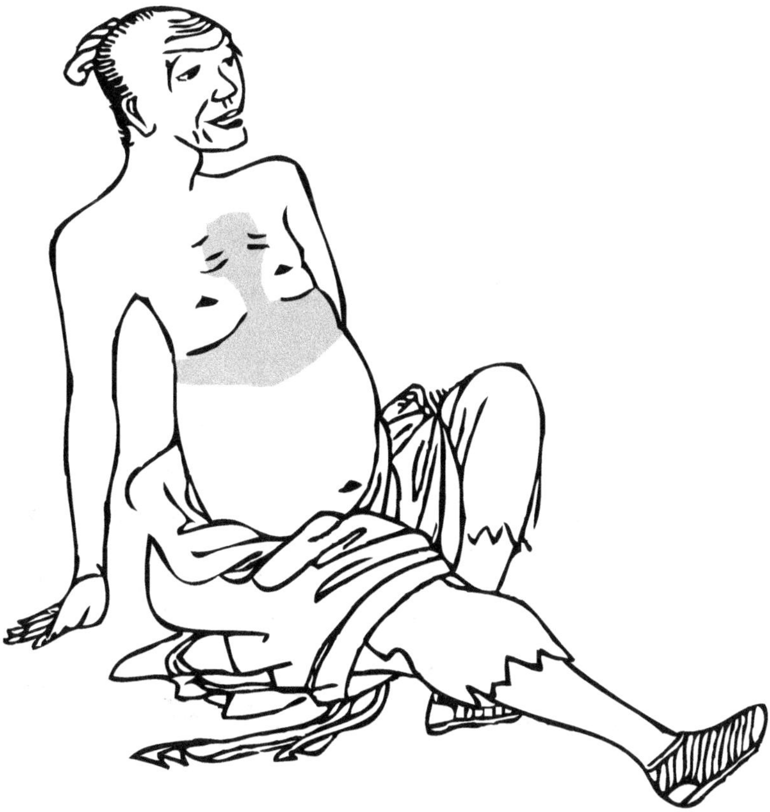

Fig. 26

舊に余、此の證の一患人有つて、此の證を誤りて、前に云ふ諸方を用ひて効を得ず。晝夜困苦して以て漸く此の方を與へ、二十餘劑を以て、數年の患人全く愈ゆ。其の後、此の證の者に逢ふごとに、數しば効を得ること、譬ふるにものなし。其の腹診の詳らかなること、口授あつて存す。

136. *Jutsu-Bōi-Kyo-Sekkō-Ka-Bukuryō-Bōshō-Tō* 朮防已去石膏加茯苓芒硝湯 (Ch: *Zhú Fáng Jǐ Qù Shí Gāo Jiā Fú Líng Máng Xiāo Tāng*; atractylodes and fangji decoction minus gypsum plus poria and mirabilite) is discussed separately in its own section in this book.
137. *Tiáo Wèi Chéng Qì Tāng* 調胃承氣湯 (Jp: *Chōi-Jōki-Tō*; stomach-regulating qì-infusing decoction) is discussed separately in its own section in this book.

In the past, I once had a patient who presented with this pattern, but I mistook it [for another pattern] and used the above-mentioned formulae, but I was unable to obtain any success [in treating the condition]. I struggled day and night [to understand the pattern], but when I eventually administered this formula, the patient was [finally] completely cured after receiving more than twenty different drugs over a period of several years. When I subsequently met patients who presented with this pattern, I obtained such successful results [in using this formula] that [the efficacy of the formula] cannot be compared to anything else. The details of the abdominal examination [for this pattern] have been handed down through oral tradition.

大黃甘草湯之證

The Pattern for Dà Huáng Gān Cǎo Tāng[138] 大黃甘草湯

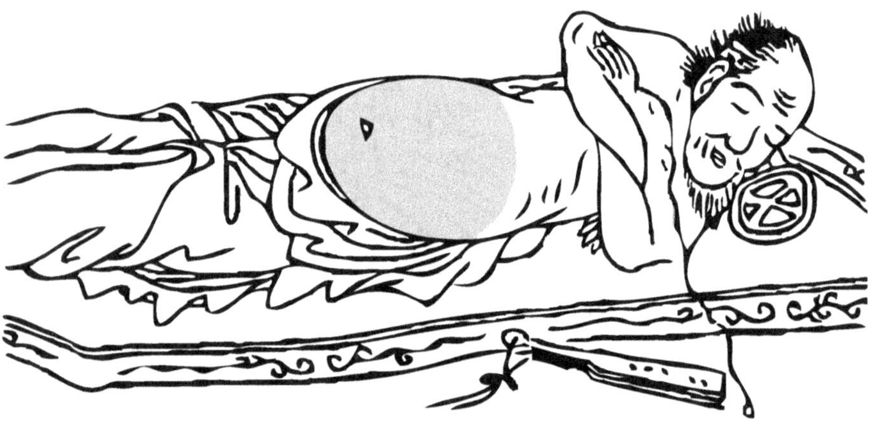

Fig. 27

圖の如く、腹滿すといへども、あへて實せず、大便閉のもの。『論』に云はく、「食已んですなはち吐するもの、大いに効あり」

138. The formula for *Dà Huáng Gān Cǎo Tāng* 大黃甘草湯 (Jp: *Daiō-Kanzō-Tō*; rhubarb and licorice decoction) was originally found in *Jīn Guì Yào Lüè*. The extract preparation of the formula is covered by the Japanese National Health Insurance program as a prescription drug, and is also commonly sold in Japanese drug stores as an over-the-counter drug. It is currently indicated by the MHLW for the amelioration of: constipation and dull headache, hot flashes, eczema, dermatitis, pimples (acne), anorexia (appetite loss), abdominal distension, abnormal intestinal fermentation, and hemorrhoids associated with constipation. This drug may be used regardless of physical strength (便祕、便祕に伴う頭重・のぼせ・濕疹・皮膚炎・ふきでもの「にきび」・食欲不振(食欲減退)・腹部膨満・腸内異常醗酵・痔などの症狀の緩和。体力に関わらず、使用できる).

。克、按ずるに、本文にいふ「食已んですなはち吐するもの」、所謂反胃・膈噎。この證、ままあり。我が門、これを用ひて、二三子、効を得。學者、用ひて以て効をしるべし。或るひは曰く、「祕閉急迫、是れ又た腹診考ふ可き也」。

As shown in the illustration, although the patient presents with abdominal fullness, it is not a case of repletion, [but rather] a fecal block. The text [of *Jīn Guì Yào Lüè*] states that "[this formula] is extremely effective in patients who vomit immediately after eating."[139] I believe that the "...patients who vomit immediately after eating" referred to in the text have what is known as stomach reflux or dysphagia-occlusion.[140] This is the pattern that matches [this formula]. My pupils have used this formula and experienced its efficacy. As the student [of abdominal patterns] uses [this formula], he will come to know its efficacy. One person has said that "[...in cases of] constipation with distress, abdominal examination [findings] should be considered [when making diagnoses]."

厚朴三物湯之證

The Pattern for Hòu Pò Sān Wù Tāng[141] 厚朴三物湯

圖の如く、臍の底、臍のほとり、龜の甲のごとく、かたきものありて、これを按ずるに、胸にこたへ、嘔氣を覺ゆるもの、これ此の症の目當てたり。又た曰く、胸腹の滿結實、或るひは痛閉の者。

139. This quotation is found in *Jīn Guì Yào Lüè*, Chapter 17, Line 17: On Identification of Pulse, Symptom Complex, and Treatment of Vomiting, Retching, and Diarrhea Chapter (Ch: *Bìng Mài Zhèng Bìng Zhì* 嘔吐噦下利病脈證治; Jp: *Ōto-Etsu-Geri-Byō-Shō-Chi*) is as follows: "食已即吐者「、用後方、」大黃甘草湯方。" (*Dà Huáng Gān Cǎo Tāng* 大黄甘草湯 [should be] used for patients who vomit immediately after eating).

140. The characters used in the original Japanese text for stomach reflux (Ch: *fǎn wèi* 反胃; Jp: *hon'i*) and dysphagia-occlusion (Ch: *gé yē* 膈噎; Jp: *kaku'i*) are normally reversed (Ch: *wèi fǎn* 胃反 and *yē gé* 噎膈, respectively). Dysphagia-occlusion refers to difficulty in swallowing with the feeling of food stuck in the throat. It is a commonly encountered symptom of esophagopathy and also can be seen in diseases involving the stomach, chest, diaphragm, heart, oral cavity, and throat in addition to impediment, flaccidity, paralysis, and stroke.

141. The formula for *Hòu Pò Sān Wù Tāng* 厚朴三物湯 (Jp: *Kōboku-Sanmotsu-Tō*; officinal magnolia bark three agents decoction) was originally found in *Jīn Guì Yào Lüè*. At present, this formula is not covered by the Japanese National Health Insurance program and is not commonly used in Japan.

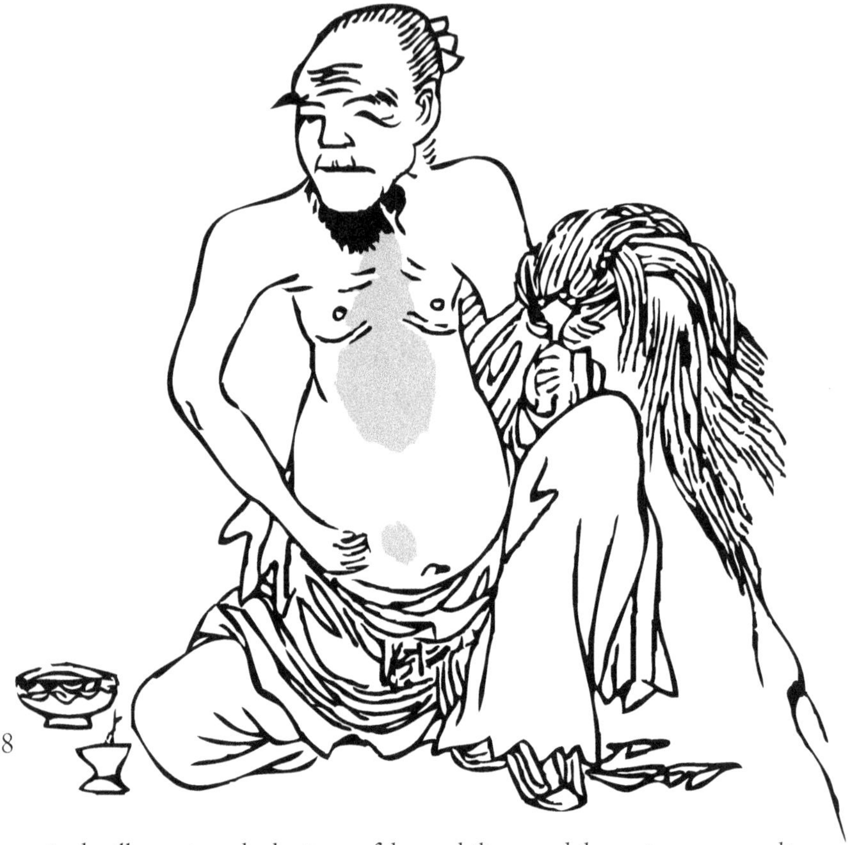

Fig. 28

As shown in the illustration, the bottom of the umbilicus and the region surrounding the umbilicus feel hard, similar to the feeling of a turtle's shell. When [the abdomen is] palpated, the patient feels a response in the chest and may feel like retching. This should be the guide for [determining] this pattern. Moreover, in some cases, the patient may have fullness and binding repletion in the chest and abdomen, and in some cases, the patient presents with a painful [fecal] block.

又た曰く、頭痛、百藥を以て治せざる者、數効を得。口授有りて存す。或るひは曰く、腹滿、心下痛んで大便通ぜざる者。又た曰く、心下滿痛、水を吐き出だす者。

I have often achieved successful results in patients who presented with a headache that could not be cured by the hundred medicinals. [The details of treatment] have been passed down by oral tradition. One person has said that patients who present with abdominal fullness, pain in the region below the heart, and fecal stoppage [are indicated for this formula. Patients who present with fullness and pain in the region below the heart and vomit water [are] also [indicated].

乾姜附子湯之證

The Pattern for Gān Jiāng Fù Zǐ Tāng[142] 乾薑附子湯

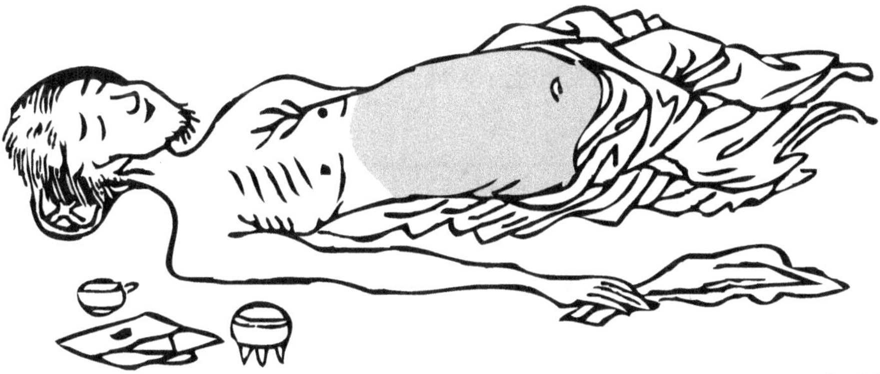

Fig. 29

圖のごとく、煩燥食せず、その狀（かたち）如何ともすべからざるもの。自ら患ふるところをしらず、一身ことごとくひへ、晝夜氣急促迫、その餘腹診傳あり。はなはだしきものは、凡そ死證なり。

As shown in the illustration, the patient presents with vexation and agitation and does not eat; it appears as if nothing can be done [to cure the patient. The patient] is unable to identify the exact region that is afflicted [by the toxin], has generalized coldness in the body, and presents with distressed rapid breathing day and night. Other abdominal [signs manifested during] examination can be found in [other] texts. Severe cases are usually death patterns.

『論』に曰く、「之れを下して後、復た汗を發す。晝日煩燥眠ることを得ず、夜にして安靜。嘔せず、渴せず、表證無く、脉沈微、身大熱無き者」。克曰く、本文、大凡そ備はれり。

142. The formula for *Gān Jiāng Fù Zǐ Tāng* 乾薑附子湯 (Jp: *Kankyō-Bushi-Tō*; dried ginger and aconite decoction) was originally found in *Shāng Hán Lùn*. At present, this formula is not covered by the Japanese National Health Insurance program and is not commonly used in Japan.

In *Shāng Hán Lùn* it is written, "...after precipitation, [the patient] will sweat again. [The patient has] vexation and agitation, and is unable to sleep during the daytime, but is quiet and tranquil at night. There is no retching, no thirst, no exterior pattern, the pulse is sunken and faint, and no great heat is present in the body."[143] In my opinion, this passage perfectly describes [this pattern].

芎歸膠艾湯及び豬苓湯之證

The Patterns for Xiōng Guī Jiāo Ài Tāng[144] 芎歸膠艾湯 and Zhū Líng Tāng[145] 豬苓湯

圖の如く、小腹に物あり、之れを按じて痛む者、即ち此の症也。然れども按じて痛む者、桃軍圓の證ありて紛れやすし。然れども桃軍圓の證は、之れを按ずるに腹底へこたへて、力ありて堅く痛む。即ち急結の二字を思ひ合はすべし。

As shown in the illustration, when something [can be felt] in the smaller abdomen [during the abdominal examination], and pain is present upon palpation, it is an example of

143. This is found in *Shāng Hán Lùn*, Line 61: On Identification of Pulse, Symptom Complex, and Treatment of Tàiyáng Diseases Chapter (Ch: *Biàn Tài Yáng Mài Zhèng Bìng Zhì* 辨太陽病脈證并治; Jp: *Ben-Taiyō-Byō-Myakushō-Hei-Chi*). The original text is as follows: "下之後、復發汗、晝日煩躁不得眠、夜而安靜、不嘔不渴、無表證、脈沉微、身無大熱者、乾薑附子湯主之."

144. The formula for *Xiōng Guī Jiāo Ài Tāng* 芎歸膠艾湯 (Jp: *Kyū-Ki-Kyō-Gai-Tō*; Chinese angelica, ass hide glue, and mugwort decoction) was originally found in *Jīn Guì Yào Lüè*. The extract preparation of the formula is covered by the Japanese National Health Insurance program as a prescription drug, and may be sold in Japanese drug stores as an over-the-counter drug. It is currently indicated by the MHLW for: bleeding hemorrhoid, anemia, abnormal menstruation, menorrhagia, metrorrhagia, and subcutaneous hemorrhage in persons with moderate or weak physical strength who have cold extremities or bleeding tendency without any gastroenteropathy (體力中等度以下で、冷え症で、出血傾向があり胃腸障害のないものの次の諸症：痔出血、貧血、月經異常・月經過多・不正出血、皮下出血).

145. The formula for *Zhū Líng Tāng* 豬苓湯 (Jp: *Chorei-Tō*, polyporus decoction) was originally found in *Jīn Guì Yào Lüè* and *Shāng Hán Lùn*. The extract preparation of the formula is covered by the Japanese National Health Insurance program as a prescription drug, and is also commonly sold in Japanese drug stores as an over-the-counter drug. It is currently indicated by the MHLW for: patients with difficulty in urinating, painful urination, sensation of incomplete bladder emptying, frequent urination, and edema in persons with urinary abnormalities who often have dry mouth. This drug may be used regardless of physical strength (體力に關わらず使用でき、排尿異常があり、ときに口が渴くものの次の諸症：排尿困難、排尿痛、殘尿感、頻尿、むくみ).

this pattern. However, it is easy to confuse this with the pattern for *Tō-Gun-En,* in which pain is [also] present upon palpation [of the abdomen]. In the case of the pattern for *Tō-Gun-En,* the depths of the abdomen spring back when palpated [deeply; the abdomen] has strength and is hard, but pain is present [upon palpation]. In this case, the two words "tense bind" should come to mind.

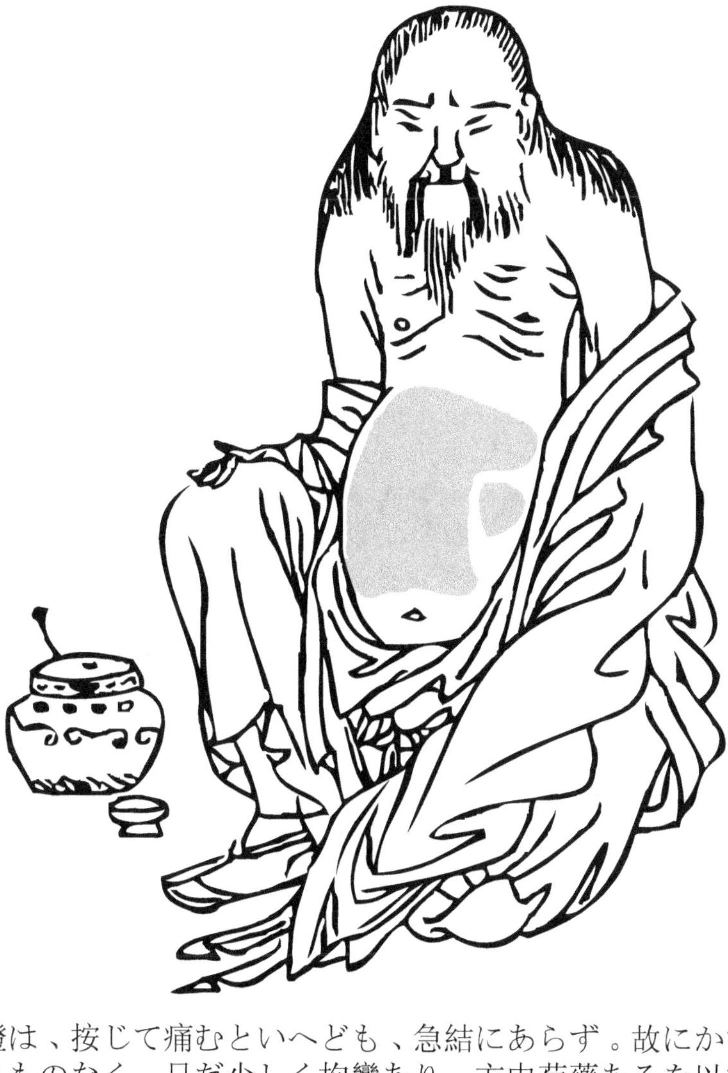

Fig. 30

此の證は、按じて痛むといへども、急結にあらず。故にかたくこたゆるものなく、只だ少しく拘攣あり。方中芍藥あるを以て思ふべし。且つ桃軍圓より多味にして、甘草の分量少なきを以て分つべし。凡そ此の證、間々腹痛むものなり。

In this pattern, although there is pain [in the abdomen] upon palpation, it is not a case of tense bind. Therefore, there is nothing [in the abdomen] that is hard and springs back [upon palpation]; only slight hypertonicity is present. It should be kept in mind that for this reason *sháo yào* is included in the formula. Moreover, [the patterns] can be differentiated by the fact that *Tō-Gun-En* is composed of many flavors and contains a smaller amount of *gān cǎo,* [whereas] in this pattern, the patient generally presents with abdominal pain.

或るひは大いに下血・漏下などすることあり。余、跋渉に勤め、大いに困しんで、此の腹證を得たり。甚だ分ちやすからず。若し桃軍圓との分ちを知り極めんと欲せば、之れを按じて痛むに、下へ引いて痛むもの、此の方の證なり。上へ引いて痛むもの、桃軍圓の證なり。上下へ引いて痛むものは、二方の證、相合するなり（兼用、解毒丸・芎黄の類考ふ可し）。

In some cases there is a great descent of blood or spotting. It was only after extensive scouring and facing great difficulties that I was able to understand this pattern. [The pattern] is extremely difficult to differentiate. If one would like to completely know the difference between [the *Xiōng Guī Jiāo Ài Tāng* pattern] and [the pattern for] *Tō-Gun-En,* the cases in which there is pain that is conducted downward upon palpation [of the abdomen] are examples of [the *Xiōng Guī Jiāo Ài Tāng*] pattern. In the pattern for *Tō-Gun-En,* pain is conducted upward. If the pain is conducted both upward and downward, then it is a pattern [formed by] two [different] formula-patterns ([Therefore] the concurrent use of formulae such as *Gedoku-Gan* or *Xiōng Huáng Sǎn* may be considered).

又た豬苓湯の腹症も圖の如く、小腹に物ありて、これを按じて痛む。是れ大いに膠艾湯の腹症に似たり。故に外證を以てこれを分つべし。然れども、外證頗る五苓散と紛るることあり。其の血證の有無を以て察すべし。豬苓湯は血症あり。冒悸して渴し、小便不利、腹中滿、これを按ずるに軟にして膠艾湯の證に似たり。

Moreover, as shown in the illustration, in the pattern for *Zhū Líng Tāng,* the patient presents with [the sensation of] something in the smaller abdomen, and pain is present upon palpation [of the region]. This [pattern] is very similar to the pattern for [*Xiōng Guī*] *Jiāo Ài Tāng.* Therefore, the external signs should be used to differentiate [the patterns]. However, in some cases, it is extremely easy to confuse the external signs [of this pattern] with [those of] the pattern for *Wǔ Líng Sǎn*.[146] [The physician] should observe the patient [and inspect] for the presence of a blood pattern. [The pattern for] *Zhū Líng Tāng* is a blood pathocondition. This pattern is similar to the pattern for [*Xiōng Guī*] *Jiāo Ài Tāng*, in that the patient presents with veiling palpitations and has thirst, inhibited urination, and fullness in the abdomen, which feels soft upon palpation.

余、この腹症を理會せざること多年。曩に三箇島(武州入間部)に遊んで、眼科鈴木良碩を主とす。一病婦あり、治を乞ふ。診して以爲へらく、「芎歸膠艾湯の證なり」と。因つて數劑を與ふるに功なし。其の後良碩、五苓散を用ひ、又た深く苦心して豬苓湯を與ふること數劑、終に全功を收む。余、これを聞いて再び三箇島に到り、良碩と共に論定して、遂にこの一證を得たり。要するに、膠艾湯の腹症に似て、腹部軟滿にして口渴し、小便不利、時々膿血を便にす。これ、その證なり。

I was unable to understand this pattern for many years. A certain time, I traveled to Mikajima (located in Bushū),[147] where I stayed with an ophthalmologist named Suzuki Ryōseki.[148] [One day,] a sick woman came asking for treatment. When I performed an examination, I thought that she had the pattern for *Xiōng Guī Jiāo Ài Tāng*, and I there-

146. The details of the formula for *Wǔ Líng Sǎn* 五苓散 (Jp: *Gorei-San*; poria five powder) are not discussed in this book. This formula was originally found in *Jīn Guì Yào Lüè* and *Shāng Hán Lùn*. The extract preparation of the formula is covered by the Japanese National Health Insurance program as a prescription drug, and is also commonly sold in Japanese drug stores as an over-the-counter drug. It is currently indicated by the MHLW for: watery diarrhea, acute gastroenteritis (however, the drug is contraindicated for cases of [what is known in Japan as] "strained abdomen"), heat stroke, headache, edema, and hangover in persons who have thirst accompanied by oliguria, dizziness, nausea, vomiting, abdominal pain, headache, or edema (this drug may be used regardless of physical strength). Note: Strained abdomen (Jp: *shiburi-bara* 澀り腹) refers to the feeling of incomplete stool evacuation and repeated desire to defecate accompanied by abdominal pain [i.e., tenesmus; also known as abdominal urgency and rectal heaviness; Ch: *lǐ jí hòu zhòng* 裏急後重; Jp: *rikyū-kōjū*] (體力に關わらず使用でき、のどが渴いて尿量が少ないもので、めまい、はきけ、嘔吐、腹痛、頭痛、むくみなどのいずれかを伴う次の諸症：水樣性下痢、急性胃腸炎「しぶり腹」のものには使用しないこと)、暑氣あたり、頭痛、むくみ、二日酔。しぶり腹とは、殘便感があり、くり返し腹痛を伴う便意を催すもののことである).

147. Mikajima 三箇島, now commonly written as 三ヶ島, is currently part of Tokorozawa City (Jp: *Tokorozawa-Shi* 所澤市). Bushū 武州 is the abbreviated form of Musashi Province (Jp: *Musashi-No-Kuni* 武藏國), which today comprises Tokyo Metropolis (Jp: *Tōkyō-To* 東京都), most of Saitama Prefecture (Jp: *Saitama-Ken* 埼玉縣), and part of Kanagawa Prefecture (Jp: *Kanagawa-Ken* 神奈川縣).

148. There are no available records concerning Suzuki Ryōseki 鈴木良碩.

fore administered numerous doses of the formula, but [the treatment] was unsuccessful. Ryōseki subsequently gave her *Wǔ Líng Sǎn*, and after much painstaking work, he decided to administer several doses of *Zhū Líng Tāng*; the treatment eventually led to complete success [in curing the pattern]. When I heard about this, I returned to Mikajima, and after some discussion with Ryōseki, we were able to understand this pattern. In summary, [this pattern] is similar to the abdominal pattern for [*Xiōng Guī*] *Jiāo Ài Tāng*, as the patient presents with soft fullness of the abdominal region, thirst, inhibited urination, and occasionally passes stools containing pus and blood.[149] These [symptoms] are [the indications for] the pattern.

嗚呼、良碩なるもの、吾が門に於いて抜群の良才なる哉。余、結髮してより、この技に刻意すといへども、一腹症を得るもの、許多の螢雪を經ざれば、定め極むることあたはず。然るに良碩は一朝にしてこの證を得たり。吾が門にしてかくの如き人才を得ること、豈に天の寵靈にあらずや。しかのみならず、良碩、眼科を業として、祖先已來、眼目を療すること、億萬何の限りあらん。良碩に至つて猶(なを)且つ安んぜず、廣く生民の疾苦を濟ふの志を起し、余を邀へて腹症を學び、いくほどならずして、其の蘊奧をきはめ、是れ等の證を理會す。實に崑山に入りて尺璧を獲るもの、亦た衹だ、積善の餘慶なる哉。

Oh, that Ryōseki! He far surpasses my other pupils in his ability [of diagnosis]! Since tying my hair back [i.e., coming of age],[150] I have made painstaking efforts to [learn] the techniques, and I was only able to understand even a single abdominal pattern after much diligent study. However, Ryōseki was able to elucidate this pattern in a single morning. It must be by the grace and favor of Heaven that I was able to have such a talented pupil in my school! Moreover, Ryōseki practiced [the family business of] ophthalmology, and there is no telling how many eyes [his family] has treated since the time of his ancestors. Even so, Ryōseki remained unsatisfied [with his past successes],

149. Stool with pus and blood (Ch: *biàn nóng xuè* 便膿血; Jp: *ben-nō-ketsu*) refers to the passage of blood, pus, and mucus together with stool, a symptom usually indicating dysentery.
150. Tying hair back (Jp: *keppatsu* 結髪) refers to the traditional Japanese coming-of-age ceremony called *genpuku* 元服, which was usually held when a boy reached the age of adulthood (the exact age ranged from 12 to 17, depending on the family tradition and time period). During the Edo period, it was common for most adult men to shave the top of their heads and tie the remaining hair, which was long and oiled, into a small queue. The queue was then folded onto the top of the head in a topknot (Jp: *chonmage* 丁髷). However, most physicians did not shave the top of their hair, and tied their hair in a characteristic ponytail called *sōhatsu* 總髮 (literally, "total hair").

and has the desire to widely save the common people from their afflictions. He invited me to come so that he could learn about abdominal patterns, and within no time, he had mastered the deep secrets [of abdominal examination] and was thus able to understand these patterns. [Ryōseki being able to obtain the patterns] is indeed [similar to] entering Mount Kun[151] and obtaining a cubit-long jewel.[152] It could also be [called a case of] reaping the benefits of past accumulated good deeds![153]

苓桂朮甘湯之證

The Pattern for Líng Guì Zhú Gān Tāng[154] 苓桂朮甘湯

圖の如く、心下に毒ありて悸し上衝し、起ればすなはち頭眩し、小便不利、あるひは心煩、あるひは欝々として、志氣安からざるもの、この證なり。何病ひを問はず、心下悸し、小便不利を準據として、此の方を用ゆべし。又た苓姜朮甘湯は、臍下悸して、身體重く、腰冷へ、水中に坐するが如し。その餘諸患ありといへども、臍下の悸を準據として苓姜朮甘湯を用ゆべし。

As shown in the illustration, there is a toxin in the region below the heart that causes palpitations, upward surging, a dizzy head upon rising, or inhibited urination. In some

151. This most likely refers to Mount Kunlun (Ch: *Kūn Lún Shān* 崑崙山; Jp: *Konron-San*), a mythological mountain in Chinese mythology. It was said to be the home of various gods and goddesses, in addition to wondrous fauna and flora.

152. A cubit (Ch: *chǐ* 尺; Jp: *shaku*) was a Chinese unit of length that was widely used in East Asia. The exact length varied depending on the time period and region in which it was used (generally 23–35cm).

153. This phrase can originally be found in the "*Kūn* 坤 (Jp: Kon) Chapter" of *Yì Jīng*《易經》(Jp: *Eki-Kyō*; I Ching/Book of Changes). The original text is as follows: "積善之家、必有餘慶。積不善之家、必有餘殃" (The family that accumulates goodness is sure to have superabundant happiness, and the family that accumulates evil is sure to have superabundant misery). This is a reference to the pre-Buddhist Chinese notion of "karma." The author apparently believes that the talent of Ryōseki is due to the past good works of his family.

154. The formula for *Líng Guì Zhú Gān Tāng* 苓桂朮甘湯 (Jp: *Ryō-Kei-Jutsu-Kan-Tō*; poria, cinnamon twig, [white] atractylodes, and licorice decoction) was originally found in *Jīn Guì Yào Lüè* and *Shāng Hán Lùn*. The extract preparation of the formula is covered by the Japanese National Health Insurance program as a prescription drug, and is also commonly sold in Japanese drug stores as an over-the-counter drug. It is currently indicated by the MHLW for: lightheadedness, dizziness, headache, tinnitus, palpitations, shortness of breath, neurosis, and neurologic hypersensitivity in persons with moderate or weak physical strength who have dizziness, lightheadedness, and occasional hot flashes or palpitations (體力中等度以下で、めまい、ふらつきがあり、ときにのぼせや動悸があるものの次の諸症：立ちくらみ、めまい、頭痛、耳鳴り、動悸、息切れ、神經症、神經過敏).

cases there is heart vexation, and in some cases there is depression and the mind qì is disquieted. These are examples of this pattern. Regardless of the name of the disease [that was diagnosed], this formula should be used for the indications of palpitations in the region below the heart and inhibited urination. Furthermore, in the pattern for *Líng Jiāng Zhú Gān Tāng*, the patient presents with palpitations in the subumbilical region, a heavy [feeling in the] body, and coldness in the lumbus, as if [the patient] is sitting in water. Although there are various other afflictions [that match the pattern, the diagnosis of] *Líng Jiāng Zhú Gān Tāng* should be based on the indication of palpitations in the subumbilical region.[155]

悸は動よりちいさく、これをしること至つて難し。診するの傳、胸より静かに手を下し、病人の膚に、指頭あたるやあたらざるやにして、之れを窺ふ。若くは臍下腹底に少しき動あり。垂れ帶の風に動いて手にさはるがごとし。手脉にたとふれば、伏沈にして遲なるがごとし。至つてかすかなり。又た面部・手足・身體、ひりつき、しやくり動くことあり。是れ肉瞤筋惕なり。或るひは振々として、地に擲たんと欲し、或るひは起れば則ち頭眩するもの、皆、悸するの毒のなす所、茯苓の主證なり。

[Subumbilical] palpitations are smaller than stirring, thus it is extremely difficult to understand [the difference between the two signs].[156] The traditional method to perform the [abdominal] examination is to softly lower the hands to the chest of the patient and search the region so lightly that the fingertips barely touch the skin. In some cases, there may be slight stirring in the bottom of subumbilical region of the abdomen.

155. The formula for *Líng Jiāng Zhú Gān Tāng* 苓薑朮甘湯 (Jp: *Ryō-Kei-Jutsu-Kan-Tō*; poria, ginger, [white] atractylodes, and licorice decoction) is found in *Jīn Guì Yào Lüè*. The extract preparation of the formula is covered by the Japanese National Health Insurance program as a prescription drug, and is also commonly sold in Japanese drug stores as an over-the-counter drug. It is currently indicated by the MHLW for: low back pain, cold sensation in the lower back, nocturnal enuresis, and neuralgia in persons with moderate or weak physical strength who have a cold sensation and ranging from the lumbus to the lower extremities, and polyuria (體力中等度以下で、腰から下肢に冷えと痛みがあって、尿量が多いものの次の諸症：腰痛、腰の冷え、夜尿症、神經痛).

156. Subumbilical stirring palpitations (Ch: *qí xià jì dòng* 臍下悸動; Jp: *seika-kidō*) generally refer to rapid throbbing or pulsations felt in the region below the umbilicus, in many cases are the same as subumbilical aortic pulsation. Stirring palpitations (Ch: *jì dòng* 悸動; Jp: *kidō*) are traditionally understood as a single concept, but the author differentiates the softer palpitations (Ch: *jì* 悸; Jp: *ki*) and the stronger stirring (Ch: *dòng* 動; Jp: *dō*).

When touched with the hands, it feels similar to a *tareobi* being blown in the wind.[157] If [the sensation] is compared to pulse taking of the wrists, it feels similar to a pulse that is hidden, sunken, and slow. It is very faint. In some cases the patient presents with tingling

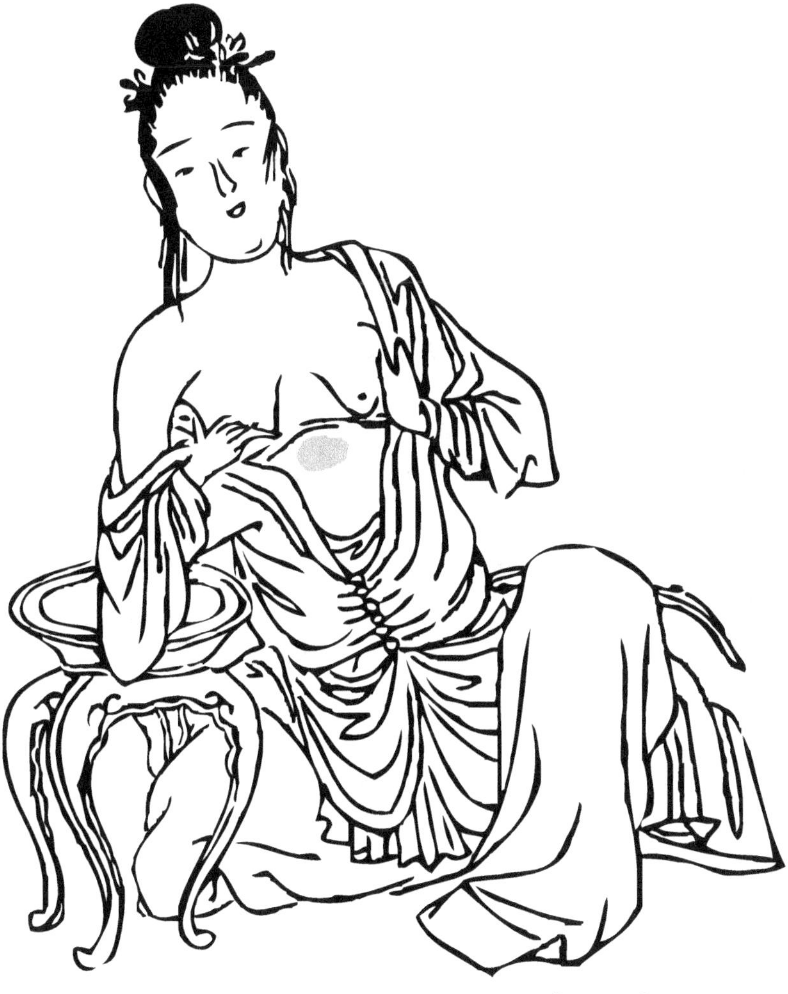

Fig. 31

and twitching of the face, extremities, and body. These are [cases of] jerking sinews and twitching flesh.[158] In some cases, [the shaking] is so great that the patient tends to be thrown down to the ground. In some cases, the patient has a dizzy head upon rising. The chief [indication] for *fú líng* is the presence of a pattern in which the patient presents with palpitations caused by a toxin.

157. *Tareobi* 垂れ帯 is a long cloth belt that is tied around the waist with the ends allowed to droop in the front. It is still used in the uniforms worn by the practitioners of karate and other Japanese martial arts.
158. Jerking sinews and twitching flesh is usually written as 筋惕肉瞤 (Ch: *jīn tì ròu rùn*; Jp: *kinteki-nikujun*). This expression collectively refers to short spastic muscular contractions.

悸の字、「心動」と訓ず。又た『詩』の「衛風」(芄の篇)に「容兮遂兮、垂帯悸兮」。朱氏注に「『悸』は帯の下り垂るの貌(かたち)なり」と。蓋し垂帯の歩むに従ひて、ひらり、はらりとする貌。これを腹症にあて考ふるに、その字義實に符合す。豈にそれ彷彿たるものならんや。誠に古人字を用ゆる、苟もせざることをみるべし。

The character for palpitation (*jì* 悸) can be interpreted as "stirring of the heart." It is also [mentioned in the poem] *Wán Lán* [found in the] "Odes of Wèi [Chapter]" of *Shī Jīng* 《詩經》(Classic of Poetry)[159]: "How easy and conceited is his manner, with the ends of his girdle hanging down as they do!"[160] The commentary by Zhū Xī[161] states that "The character *jì* 悸 shows the appearance of a girdle that is drooping down." This is the appearance of a *tareobi* that is fluttering lightly and gently as one walks. If we apply this [concept] to abdominal patterns, then the meaning of the character does indeed match [this pattern]. How this character resembles [the pattern]! We can see that the ancients indeed paid careful attention to each character that they used.

又た苓桂甘棗湯は、心下及び臍下に悸ありて、攣急上衝するものなり。唯だこの三方のみにあらず、『傷寒論』にのするところ、茯苓ある方はみな心下悸、あるひは肉瞤筋惕等、方意をあきらかにして、詳らかに察すべし。故にここに略す。按ずるに、苓桂朮甘湯は、芎黄散・三黄丸・解毒丸の類、かんがへ兼用すべし。苓姜朮甘湯は平水丸兼用考ふべし。

159. *Shī Jīng*《詩經》(Jp: *Shi-Kyō*; Classic of Poetry) is the oldest existing collection of Chinese poetry, comprising 305 works dating from the 11th to 7th centuries BCE. It is one of the Confucian classics, and was widely studied and memorized by the literati of East Asia.

160. The original text of the poem *Wán Lán* 芄蘭 (Jp: *Gan-Ran*; Sparrow-Gourd) as found in the Odes of Wèi Chapter (Ch: *Wèi Fēng* 衛風; Jp: *Ei-Fū*) and translation by the famous Sinologist James Legge (1815–1897 CE) are as follows: "芄蘭之支、童子佩觿。雖則佩觿、能不我知、容兮遂兮、垂帶悸兮。" (There are the branches of the sparrow-gourd; There is that lad, with the spike at his girdle. Though he carries a spike at his girdle, he does not know us. How easy and conceited is his manner, with the ends of his girdle hanging down as they do).

161. Zhū Xī 朱熹 (1130–1200 CE) was the most influential rationalist Neo-Confucian scholar of the *Sòng* (宋) dynasty. His commentaries on the Confucian classics formed the basis of civil service examinations in China until the modern period. The original text of the commentary is as follows: "悸、帶下垂貌。"

Furthermore, in the pattern for *Líng Guì Gān Zǎo Tāng*,[162] the patient presents with palpitations in the region below the heart and the subumbilical region, hypertonicity, and upward surging. According to *Shāng Hán Lùn*, not only these three formulae, but all formulae containing *fú líng* are indicated for [symptoms] such as heart palpitations or jerking sinews and twitching flesh. [Based on this, the physician] should elucidate the meaning of the formulae and carefully inspect [the patterns]. Therefore, I will omit [the details] here. I believe that formulae such as *Xiōng Huáng Sǎn, Sān Huáng Wán*, or *Gedoku-Gan* may be considered for concurrent use with *Líng Guì Zhú Gān Tāng*.[163] The concurrent use of *Píng Shuǐ Wán* may be considered [when administering] *Líng Jiāng Zhú Gān Tāng*.

大黃牡丹皮湯之證
The Pattern for Dà Huáng Mǔ Dān Pí Tāng[164] 大黃牡丹皮湯

附臍下之毒、診察之論
The Method of Examination of a Toxin That Is Attached to the Subumbilical Region

162. The formula for *Líng Guì Gān Zǎo Tāng* 苓桂甘棗湯 (Jp: *Ryō-Kei-Kan-Sō-Tō*; poria, cinnamon twig, jujube, and licorice decoction) was originally found in *Shāng Hán Lùn*. The extract preparation of the formula is approved by the MHLW to be sold in Japanese drug stores as an over-the-counter drug. It is currently indicated by the MHLW for: palpitations and anxiety in persons with moderate or weak physical strength who experience hot flashes or palpitations and severe nervousness (體力中等度以下で、のぼせや動悸があり神經がたかぶるものの次の諸症：動悸、精神不安).

163. There are several different Chinese formulae with the name *Xiōng Huáng Sǎn* 芎黃散 (Jp: *Kyū-Ō-San*; chuanxiong and rhubarb decoction). Because the details of this formula are not discussed in this work, it is unclear which formula the author refers to. However, in Japan, *Xiōng Huáng Sǎn* is often used as an alternative name of *Yìng Zhōng Sǎn* 應鐘散 (Jp: *Ōshō-San*; bell powder), which is a simple formula comprising *chuān xiōng* 川芎 (2 *liǎng*) and *dà huáng* 大黃 (6 *liǎng*), although the exact quantities of the ingredients may vary. *Yìng zhōng* 應鐘 is the name of the twelfth note of the Chinese twelve-note musical scale (Ch: *shí èr lǜ* 十二律).

164. The formula for *Dà Huáng Mǔ Dān Pí Tāng* 大黃牡丹皮湯 (Jp: *Daiō-Botanpi-Tō*; rhubarb and moutan decoction) was originally found in *Jīn Guì Yào Lüè*. The extract preparation of the formula is covered by the Japanese National Health Insurance program as a prescription drug, and is also commonly sold in Japanese drug stores as an over-the-counter drug. It is currently indicated by the MHLW for: irregular menstruation, dysmenorrhea, menstrual pain, constipation, and hemorrhoids in persons with moderate or strong physical strength who have lower abdominal pain and tend to experience constipation (體力中等度以上で、下腹部痛があって、便祕しがちなものの次の諸症：月經不順、月經困難、月經痛、便祕、痔疾).

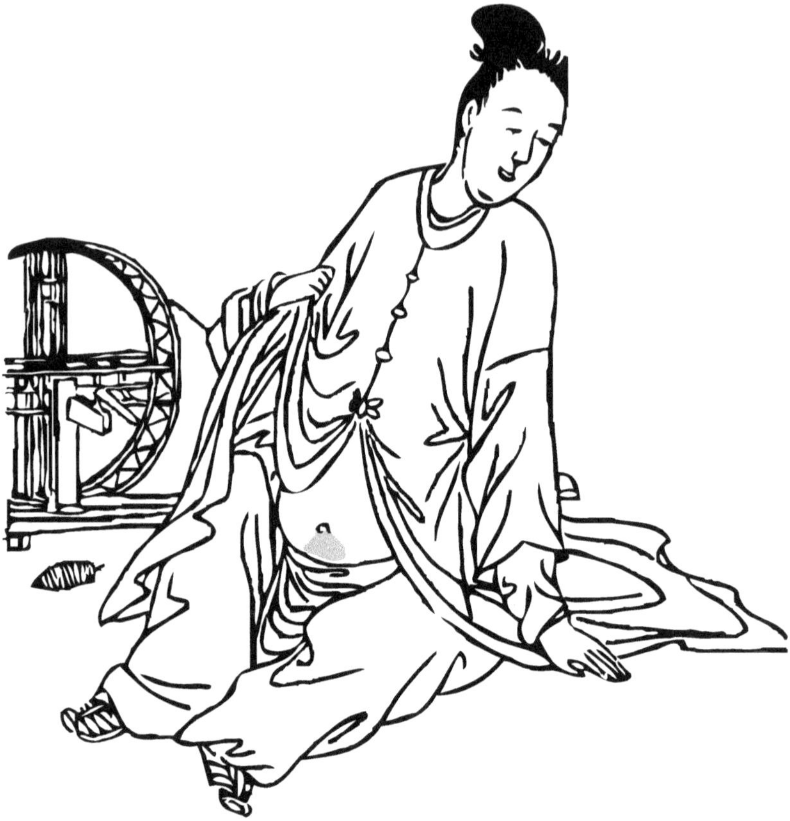

Fig. 32

圖の如く、臍下に毒有りて、之れを按じて痛むもの、即ちこの證なり。所謂經閉、血塊の類。或るひは乳岩、男女諸惡瘡を發し、腐爛するものの類に、此の證多し。其の餘、何病ひを問はず、臍下堅塊あり。之れを按じて痛むものは、みな此の證なり。

As shown in the illustration, when the patient has a toxin in the subumbilical region that causes pain upon palpation, it is this pattern. Common examples of this pattern are conditions such as what are known as a "menstrual block" or blood clot. In many other cases, [female patients] often present with a mammary rock, or putrid malign sores that may develop in either male or female [patients]. In other cases, there is a hard lump in the subumbilical region, regardless of [the name of] the disease. Any case in which pain is present upon palpation of this [region] is this pattern.

又た此の方のみに限らず、桃軍圓、或るひは癥痼圓、或るひは芎歸膠艾湯、或るひは葛根加大黄湯の類の諸證に、世にいはゆる腐骨疽・乳岩の類、難治と稱するもの。其の餘諸般の惡瘡腐爛するもの多し。ここに於いては、皆、丸・散兼用、證に隨つて用ゆること、忽せにすべからず。

Furthermore, not limited to [the pattern matching] this formula, but also [in other patterns such as the patterns for] *Tō-Gun-En, Chōko-En, Xiōng Guī Jiāo Ài Tāng*, or *Gé Gēn Jiā Dà Huáng Tāng*,[165] the patient [presents with] what are commonly referred to as intractable diseases such as putrid bone abscess[166] or mammary rock.[167] In many other cases, the patient presents with various types of putrid malign sores. In any of these cases, [the physician] must not disregard [the importance of] the concurrent use of [the appropriate] pills or powder according to the pattern that is presented.

たとへば惡瘡腐爛するものならば、まづ腹證を審らかにして、本劑を與ふること四、五日。毎夜伯州散二戔、或るひは三戔を兼用し、時々梅肉散を以て攻むること、毒の厚薄に隨つて、或るひは二分、三分より五、六分。甚だしきものは、一戔以上に至り、これを用ゆ。若くは其の毒大いにして腐爛はなはだしく、膿汁出づるものの類は、雲龍散に輕粉を加倍してこれを與へ、口中腐爛し、食することあたはざること、一旬、或るひは二旬にして治す可し。尚愈へざるものは、口中腐爛止んで後、又た前方を用ひ、毒の愈ゆるを度とすべし。然れども、大黄牡丹皮湯を服するうちは、本劑に大黄・芒硝あるゆへ、兼用の方を投ずべからず。

For example, if the patient presents with putrid malign sores, [the physician] must first discern the abdominal pattern and then administer this formula for four or five days.

---

165. There are many different formulae using *Gé Gēn Tāng* 葛根湯 as the base formula with additional ingredients. The formula for *Gé Gēn Jiā Dà Huáng Tāng* 葛根加大黄湯 (Jp: *Kakkon-Ka-Daiō-Tō*; pueraria decoction plus rhubarb), as found in *Wada-Kahō-Kan* 《和田家方函》 (Coffer of Formulae of the Wada Family), appears to have been an invention of Wada Tōkaku 和田東郭 (1744–1803 CE), an esteemed physician who studied under Yoshimasu Tōdō 吉益東洞. At present, this formula is not covered by the Japanese National Health Insurance program and is not commonly used in Japan.

166. Putrid bone abscess (Ch: *fǔ gǔ jū* 腐骨疽; Jp: *fukosso*) is normally called bone flat-abscess (Ch: *fù gǔ jū* 附骨疽; Jp: *fukosso*) and refers to suppurative osteomyelitis, a suppurative inflammatory disease of bone, marked by local death and separation of tissue.

167. Mammary rock (Ch: *rǔ yán* 乳巖; Jp: *nyūgan* 乳岩) refers to a rocky mass in the breast, (i.e., malignant tumor occurring in the mammary region).

Each night, two or three *qián* of *Hakushū-San*[168] may be concurrently used, and *Bainiku-San*[169] may be occasionally used to attack [the pattern]. Depending on the depth of the toxin, in some cases two, three, or up to five or six *fēn* may be used. In severe cases, use one *qián* or more. In cases in which the toxin is great and the patient presents with severe putrefaction, *Unryū-San*[170] should be administered with the quantity of *qīng fěn* doubled. Patients who have putrid oral [sores] and are unable to eat will be cured after ten or twenty days. In the case that [the patient] is still not cured, after the putrid oral [sores] have ceased, the above-mentioned formula should be administered again with the aim of curing the toxin. However, because *dà huáng* and *máng xiāo* are included in this formula, the concurrent administration [of this formula] with *Dà Huáng Mǔ Dān Pí Tāng* should be avoided.

若し右の如く傍ら兼用の證あるときは、本剤を止めて用ゆべし。しかしながら、伯州散は本剤に同じき藥なきゆへ、毎夜兼用して可なり。梅肉散は峻き剤なれば、五日若しくは七日を隔てて用ゆ可し。

If [the patient] presents with a concurrent pattern as earlier mentioned, this formula should be discontinued. Nevertheless, because *Hakushū-San* is not the same as this formula, concurrent use each night is permissible. Because *Bainiku-San* is a drastic [i.e., powerful] drug, it should be used with intervals of five to seven days between doses.

168. *Hakushū-San* 伯州散 (Ch: *Bó Zhōu Sǎn*; Hōki Province powder) takes its name from Hakushū 伯州, the abbreviated name of Hōki Province (Jp: *Hōki-No-Kuni* 伯耆國), the area that currently comprises the western part of Tottori Prefecture 鳥取縣. The history of the formula is unclear. It appears to have been an ancient folk remedy from Hōki Province that was listed under the name *Hōki-yaku* 伯耆藥 (Ch: *Bó Zhōu Sǎn*; Hōki Province medicinal) in *Daidō-Ruijuhō* 《大同類聚方》(Ch: *Dà Tóng Lèi Jù Fāng*; Classified Assemblage of Prescriptions of the Daidō Era; published by imperial decree in 808 CE), the earliest Japanese medical text. It was later popularized during the Edo period by Yoshimasu Tōdō 吉益東洞 in *Tōdō-Sensei-Kajuku-Hō* 《東洞先生家塾方》(Master Tōdō's Family Formulary). The formula was nicknamed "surgeon overthrower" (Jp: *geka-taoshi* 外科倒し) due to its reported efficacy in treating toxic sores. Although there are several variations of the formula, the standard preparation contains the following three ingredients charred and mixed together in equal quantities: *fǎn bí* 反鼻, *xiè* 蟹 (usually Eriocheir japonica), and *lù jiǎo* 鹿角. At present, this formula is not covered by the Japanese National Health Insurance program and is not commonly used in Japan, although it can be bought online from several pharmacies specializing in Kampō medicine.

169. The details of *Bainiku-San* 梅肉散 (Ch: *Méi Ròu Sǎn*; mume powder) are given in the final section of this work.

170. The formula for *Unryū-San* 雲龍散 (Ch: *Yún Lóng Sǎn*; cloud dragon powder) is not explained in the this work, and the details of the formula appear to be lost.

按ずるに、右の外、臍下に毒あるもの、前に云ふところの苓姜朮甘湯及び赤石脂禹餘糧湯・八味丸等なり。赤石脂禹餘糧湯は、臍下を按ずるに軟にして痛み、下痢或るひは膿血を便するものなり。又た臍の上下・左右、按じてみな痛むものもあり。八味丸は、臍下不仁して、小便不利なるもの、是れなり。

I believe that in addition to the aforementioned cases, when the patient presents with a toxin in the subumbilical region, it is the pattern for [a formula] such as *Líng Jiāng Zhú Gān Tāng*, *Chì Shí Zhī Yǔ Yú Liáng Tāng*,[171] or *Bā Wèi Wán*.[172] [In the pattern for] *Chì Shí Zhī Yǔ Yú Liáng Tāng*, the subumbilical region is soft, pain is present upon palpation, and the patient has dysentery or passes stools containing pus and blood. Furthermore, pain is present in [the areas] superior, inferior, left, and right of the umbilicus. In the pattern for *Bā Wèi Wán*, the subumbilical region is insensitive, and the patient has inhibited urination.

癥痼圓之證

The Pattern for Chōko-En[173] 癥痼圓

圖の如く、臍を遶りて動あり。これ所謂「胎動」なり。天下の人、十に六、七は此の患へあらざることなし。病ひ未だ發せざるうちは、さまでに患へ煩ふことなけれども、若し此の病ひ發するときは、世に所謂「中風」・「勞瘵」等の患へをなす。欝々として心煩上衝し、起くれば則ち頭眩し、或るひは肉瞤筋惕、小便不利、血證等の諸症を顯はす。一に皆、胎動を以て準據として、此の症を極むべし。

171. The formula for *Chì Shí Zhī Yǔ Yú Liáng Tāng* 赤石脂禹餘糧湯 (Jp: *Shakusekishi-Uyoryō-Tō*; halloysite and limonite decoction) was originally found in *Shāng Hán Lùn*. The formula itself is quite simple, consisting of *chì shí zhī* 赤石脂 and *yǔ yú liáng* 禹餘糧, albeit classical physicians were not in agreement concerning the quantities of said ingredients. At present, this formula is not covered by the Japanese National Health Insurance program and is not commonly used in Japan.

172. *Bā Wèi Wán* 八味丸 (Jp: *Hachimi-Gan*; eight-ingredient pill) is discussed in its own section in this work.

173. The source of the formula for *Chōko-En* 癥痼圓 (Ch: *Zhēng Gū Yuán*; intractable concretion pill) is unclear. At present, the formula is not covered by the Japanese National Health Insurance program and is not well known in Japan.

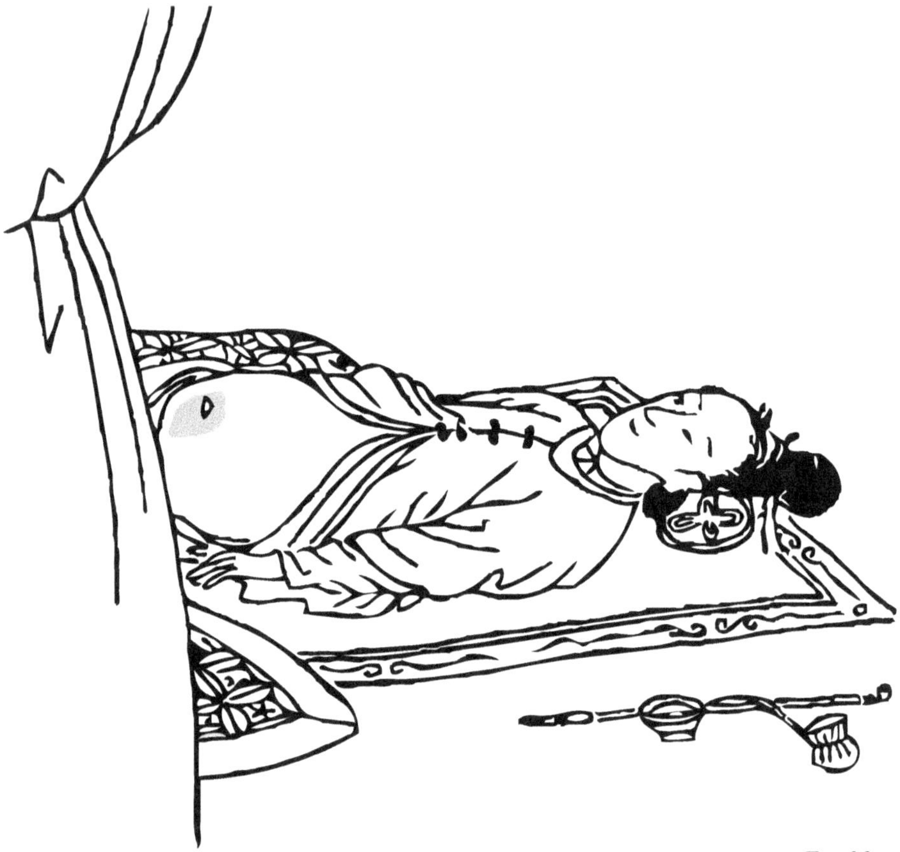

Fig. 33

As shown in the illustration, stirring is present in the regions surrounding the umbilicus. It is what is known as "stirring fetus."[174] As many as six or seven out of every ten patients present with this affliction. When this disease has not yet arisen, [the patient] does not suffer and is not vexed. However, once the disease arises, it causes afflictions such as what are commonly referred to as "wind strike" and "consumption." The patient presents with a depressive heart vexation that surges upward, causing a dizzy head upon rising. In some cases, various symptoms such as twitching flesh and jerking sinews, inhibited urination, or a blood pattern may be apparent. In all cases, [the presence of] stirring fetus should be used as the indication to determine this pattern.

174. Stirring fetus (Ch: *tāi dòng* 胎動; Jp: *taidō*; also known as *tāi dòng bù ān* 胎動不安; Jp: *taidō-fuan*) refers to frequent fetal movement usually accompanied with abdominal pain, bearing-down sensation, lumbago, or mild vaginal bleeding. The condition is a sign of possible miscarriage.

甚だしきものは、胎動上りて心胸に迫るを覺ふ。是れ所謂「奔豚氣」なり。之れを診ふの傳、中指の本節を臍穴にあて、指頭をかけて按ずること、或るひは重く、或るひは輕くすれば、胎動なる者、臍底より到るを考ふべし。

In severe cases, there is a feeling of a stirring fetus ascending, which causes distress in the heart and chest. This is what as known as "running piglet qì."[175] The traditional [method] to examine [the abdomen to determine the pattern] is to place the base joint [i.e., the fingertip] of the middle finger into the hole of the umbilicus and palpate [the umbilical region] using the fingertips. [The physician] should sometimes [press] strongly and sometimes [press] lightly to determine if the stirring fetus has reached the bottom of the umbilicus.

胸腹之毒、凝結して背に着く（二圖）

Two Illustrations of a Chest and Abdominal Toxin that has Congealed and Become Affixed to the Back[176]

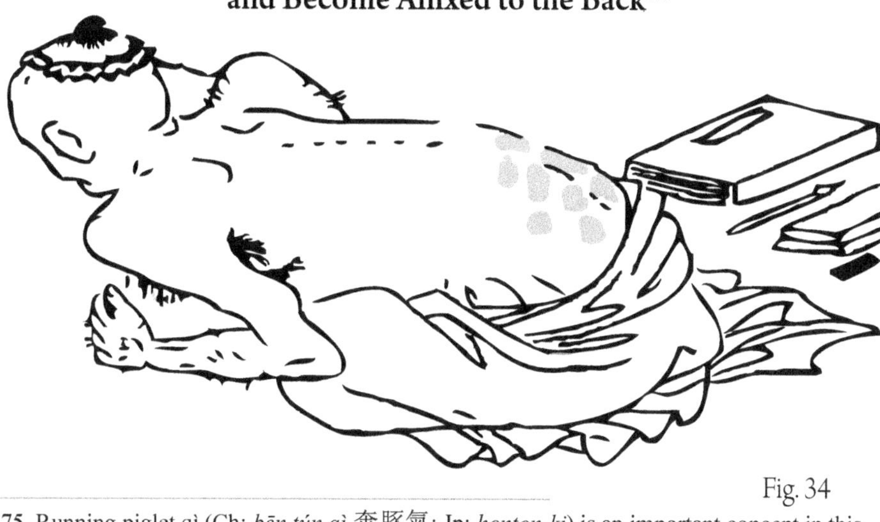

Fig. 34

175. Running piglet qì (Ch: *bēn tún qì* 奔豚氣; Jp: *honton-ki*) is an important concept in this work. It refers to a subjective sensation of upsurging from the lower abdomen to the chest, epigastrium, and throat. This sensation is typically accompanied by gripping abdominal pain, chest oppression, rapid breathing, dizziness, heart palpitations, or heart vexation.

176. This is one of the two sections of the book to discuss moxibustion. By the middle of the Edo period (1603–1868 CE), physicians of Kampō medicine had largely turned their interest toward internal medicine (herbology and pharmacology). Internists (known as *hondō-i* 本道醫 [literally, "main path physicians"]) were the most respected physicians, followed by surgeons, and then acupuncturists. Acupuncture, moxibustion, and massages were widely performed by blind people, and it appears that many internists of the time may have had insufficient knowledge of specific techniques related to moxibustion.

いづれの證によらず、腹證を診ふて、毒の厚深凝結したるものは、みな背につくなり。これを治するの法、まづ腹證を按じて、毒の在る所をしり、その凝結するところに假り點をうち、紙線を以て背後へまわし、脊骨の中央にまた假點をうち、これにならひて、左右若干所を指頭をもつてこれを按すに、腹中にこたゆるところあり。すなはちその上に點じ、灸すること、一穴五十壯づつ。七日あるひは二七日、又たは三七日にいたるときは、その毒動きて腹張りいづるものなり。この時、證にしたがひて藥劑を投じて、これを攻むべし。

When abdominal pattern diagnosis has revealed the presence of any thick, deep toxin that has congealed, the said toxin becomes affixed to the back, regardless of the pattern presented. The method to cure [the toxin] is to first palpate the abdominal pattern [presented] in order to understand the location of the toxin, and then place temporary markings on each point of congealment. After that, [starting from each marked point,] wrap a paper thread around the waist to the center of the spine and again place temporary markings on the center of spine [where the string touches]. Palpate the regions to left and right [of the spinal markings] using the fingertips, and there will be places on the abdomen that respond upon being pressed. [After doing so,] place and burn fifty cones of moxa on each point [of congealment on the back]. When [moxibustion is performed] for a seven-day period, or two seven-day periods [i.e., fourteen days], or three seven-day periods [i.e., twenty-one days], the toxin stirs and the abdomen feels tense. At this time, [the physician] should continue to attack [the toxin] by administering the formula according to the pattern presented.

もしうごかざるときは、又た灸してやまず。うごくに乗じてこれを攻む。これいにしへの法なり。かくのごとくにして、病毒うごかざることなし。然れども腹證をみること、つまびらかならざるときは、法のごとく灸すとも功なし。醫者、豈に腹症をゆるがせにすべけんや。

If [the toxin] does not stir, [the physician should] perform moxibustion again without ceasing, and continue to attack [the toxin] until it stirs. This is the ancient method [to treat the pattern]. If performed in this way, there will be no pathogenic toxin that remains unstirred. However, if the abdominal pattern is unclear after examination [of the patient], moxibustion performed in accordance with the [above] method will not be successful. [For this reason,] how can any physician neglect abdominal patterns?

The Second Illustration

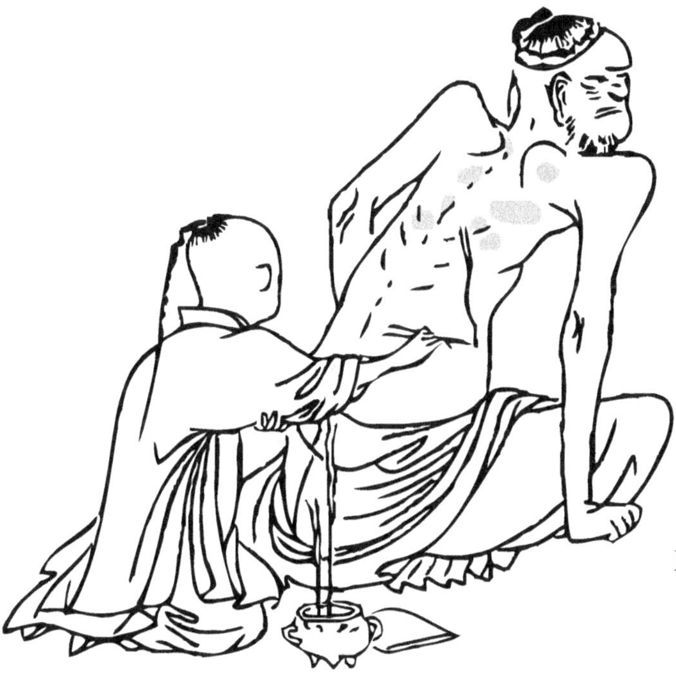

Fig. 35

又た一證、圖の如く、胸毒深厚にして動かざるもの、或るひは心痛背に徹して痛むもの。其の毒の凝るところへ、假點をうち、是れに傚ひて右の法の如く、指頭を以て之れを按じ、痛む處へ點をうち、灸をすること。亦た前の法の如くして、後、本劑兼用、丸・散等を以て之れを攻むべし。

In another pattern, as shown in the illustration, the chest toxin is deep, thick, and is not stirred. In some cases, the patient presents with heart pain stretching through to the back. [The physician] should place temporary markings on the locations where the toxin has congealed and then follow the method outlined above by palpating the region [proximal to the marked points] using the fingertips, place markings on the locations where pain is present, and then perform moxibustion. As mentioned in the previously mentioned method, [the physician] should then simultaneously attack [the pattern] using this formula in pill, powder, or other form.

是れを定むるの傳、指の横はらの頭にていろひ按すに、自然に凹なる所あり。是れを愈位とす。又た徹して痛みこたゆる所を愈位とす。是れ其の毒の所在なり。且つ夫れ古昔の經絡・愈穴・禁穴あることなし。『靈樞』に云はく、「痛を以て愈位と爲す」と。是れ乃ち天然自然にして、愈位有る者なり。故に是れを「天應の穴」と云ふなり。疾醫家、知らざる可からず。

The traditional method to determine [the moxibustion points] is to palpate [the back] using the bottom of finger tips and feel for natural pits. These [pits] are [moxibustion] points. Regions where pain is present are also [moxibustion] points. These are the locations of where the toxin resides. In ancient times, there were no [concepts of] channels, network vessels, [acupuncture] points, or contraindicated points. The *Líng Shū* states that "pain indicates the [acupuncture] point [to be needled]."[177] The cases [above] are cases of patients having natural [moxibustion] points. Therefore these are called "natural reaction points." The physician who specializes in [treating] diseases must understand this [concept].

薏苡附子敗漿散之證

The Pattern for Yì Yĭ Fù Zĭ Bài Jiàng Săn[178] 薏苡附子敗醬散

圖の如く、腹腫るること脹滿に似たり。其の膚甲錯、腹皮急。之れを按ずるに軟なり。甲錯は、たが子の錯りたるごとく、手にあたりてあらきものなり。此の證、世に間々あり。方證相對して攻めざるときは、年月を經るといへども治せず。

177. *Líng Shū*《靈樞》(Jp: *Reisū*; The Magic Pivot) is an ancient Chinese medical text (thought to be compiled in the 1st century BCE). It is one of two parts of a larger medical work known as the *Huáng Dì Nèi Jīng*《黃帝内經》(Jp: *Kōtei-Daikei*; The Yellow Emperor's Inner Canon), which forms the theoretical and practical basis for much of traditional Chinese medicine (TCM) and other Asian systems of medicine such as Kampō medicine. The original quote as found in the "Channel Sinews Chapter (Ch: *Jīng Jīn*《經筋》; Jp: *Kei-Kin*) of *Líng Shū* is as follows: "以知爲數、以痛爲輸。"

178. *Bài jiàng* 敗漿 (Jp: *haishō*) is normally written as 敗醬. The formula for *Yì Yĭ Fù Zĭ Bài Jiàng Săn* 薏苡附子敗醬散 (Jp: *Yokui-Bushi-Haishō-San*; coix, aconite, and patrinia powder) was originally found in *Jīn Guì Yào Lüè*. The extract preparation of the formula is approved by the MHLW to be sold in Japanese drug stores as an over-the-counter drug. It is currently indicated by the MHLW for: lower abdominal pain that is not accompanied by fever, eczema, dermatitis, skin roughening, and warts in persons with weak physical strength (體力虛弱なものの次の諸症：熱を伴わない下腹部の痛み、濕疹・皮膚炎、肌あれ、いぼ).

As shown in the illustration, the abdomen is swollen, similar to [a case of] distention and fullness. [The patient presents with] squamous dry skin and tense abdominal skin.[179] When palpated, [the abdomen] is soft. Encrustation [of skin] is readily apparent

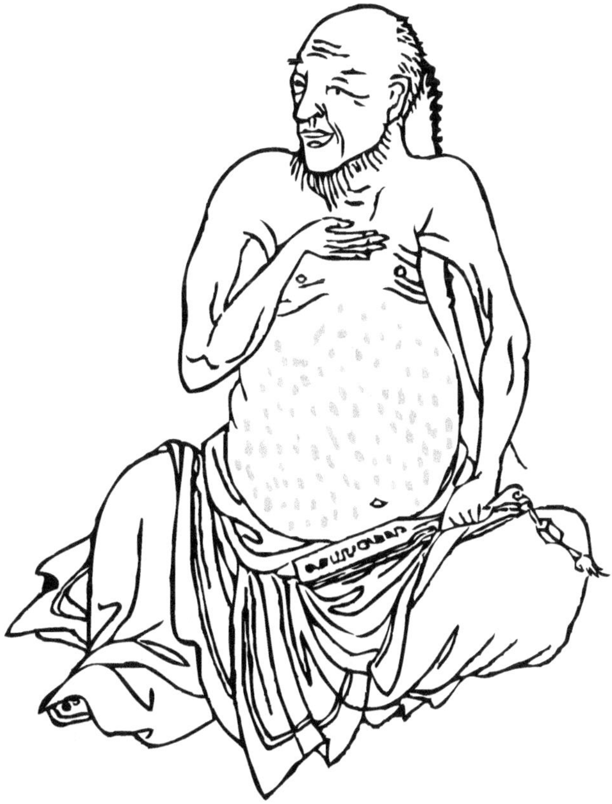

Fig. 36

when pressed with the hands, and cannot be mistaken, any more than [a parent] would mistake [his or her child] for another child. This pattern can be [commonly] found in the world. Unless the [appropriate] formula is matched to the pattern, [the disease] will not be cured, even after years of treatment.

往年、浪華・谷街某の妻、歳二十六、七、此の證あり。治せざること三年、衆醫みな手を束ねて、治療の術を失ふ。後、余に治を請ふ。往きて診するに、腹滿して身重く胎孕の如く、必ず蓐臥することなけれども、心煩して歩行することあたはず。

179. Squamous dry [skin] (Ch: *jiǎ cuò* 甲錯; Jp: *kōsaku*), also known as encrustation [of skin], refers to dried, roughened, and scaling skin, often indicating chronic blood stasis.

Years ago, the wife of a certain man in the Tanimachi area of Naniwa presented with this pattern.[180] [Her condition] could not be cured after three years [of treatment]; a multitude of physicians folded their arms [i.e., gave up on her] and were at a loss for a method of treatment. She later asked me to treat her. When I went to examine her, she presented with abdominal fullness and generalized heaviness;[181] it appeared as if she were pregnant. Although she was not necessarily bedridden, she had heart vexation and could not walk.

余、その頃、腹診未熟なるゆへ、誤つて腹満なるものとして、大承氣湯を以てこれを攻むるに、功なし。因つて大柴胡湯を與ふること、凡そ半年餘にして、始めにかはることなし。是こに於いて病家、その功なきを以て憮然として謂つて曰く、「足下、平常大言を吐く。然れども今その驗なし。然るときは、他醫亦たいづくんぞ治すべけん乎。生涯廢人たらんこと疑ひなし。嗚呼、悲歎に堪へず」と。

At that time, I was still unskilled in abdominal examination, and for this reason, I erroneously gave her a diagnosis of abdominal fullness, and attacked the pattern with *Dà Chéng Qì Tāng*, but there was no effect. I then [switched medicinals and] gave her *Dà Chái Hú Tāng* for a little longer than half a year, but her condition remained the same as it first was. The patient therefore glumly said to me, "Sir, you often boast [of your skills], but even now [after all this time, your treatment] has no effect. At this rate, how can any other physician cure me? I will undoubtedly be a cripple for the rest of my life. Oh! I can no longer control my grief!"

余、これを聞いて、其の言行一致せざることを愧ぢて、余が先師鶴先生に告ぐ。先生乃ち往いて之れを診し、大いに余を責めて曰く、「汝、古醫の術、未練なるが故に、病者あらば必ず我に告げて、而うして後に治療を施すべし」と云ひをけり。然るに汝、我が言を用ひず、自是として其の腹證を審らかにせず、妄りに是くの如き峻劑を投じて病者を苦しましむ。術を慎まず、師を侮るの罪、大い矣。世に汝がごとき拙技の者ありて、大いに我が古醫道をみだる。惡むべく、哀しむべきの甚だしい哉」と。

180. Naniwa 浪華 (more commonly written as 浪速) is the former name of Ōsaka 大阪.

181. Generalized heaviness (Ch: *shēn zhòng* 身重; Jp: *mi-omo*) refers to the subjective sensation of heaviness in the body with difficult movement.

When I heard this, I was ashamed that my deeds did not match my words and therefore reported the case to my master, Kaku-Sensei. [Kaku-]Sensei then went to examine her, and severely criticized me saying, "I previously told you that you were still unskilled in the techniques of the ancient physicians. Hence, without fail, you were to inform me before you started to perform any sort of treatment. However, in this case, you did not listen to my words and trusted yourself without making the pattern clear. By recklessly administering such a drastic [i.e., strong] drug as this to the patient, you have caused the patient to suffer. You have committed a grave transgression by being careless about treatment and dishonored your master! It is because of people with poor skills such as you that have greatly caused this ancient way of medicine to become corrupted. [Your actions] have both angered and saddened [me] a great deal."

因つて教へて曰く、「此の證、膚甲錯、腹皮急、之れを按じて軟なる者、是れ薏苡附子敗漿散の證なり。汝が先に用ゆる所の大承氣湯・大柴胡湯の症、何くにか在る哉。汝、これを以て後來の誡めとし、輕忽を謹しむべし」と。余、大いに其の罪を謝し、教に從つて右の方を與ふ。纔かに二旬許りにして其の疾ひ、頓に愈ゆ。余よつて深く腹診の易々ならざるを曉り、玆れ自りますます精研して、後來、大いに術に進むことを得たり。

He then explained to me, "This pattern, in which the patient presents with squamous dry skin [i.e., encrusted skin], tense abdominal skin, and a soft [abdomen] upon palpation, is the pattern for *Yì Yĭ Fù Zĭ Bài Jiàng Săn*. Where are the patterns for the formulae of *Dà Chéng Qì Tāng* or *Dà Chái Hú Tāng* that you used? You must use this [experience] as a warning for the future, and be careful to never do such a careless thing again."

I greatly apologized for my error and administered the above-mentioned formula according to the instruction [that I had received]. After approximately two ten-day periods (i.e., twenty days), the disease was suddenly cured. I then deeply understood that performing abdominal examinations was no easy task and therefore studied even more diligently, thenceforth making great strides in the art [of performing examinations].

四逆湯之證

The Pattern for Sì Nì Tāng[182] 四逆湯

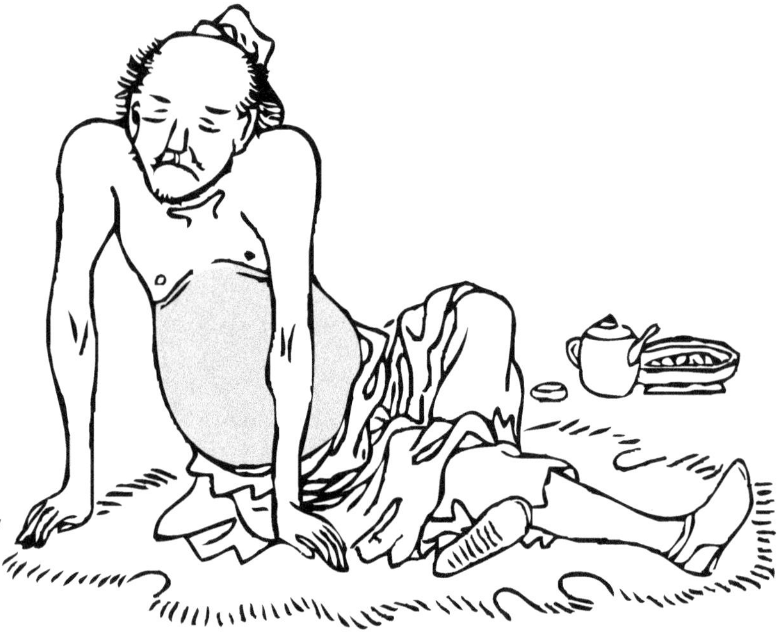

Fig. 37

圖の如く、腹滿して軟。これを按ずるにちからなく、腹體、あるひは心下底にこたゆるの毒なく、又た肌膚はうるほひなく、甲錯して、俗にいふ「さめはだ」のごとく。手足逆冷、あるひは厥逆、且つ腹底ひえ、あるひは臍下關元の邊不仁にして、腹底にちからなし。又た云はく、腹底攣急、或るひは下痢清穀、或るひは小便不利。その餘、本文を以て考ふべし。

As shown in the illustration, the abdomen is full and soft. Palpatory findings reveal a lack of [abdominal] strength, and there is no toxin that springs back [when pressed] present in the bottom of the abdominal body or the region below the heart. Furthermore,

182. The formula for *Sì Nì Tāng* 四逆湯 (Jp: *Shigyaku-Tō*; counterflow cold decoction) was originally found in *Jīn Guì Yào Lüè* and *Shāng Hán Lùn*. The extract preparation of the formula is covered by the Japanese National Health Insurance program as a prescription drug, and may be sold in Japanese drug stores as an over-the-counter drug. It is currently indicated by the MHLW for: the common cold, acute or chronic gastroenteritis, diarrhea, and nausea in persons with weak physical strength or physically exhausted persons who have cold extremities (體力虛弱あるいは體力が消耗し、手足が冷えるものの次の諸症：感冒、急・慢性胃腸炎、下痢、はきけ).

the skin has no moisture and is squamous and dry; it [feels exactly] like its colloquial nickname of "shark skin." The patient [also] presents with counterflow cold of the limbs. In some cases [the patient presents with] reverse flow, and the depths of the abdomen are cold. In some cases, the subumbilical region surrounding *Guān Yuán* (Jp: *Kangen*; CV-4) is insensitive, and there is a lack of strength in the depths of the abdomen.[183] Furthermore, hypertonicity [may be felt] in the depths of the abdomen. In some cases, the patient presents with clear-food diarrhea,[184] and in some cases the patient presents with inhibited urination. The text [of this section] should be referred to in other [similar cases].

灸治法

The Method of Treatment Using Moxibustion

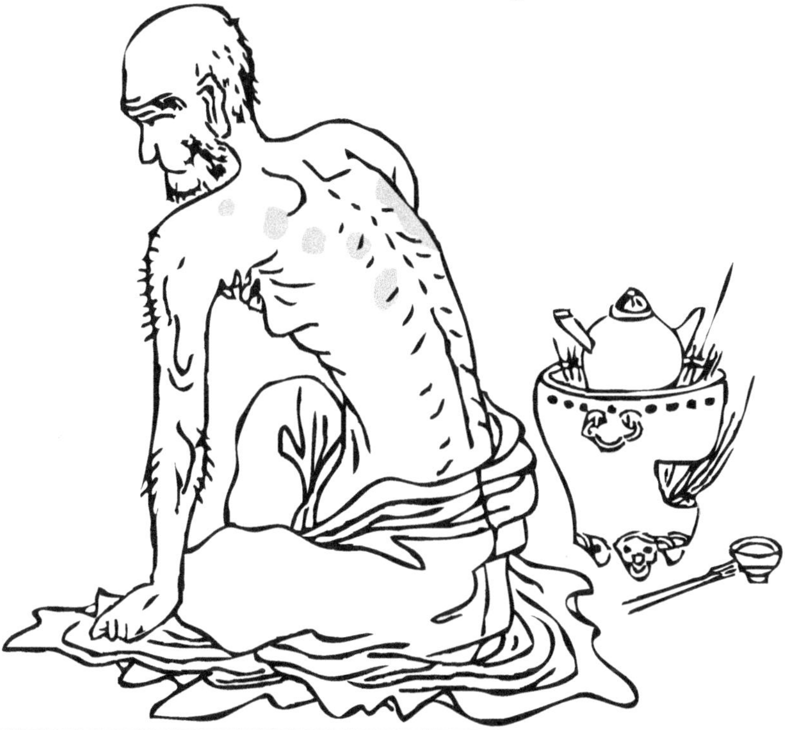

Fig. 38

183. *Guān yuán* 關元 is commonly called *tanden* 丹田 (Ch: *dān tián*) in Japan, although the term often does not refer only to the acupuncture point itself, but the entire surrounding region, including points such as *qì hǎi* 氣海 (Jp: *kikai*; CV 6). Not only is the region a major focus of Japanese abdominal diagnosis, but it is also the focal point of zazen (Jp: *zazen* 坐禪; Ch: *zuò chán*) meditation in Zen Buddhism and is considered to be the center of balance and *ki* 氣 (Ch: *qì*) in Japanese martial arts.

184. Clear-food diarrhea (Ch: *xià lì qīng gǔ* 下痢清穀; Jp: *geri-seikoku*) refers to frequent discharge of fluid stools containing undigested food, the same as undigested food diarrhea.

圖の如く、項背の若干凸して拘攣、或るひは項背強急。これみな胸毒はなはだしくして、諸藥方證相對すといへども、全く治せざるものままあり。その毒深きを以て背につく。いはゆる毒陰文につくものこれなり。

As shown in the illustration, [the patient presents with] a number of bulges on the nape and back [accompanied by] hypertonicity. In some cases, [the patient presents with] stiffness of the nape and back. These are all cases of severe chest toxins; [hence,] even if [the physician attempts to] match the formulae of various medicinals according to the pattern presented, the patient will not be completely cured. [In such cases,] the toxin is deep and has become attached to the back. What is known as an "engraved toxin" is referring to this.[185]

これに灸するの法、その凸なるところ、骨をはづれて、指の腹を以てこれを按ずるに、病者こたゆるところ、みな毒なり。指頭の陥沒徹底するところ、これにみな灸すること。一穴に二、三十壯。あるひは七日、あるひは二十一日。灸して以て證に從ひ、方劑を以てこれを攻む。治せざることなし。

The method to perform moxibustion [on these points] is to feel for bulges using the "belly" of the fingertips while disregarding any bony [landmarks]. Any spot that the patient reacts to when palpated contains a toxin. Any spot in which the fingertips are able to completely sink into, is a location where moxibustion should be performed. Twenty to thirty cones of moxa should be used on each point. In some cases, [the treatment should continue] seven days, and in some cases, [treatment should continue up to] twenty-one days. If [the physician] performs moxibustion and administers [the appropriate] formula according to the pattern, there will be no [patient] that cannot be cured.

185. The word "engraved" (Jp: *inbun* 陰文; Ch: *yīn wén*) was originally used to describe the carvings made on stone and metal monuments.

抵當湯或抵當丸之證
The Pattern for Dǐ Dāng Tāng 抵當湯 or Dǐ Dāng Wán[186] 抵當丸

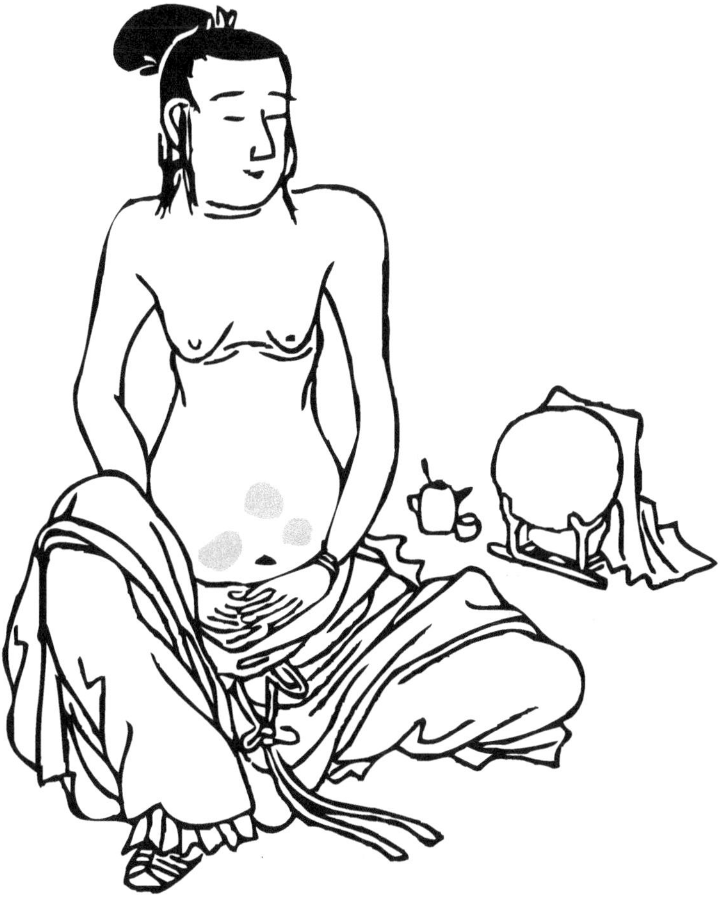

Fig. 39

圖のごとく、腹中軟滿にして物あり。雞子殼のごときもの、水中にうかみてあるがごとく、これを按じてすなはち沈み、手を去つてしたがつて浮かむ。あるひはこれを按じて傍らへ去り、その數、あるひは一、二、あるひは五、六。その人、面顏唇手足ともに青白色すきとをるごとくして、つやなし。

186. The formulae for *Dǐ Dāng Tāng* 抵當湯 (Jp: *Teitō-Tō*; dead-on decoction) and *Dǐ Dāng Wán* 抵當丸 (Jp: *Teitō-Gan*; dead-on pill) were originally found in *Shāng Hán Lùn*. At present, these formulae are not covered by the Japanese National Health Insurance program and are not well known in Japan.

As shown in the illustration, the abdomen is soft and full, [feeling as if] there are objects [inside of it. These objects feel] like eggshells floating in the water. When palpated, they sink, and when the hand is released, they float again to the surface. In some cases, when [the physician] palpates laterally, one, two, or in some cases five or six [items can be felt]. The person [who presents with this pattern] has an unhealthy complexion; the face, lips, and extremities all have a pale green-blue color that appears almost transparent and lacks luster.

あるひは黄色なるかたち、勞瘵の如し。小便快利、大便硬反つて易く。その色黒く、あるひは塊物、臍下・臍傍、あるひは陰門、あるひは陰莖邊、あるひは小腹、或るひは腹中來去遊走のもの。又た本文の如く、腹滿せず、其の人、「我は滿す」と言ふ者。

In some cases, the patient presents with a yellow [complexion], similar to [that seen in cases of] consumption. Urination is free and uninhibited, and stools are hard and easy [to pass] and [appear] dark in color. In some cases, the patient presents with lumps in the subumbilical region and regions lateral to the umbilicus. In some cases, there may be a feeling of something arriving and departing, as if wandering throughout the yīn door [i.e., vulva], yīn stem [i.e., penis], smaller abdomen, or abdominal region. [This formula may be used even] in cases in which the patient does not present with abdominal fullness as described in this chapter, yet the patient still says, "I have [a sensation of] fullness [in the abdomen]."

梔子豉湯之證

The Pattern for Zhī Zǐ Chǐ Tāng[187] 梔子豉湯

圖の如く、心下空。これを按ずれば、軟。心中窒結痛、時々煩熱し手足温。もしくは甚しきものは心中懊憹。その餘、傳有つて存す。

187. The formula for *Zhī Zǐ Chǐ Tāng* 梔子豉湯 (Jp: *Shishi-Shi-Tō*; gardenia and fermented soybean decoction) was originally found in *Jīn Guì Yào Lüè* and *Shāng Hán Lùn*. Although the formula is not well known in Japan at present, the extract preparation of the formula is approved by the MHLW to be sold in Japanese drug stores as an over-the-counter drug. It is currently indicated by the MHLW for: insomnia, stomatitis, glossitis, sore throat, eczema, and dermatitis in persons with moderate or weak physical strength who have a painful sensation of blockage in the chest and have a sensation of heat (體力中等度以下で、胸がふさがり苦しく、熱感があるものの次の諸症：不眠、口内炎、舌炎、咽喉炎、濕疹・皮膚炎).

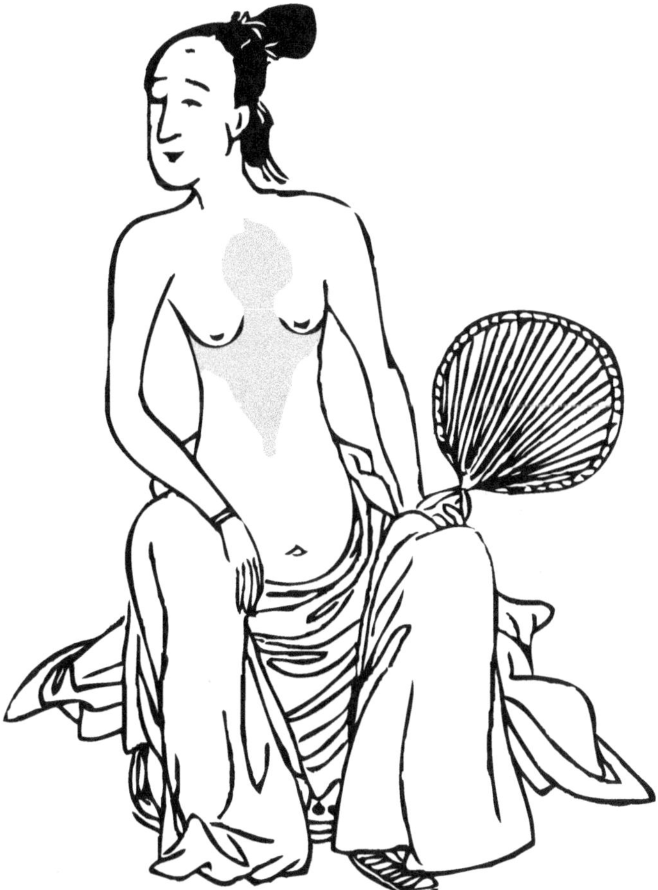

Fig. 40

As shown in the illustration, [the patient presents with] emptiness in the region below the heart. [The abdomen] is soft upon palpation. The patient has gripping pain in the heart, and occasionally presents with heat vexation and warm extremities.[188] In severe cases, the patient may present with heart anguish.[189] Further [details concerning this pattern] exist in other records.

又た曰く、梔子甘草豉湯の證、梔子豉湯の證に而て氣息吸々して將に絶せんとするの狀の如き者。其の餘、梔子生姜豉湯、あるひは枳實梔子豉湯・梔子大黄豉湯、みな前の梔子豉湯の證を以てこれを推す。然りといへども、豉の分量、梔子の分量有無、餘藥の有無、以てつつしんで考ふべし。自づからその正證を得。

188. Heat vexation (Ch: *fán rè* 煩熱; Jp: *han-netsu*) generally refers fever accompanied by uneasiness or restlessness, also known as irritable heat sensation.

189. Heart anguish (Ch: *xīn zhōng ào náo* 心中懊憹; Jp: *shinchū-ōnō*) generally refers to heat vexation and oppression in the region of the heart and chest.

Furthermore, the patterns for *Zhī Zǐ Gān Cǎo Chǐ Tāng* and *Zhī Zǐ Chǐ Tāng*, in which the patient presents with conditions such as heavy breathing that verges on expiration, or other patterns [matching formulae] such as *Zhī Zǐ Shēng Jiāng Chǐ Tāng*, *Zhǐ Shí Zhī Zǐ Chǐ Tāng*, or *Zhī Zǐ Dà Huáng Chǐ Tāng* should be determined based on the pattern for the aforementioned *Zhī Zǐ Chǐ Tāng*. However, [the physician] should carefully consider the quantity of *chǐ* [to be used], as well as the addition or subtraction of *zhī zǐ* or other drug [ingredients.[190] Having done so the physician can] naturally understand the true pattern that the patient has.

Another Illustration of the Pattern for Zhī Zǐ Chǐ Tāng 梔子豉湯

圖の如く、小腹に簾をあみたるごとく、横に筋隠起するあり。名づけて「簾腹」といふ。其の證、小腹滿。時に腹痛し、或るひは鼓脹とならんとするものの如し。此れ寸白蟲也。俗に「真田蟲」といふ。又た腹狀にあらわれずといへども、偶たま此の蟲を下すことあり。綿々として長きこと二、三丈なるものあり。若しくは腹狀にあらはるるときは左の方用ゆべし（此の腹狀に似て竪に筋をあらはし、且つ筋の色青きものはこの証にあらず）。

As shown in the illustration, the patient presents with prominent blood vessels on the smaller abdomen that appear as if they were woven together to form a curtain [made of bamboo strips.[191] The condition] is called "curtain belly." In this pattern, [the patient pres-

190. *Zhī Zǐ Gān Cǎo Chǐ Tāng* 梔子甘草豉湯 (Jp: *Shishi-Kanzō-Shi-Tō*; gardenia, licorice, and fermented soybean decoction), *Zhī Zǐ Shēng Jiāng Chǐ Tāng* 梔子生薑豉湯 (Jp: *Shishi-Shōkyō-Shi-Tō*; gardenia, fresh ginger, and fermented soybean decoction), and *Zhī Zǐ Dà Huáng Chǐ Tāng* 梔子大黄豉湯 (Jp; *Shishi-Daiō-Shi-Tō*; gardenia, rhubarb, and fermented soybean decoction) are all variant formulas of *Zhī Zǐ Chǐ Tāng* 梔子豉湯 that are found in *Shāng Hán Lùn*. However, at present, these formulae are not covered by the Japanese National Health Insurance program and are not commonly used in Japan. Instead, the extract preparation of *Zhī Zǐ Bǎi Pí Tāng* 梔子柏皮湯 (Jp: *shishi-hakuhi-tō*; gardenia and phellodendron decoction), found in *Shāng Hán Lùn* under the name *Zhī Zǐ Bò Pí Tāng* 梔子蘗皮湯, is covered by the Japanese National Health Insurance program as a prescription drug, and may be sold in Japanese drug stores as an over-the-counter drug. It is currently indicated by the MHLW for: eczema, dermatitis, itchiness, and bloodshot eyes in persons with moderate or weak physical strength who do not have cold extremities and experience itchiness (體力中等度で、冷えはなく、ときにかゆみがあるものの次の諸症：濕疹・皮膚炎、かゆみ、目の充血).

191. The traditional Japanese curtain (Jp: *sudare* 簾) mentioned in this section is made of horizontal slats of decorative wood, bamboo, or other natural material woven together with simple string, or colored yarn to make nearly solid blinds, and could be rolled up easily when needed.

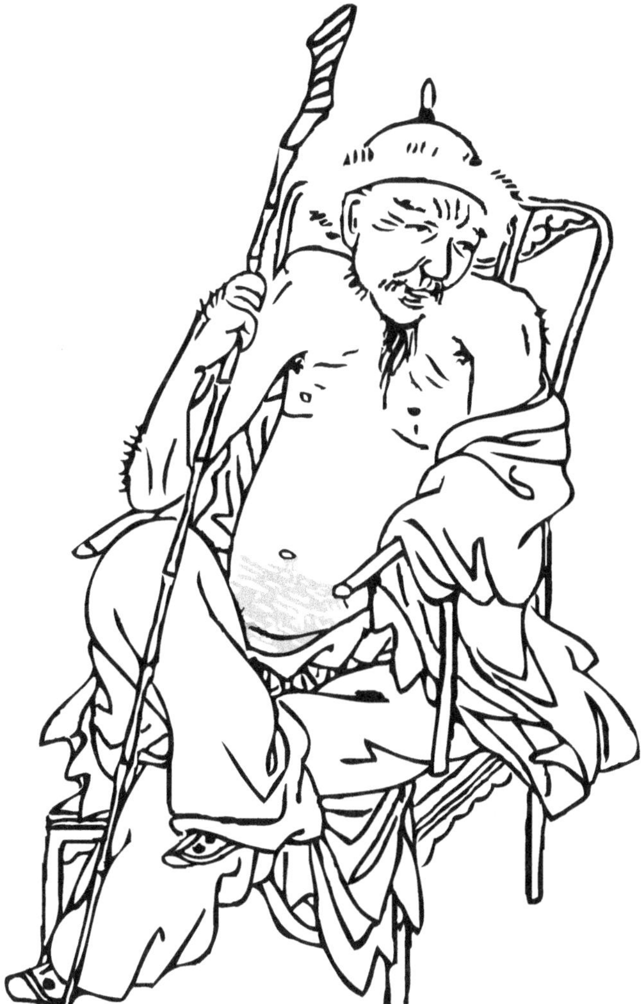

Fig. 41

ents with] fullness in the smaller abdomen. The patient often presents with abdominal pain, or in some cases, drumlike abdominal distention. This is [caused by] a tapeworm. It is colloquially referred to as "*sanada-mushi*."[192] Moreover, even if [the presence of a tapeworm] is not apparent from the appearance of the abdomen, this worm may descend in some patients. Some [tapeworms] can reach up to two or three *jō* in length.[193] When the abdominal [pattern] is apparent from its appearance, the following formula should

192. Tapeworms are commonly called *sanada-mushi* 真田蟲 (literally, "Sanada insect") in Japan because of their resemblance to *sanada-himo* 真田紐, a type of decorative fabric strap used to fasten items such as boxes and armor.
193. A *jō* 丈 is a traditional Japanese unit of length. During the Meiji 明治 period, the length of one *jō* 丈 was standardized as 3.03 meters.

be used (another pattern in which [the patient presents with] prominent green-blue abdominal blood vessels running vertically is not this pattern).

榧實（ 穀を去りて 、百六十戔を用ゆ ）

Fěi shí 榧實 (remove the husks and use 160 *qián*)

右 、分かつて十五服として 、十五日に吃し盡くす 。其の日より二 、三日の間に糞道より細長き蟲を下すこと三丈餘に及ぶものあるべし 。其の蟲出づるときは 、板片の類に巻きて 、絲をまくごとくにして 、徐々に引き出だすべし 。強くひく時は半ばにしてきれやすし 。此の方 、余 、遊歴中 、尾州名古屋に於いて 、某醫の傳ふるところなり 。奇なりといふべし 。

The [above] formula should be divided into fifteen doses and administered to the patient [over a period of] fifteen days until completely consumed. Within two or three days after the [final] day [of administration], a thin long worm that may reach up to three *jō* in length will be precipitated from the anus. When the worm starts to come out, it should be wrapped around an object such as a piece of wood in the way that one would wrap thread around a [spool. The worm] should then be slowly pulled out. If pulled too strongly, [the tapeworm] will easily break in the middle. I was taught this method by a certain physician during my travels around Nagoya in Bishū.[194] It is indeed extraordinary!

194. Bishū 尾州 is the abbreviated name of Owari Province (Jp: *Owari-No-Kuni* 尾張國), a province of Japan in the area that today comprises the western half of Aichi Prefecture (Jp: *Aichi-Ken* 愛知縣), including the city of Nagoya 名古屋.

諸症毒交發する者の圖
Illustration [Comparing] Various Patterns Caused by Toxins

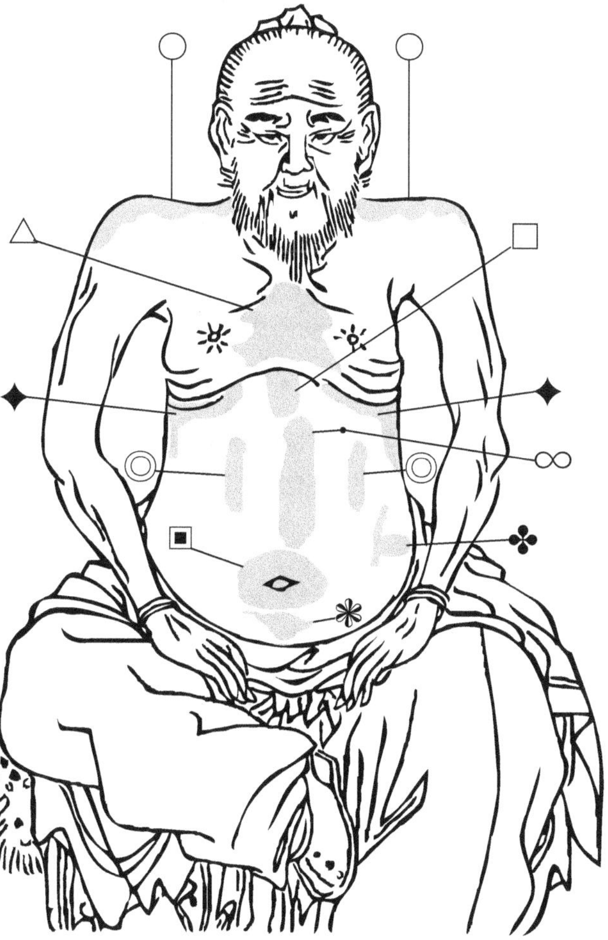

Fig. 42

○葛根湯、或るひは括蔞薤白白酒湯、或るひは茯苓杏仁甘草湯
△小陷胸湯、大陷胸湯、或るひは大陷胸丸
□桂枝人參湯、或るひは德本家理中湯
✦小柴胡湯、或るひは亦た大柴胡湯
∞大承氣湯
◎柴胡加芒硝湯
✤桃軍圓
▣癥瘤圓
❋大黄牡丹皮湯

○[The pattern for] *Gé Gēn Tāng, Guā Lóu Xiè Bái Bái Jiŭ Tāng,* or *Fú Líng Xìng Rén Gān Căo Tāng.*
△[The pattern for] *Xiăo Xiàn Xiōng Tāng, Dà Xiàn Xiōng Tāng,* or *Dà Xiàn Xiōng Wán.*
□[The pattern for] *Guì Zhī Rén Shēn Tāng* or Tokuhon's *Richū-Tō.*[195]
✦[The pattern for] *Xiăo Chái Hú Tāng* or *Dà Chái Hú Tāng.*
∞[The pattern for] *Dà Chéng Qì Tāng.*
◎[The pattern for] *Chái Hú Jiā Máng Xiāo Tāng.*
✤[The pattern for] *Tō-Gun-En.*
▣[The pattern for] *Chōko-En.*
❃[The pattern for] *Dà Huáng Mŭ Dān Pí Tāng.*

右の方書者、世に知らるる所。古方分量考、或るひは古方便覧等を以て知るべし

The above-shown formulae are well known in the world. They can be known [i.e., studied] in treatises concerning the quantities of the ancient formulae or from manuals concerning ancient formulae.

右、圖のごとく、諸證毒いちどに發するもの、かならず死す。

If various toxin-patterns simultaneously occurred as shown in the illustration, [the patient] would surely die.

此の書にあげざる所の腹症、並びに甲斐州德本翁十九方の傳、其の他諸州游歴中得るところの諸名家の奇方、他日を待つて後篇に出だす。

It is my hope to publish abdominal patterns not listed in this book or *Tokuhon-Ō-Jūku-Hō*《德本翁十九方》(Nineteen Prescriptions of the Venerable Tokuhon), written

195. *Richū-Tō* 理中湯 (Ch: *Lĭ Zhōng Tāng*; center-rectifying decoction), also known as *Richū-San* 理中散 (Ch: *Lĭ Zhōng Săn*; center-rectifying powder) in *Tokuhon-Ō-Jūku-Hō*《德本翁十九方》(Nineteen Prescriptions of the Venerable Tokuhon), is not discussed in this work. Although it is an original formula of Tokuhon, it is essentially the same as previously mentioned *Rén Shēn Tāng* 人參湯, albeit with different quantities of ingredients and the addition of *fú líng* 茯苓. The formula for *Richū-San* 理中散 as found in the received text of *Tokuhon-Ō-Jūku-Hō* is as follows: *fú líng* 茯苓 (1 *qián*), *rén shēn* 人參, [*bái*] *zhú* [白]朮 (6 *fēn* each), *guì zhī* 桂枝, *gān jiāng* 乾薑, *gān căo* 甘草 (4 *fēn* each).

by Tokuhon of Kai Province, and other wondrous formulae that I have collected during my travels around various provinces in a future volume.

湖南稲葉意仲克文禮著
Written by Konan Inaba Ichū Bunrei[196]

吉備旭江戸淵白龜畫
Illustrated by Fuchigami Kyokkō Byakki[197] of Kibi Province[198]

寛政十二庚申夏五月
[Written in] the fifth month of the twelfth year of the Kansei era[199] (*gēng shēn* year [of the sexagenary cycle]) [i.e., June 1800 CE][200]

享和元年酉七月
[Published in] the seventh month of the first year of the Kyōwa era [i.e., August 1801].

高田 和州書林 本屋源左衛門
Takada [City] Washū Shorin [Bookstore], Hon'ya Genzaemon [Publisher][201]

196. Similar to most men of the literati class of pre-modern East Asia, the author had several names that were used depending on the social situation: his family name was Inaba 稲葉, courtesy name was Bunrei 文禮, birth name was Katsu 克, alias was Ichū 意仲, and pen name was Konan 湖南.
197. Fuchigami Kyokkō 淵上旭江 (courtesy name: Byakki 白龜; 1753–1816 CE) was a famous illustrator of the Edo period.
198. Kibi Province (Jp: *Kibi-No-Kuni* 吉備國) was an ancient region of Japan that comprised modern-day Okayama Prefecture (Jp: *Okayama-Ken* 岡山縣) and eastern Hiroshima Prefecture (Jp: *Hiroshima-Ken* 廣島縣). It was later divided into three provinces: Bizen 備前, Bitchū 備中, and Bingo Provinces 備後 (literally, "near Kibi," "middle Kibi," and "far Kibi," respectively) according to their distance from the Kyōto, the capital of the time. Fuchigami was from Bizen.
199. The Kansei 寛政 era lasted from 1789 to 1801 CE.
200. *Gēng shēn* 庚申 (Jp: *kanoesaru* or *kōshin*) is the fifty-seventh year of the traditional sixty year calendar cycle.
201. Washū 和州 is the abbreviated name refers to Yamato Province (Jp: *Yamato-No-Kuni* 大和國), which corresponds to present-day Nara Prefecture (Jp: *Nara-Ken* 奈良縣). Many bookstores (Jp: *shorin* 書林) during the Edo period also published books.

心齋橋通北久太郎町河内屋喜兵衛
Shinsaibashi-Dori [Street], Kita Kyūtarō Machi [Town], Kawachiya Kihei [Publisher]

大坂書林同東久寶寺町鹽屋平助
Ōsaka Shorin [Bookstore], Higashi Kyuhōji Machi [Town], Shioya Heisuke [Publisher][202]

202. There is no information concerning Hon'ya Genzaemon, Kawachiya Kihei, or Shioya Heisuke. They appear to have been famous publishers in the Kansai region during the Edo period.

腹證奇覧上冊分量考

Quantities [of Ingredients in the Formulae Found] in the First Half of *Fukushō-Kiran* 《腹證奇覽》 (Extraordinary Views of Abdominal Patterns)

古より倭醫の分量考多しといへども、痼疾重病を療するに至りては、大服濃煎に非ざれば効無し。故に予の分量考は病重き者は必ず増して用ゆ。輕き者は略して之れを處しても効あり。是れ則ち古人處劑の意なり。

Since ancient times, Japanese physicians have used greater quantities [of medicinals in comparison with physicians in China]: when treating intractable or severe diseases, unless a large quantity of a concentrated decoction [is used, the treatment] will be ineffective.[203] Thus, the quantities that I have listed here must absolutely be increased when used in patients who present with a severe disease. [The quantities listed here are] generally effective when administered to patients who present with mild [symptoms]. This [principle] is [in line with] how the ancients thought when administering medicinals.[204]

桂枝湯之方

Guì Zhī Tāng

桂枝・生姜・大棗・芍藥（各九分）・甘草（六分）。

guì zhī	桂枝	9 fēn
shēng jiāng	生薑	9 fēn
dà zǎo	大棗	9 fēn
sháo yào	芍藥	9 fēn
gān cǎo	甘草	6 fēn

203. At present, the doses of traditional Japanese Kampō drugs as well as modern drugs are usually significantly smaller than those used in China, Korea, the United States, and other countries due to safety concerns of the MHLW.

204. In modern Japan, due to MHLW guidelines concerning the ingredients and dosage of Kampō drugs, and the fact that extract granules or tablets are generally used in clinical practice, it is not common to increase the quantity of ingredients or dose of Kampō drugs. In the case of intractable or severe diseases, two different Kampō drugs are administered concurrently or a Kampō drug is administered concurrently with a modern drug.

右、水一盞四分を以て、六分に煮取り、一度に服す。

Boil the above [ingredients] in one cup and four *fēn* of water to make six *fēn* of the decoction; take in a single dose.

小柴胡湯之方
Xiǎo Chái Hú Tāng

柴胡（一戔）・黄芩・人參・甘草・生姜・大棗（各四分強）・半夏（一戔強）。

chái hú	柴胡	1 qián
huáng qín	黃芩	a little more than 4 fēn
rén shēn	人參	a little more than 4 fēn
gān cǎo	甘草	a little more than 4 fēn
shēng jiāng	生薑	a little more than 4 fēn
dà zǎo	大棗	a little more than 4 fēn
bàn xià	半夏	a little more than 1 qián

右、水二盞四分を以て、一盞二分に煮取り、滓を去てて、再び煎じ六分にとり、一度に服す。

Boil the above [ingredients] in two cups and four *fēn* of water to make one cup and two *fēn* of the decoction. Remove the dregs and boil again to make six *fēn* of the decoction; take in a single dose.

大柴胡湯之方
Dà Chái Hú Tāng

柴胡（一戔）・黄芩・芍藥・大棗（各四分）・半夏（一戔二分）・枳實（五分強）・生姜（六分強）・大黄（三分強）。

chái hú	柴胡	1 qián
huáng qín	黃芩	4 fēn
sháo yào	芍藥	4 fēn

dà zǎo	大棗	4 fēn
bàn xià	半夏	1 qián and 2 fēn
zhǐ shí	枳實	a little more than 5 fēn
shēng jiāng	生薑	a little more than 6 fēn
dà huáng	大黄	a little more than 3 fēn

右、水、小柴胡湯と同じ。傳に云はく、大柴胡の證にして、下利の者は大黄を去る。

The [quantity of] water [should be] the same as [in the formula for] *Xiǎo Chái Hú Tāng*. [One] text says that when the patient presents with the pattern for *Dà Chái Hú Tāng* and has diarrhea, *dà huáng* should be removed [from the formula].

柴胡加芒硝湯之方
Chái Hú Jiā Máng Xiāo Tāng

柴胡（一戔）・黄芩・芍藥・大棗（各四分半）・半夏（一戔二分）・枳實（五分半）・生姜（六分半）・大黄（三分強）・芒硝（七分半）。

chái hú	柴胡	1 qián
huáng qín	黄芩	4.5 fēn
sháo yào	芍藥	4.5 fēn
dà zǎo	大棗	4.5 fēn
bàn xià	半夏	1 qián and 2 fēn
zhǐ shí	枳實	5.5 fēn
shēng jiāng	生薑	6.5 fēn
dà huáng	大黄	a little more than 3 fēn
máng xiāo	芒硝	7.5 fēn

水、小柴胡湯と同じ。

The [quantity of] water [should be] the same as [in the formula for] *Xiǎo Chái Hú Tāng*.

呉茱萸湯之方
Wú Zhū Yú Tāng

呉茱萸（二箋強）・人參・大棗・生姜（各一箋半）。

wú zhū yú	呉茱萸	a little more than 2 qián
rén shēn	人參	1.5 qián
dà zǎo	大棗	1.5 qián
shēng jiāng	生薑	1.5 qián

右、水一盞四分を以て、四分に煮とり、一度に服す。

Boil the above [ingredients] in one cup and four *fēn* of water to make four *fēn* of the decoction; take in a single dose.

人參芎軍桃花湯之方
Rén Shēn Xiōng Jūn Táo Huā Tāng

桃花（二箋五分、白桃花半開に非ざれば効うすし）・大黄（一箋）・人參・川芎（各四分半）。

táo huā	桃花	2 qián and 5 fēn	unless bái táo huā 白桃花 that is in half bloom is used, the efficacy [of the drug] is poor.
dà huáng	大黃	1 qián	
rén shēn	人參	4.5 fēn	
chuān xiōng	川芎	4.5 fēn	

右、水一盞半を以て、六分に煮取り、一度に服す。

Boil the above ingredients in one and one-half cups of water to make six *fēn* of the decoction; take in a single dose.

桃軍圓之方
Tō-Gun-En

大黄（ 二十戔 ）・桃仁・桂枝・甘草（ 各十戔 ）・芒硝（ 十二戔 ）・蕎麥（ 五戔 ）。

dà huáng	大黄	20 qián
táo rén	桃仁	10 qián
guì zhī	桂枝	10 qián
gān cǎo	甘草	10 qián
máng xiāo	芒硝	12 qián
qiáo mài	蕎麥	5 qián

右、末となし、練蜜に和して丹となす（ 此の方は『 傷寒論 』に云はく、「 桃仁承氣湯也 」、此くの如くにして其の効ある故に丹にするなり ）。

Grind the above [ingredients] into a powder and mix with *liàn mì* 煉蜜 to make an elixir (this formula is called *Táo Rén Chéng Qì Tāng*[205] in *Shāng Hán Lùn*. Because it of its efficacy, I have listed it here as an elixir).

栝蔞薤白白酒湯之方
Guā Lóu Xiè Bái Bái Jiǔ Tāng

栝蔞仁（ 四分半 ）・薤白（ 二戔九分 ）・白酒（ つねの酒なり ）。

guā lóu rén	瓜蔞仁	4.5 fēn
xiè bái	薤白	2 qián and 9 fēn
bái jiǔ	白酒	commonly available sake

右、水一盞と酒一盞とを以て、六分に煮とり、一度に服す。

Boil the above [ingredients] in one cup of water and one cup of sake to make six *fēn* of the decoction; take in a single dose.

205. The actual name of the formula as found in *Shāng Hán Lùn* is *Táo Hé Chéng Qì Tāng* 桃核承氣湯.

磁石丸之方
Jishaku-Gan

磁石・大黄（各十二戔）・浮石・桃仁（各六戔）。

cí shí	磁石	12 qián
dà huáng	大黄	12 qián
fú shí	浮石	6 qián
táo rén	桃仁	6 qián

右、末となし、小豆の大きさの如く丸す。毎夜一戔、或るひは一戔半を、白湯を以て送下す。（右、徳本家の藥品分量と少しくたがへり、効多し）。

Make the above [ingredients] into a powder to make balls the size of small [adzuki] beans. Take one *qián* or one and one-half *qián* of the decoction with hot water each night (the quantities of ingredients in the above formula are slightly different from those found in Tokuhon's version of the medicinal, but [this version] has stronger efficacy).

橘皮大黄芒硝湯之方
Jú Pí Dà Huáng Máng Xiāo Tāng

橘皮（七分半）・大黄・芒硝（各一戔四分）。

jú pí	橘皮	7.5 fēn
dà huáng	大黄	1 qián and 4 fēn
máng xiāo	芒硝	1 qián and 4 fēn

右、水一盞八分を以て、六分に煮とり、一度に服す。

Boil the above [ingredients] in one cup and eight *fēn* of water to make six *fēn* of the decoction; take in a single dose.

六君子湯之方
Liù Jūn Zǐ Tāng

人參（ 蔓人參可なり ）・白朮・茯苓・半夏・陳皮（ 各一戔二分 ）・甘草（ 四分 ）。

rén shēn	人參	1 qián and 2 fēn	màn rén shēn 蔓人參 may also be used.
bái zhú	白朮	1 qián and 2 fēn	
fú líng	茯苓	1 qián and 2 fēn	
bàn xià	半夏	1 qián and 2 fēn	
chén pí	陳皮	1 qián and 2 fēn	
gān cǎo	甘草	4 fēn	

右、水一盞半を以て六分に煮取り、一度に服す。

Boil the above [ingredients] in one and one-half cups of water to make six *fēn* of the decoction; take in a single dose.

甘草乾姜湯之方
Gān Cǎo Gān Jiāng Tāng

甘草（ 二戔 ）・乾姜（ 一戔一分 ）。

gān cǎo	甘草	2 qián
gān jiāng	乾薑	1 qián and 1 fēn

右、水一盞半を以て、六分に煮とり、一度に服す。

Boil the above [ingredients] in one and one-half cups of water to make six *fēn* of the decoction; take in a single dose.

大黄甘遂湯之方
Dà Huáng Gān Suì Tāng

大黄（ 二戔四分 ）・甘遂・阿膠（ 明の硯出に非ざれば 、効うすし ）（ 各一戔二分 ）。

dà huáng	大黄	2 qián and 4 fēn	
gān suì	甘遂	1 qián and 2 fēn	
ē jiāo	阿膠	1 qián and 2 fēn	types other than that used for Ming ink stones have weak efficacy

右 、水一盞八分を以て 、六分に煮取り 、滓を去て 、阿膠を入れ消へしめ 、少しく冷まし 、甘遂の末を入れ 、頻りに服す 。

Boil the above [ingredients] in one cup and eight *fēn* of water to make six *fēn* of the decoction. Remove the dregs, add *ē jiāo* and dissolve [into the decoction]. After [the decoction] has been cooled somewhat, add *gān suì mò* and administer repeatedly.

大承氣湯之方
Dà Chéng Qì Tāng

大黄（ 一戔二分 ）・厚朴（ 二戔四分 ）・芒硝（ 六分 ）・枳實（ 一戔五分 ）。

dà huáng	大黄	1 qián and 2 fēn
hòu pò	厚朴	2 qián and 4 fēn
máng xiāo	芒硝	6 fēn
zhǐ shí	枳實	1 qián and 5 fēn

右 、水三盞を以て 、二物を煮 、一盞半に取り滓を去て 、大黄を入れ 、六分に煮取り 、滓を去て 、芒硝を入れ消へしめ 、一度に服す 。

Boil the above two ingredients [i.e., *hòu pò* and *zhǐ shí*] in three cups of water to make one and one-half cups of the decoction. Remove the dregs, add *dà huáng* to make six *fēn*. Remove the dregs, add *máng xiāo* and dissolve [in the decoction]. Take in a single dose.

小建中湯之方
Xiǎo Jiàn Zhōng Tāng

芍藥（ 一戔四分 ）桂枝・甘草・大棗・生姜（ 各八分 ）・飴（ 三戔五分 ）。

sháo yào	芍藥	1 qián and 4 fēn
guì zhī	桂枝	8 fēn
gān cǎo	甘草	8 fēn
dà zǎo	大棗	8 fēn
shēng jiāng	生薑	8 fēn
yí táng	飴糖	3 qián and 5 fēn

右、水一盞四分を以て、六分に煮て滓を去て、飴を入れ消へしめ、一度に服す。

Boil [the ingredients] in one cup and four *fēn* of water to make six *fēn* of the decoction. Remove the residue, add *yí táng* and dissolve [in the decoction]. Take in a single dose.

桂姜棗草黄辛附湯之方
Guì Jiāng Zǎo Cǎo Huáng Xīn Fù Tāng

桂枝・生姜・大棗（ 各八分 ）・麻黄・細辛・甘草（ 各五分半 ）・附子（ 一戔三分半 ）。

guì zhī	桂枝	8 fēn
shēng jiāng	生薑	8 fēn
dà zǎo	大棗	8 fēn
má huáng	麻黄	5.5 fēn
xì xīn	細辛	5.5 fēn
gān cǎo	甘草	5.5 fēn
fù zǐ	附子	1 qián and 3.5 fēn

右、水二盞四分を以て、六分に煮とり、一度に服す。

Boil the above [ingredients] in two cups and four *fēn* of water to make six *fēn* of the decoction; take in a single dose.

大陷胸湯之方
Dà Xiàn Xiōng Tāng

大黃（ 一戔二分 ）・芒硝（ 六分 ）・甘遂（ 五分 ）。

dà huáng	大黃	1 qián and 2 fēn
máng xiāo	芒硝	6 fēn
gān suì	甘遂	5 fēn

右、水一盞八分を以て大黃を入れ、六分に煎じ滓を去て、芒硝を入れ、一、二沸して解けて後、甘遂の末を入れ、一度に服す。

Add *dà huáng* to one cup and eight *fēn* of water and boil to make six *fēn* of the decoction. Remove the dregs and add *máng xiāo*. After boiling one or two times to dissolve [the ingredients], add *gān suì mò* and take in a single dose.

大陷胸丸之方
Dà Xiàn Xiōng Wán

大黃（ 八戔 ）・葶藶・芒硝（ 各十六戔 ）・杏仁（ 六戔、右、末となし彈丸の大きさの如く丸す、但し四戔也 ）・甘遂末（ 一戔 ）・白蜜（ 三戔九分 ）。

dà huáng	大黃	8 qián	
tíng lì	葶藶	16 qián	
máng xiāo	芒硝	16 qián	
xìng rén	杏仁	6 qián	grind the above ingredients in to a powder and make balls the size of bullets. However, they should be 4 qián in quantity.
gān suì mò	甘遂末	1 qián	
bái mì	白蜜	3 qián and 9 fēn	

右、水一盞二分を以て六分に煎じ、滓を去て、甘遂末を入れ、一度に服す。

Boil the above [ingredients] in one cup and two *fēn* of water to make six *fēn* of the decoction. Remove the dregs, add *gān suì mò*, and take in a single dose.

東洞按ずるに、大陥胸丸の方、大黄（一戔六分）・杏仁・芒硝（各一戔）・甘遂（二戔）。曰く、「葶藶眞贋分ざるを以て甘遂を倍加す。右、末となし練蜜を以て丹とす」。克案ずるに、葶藶の眞贋分ざるを以て、白芥子にかへて可なり。古方控涎丹に白芥子を用ゆるを以て考ふべし。

According to [Yoshimasu] Tōdō, the formula for *Dà Xiàn Xiōng Wán* is as follows:

dà huáng	大黄	1 qián and 6 fēn
xìng rén	杏仁	1 qián
máng xiāo	芒硝	1 qián
gān suì	甘遂	2 qián

He has said, "the quantity of *gān suì* should be increased if the authenticity of *tíng lì* cannot be confirmed. Make the above [ingredients] into a powder and [mix] with *liàn mì* to make an elixir."[206] I believe that if the authenticity of *tíng lì* cannot be confirmed, *bái jiè zǐ* may be substituted. My reasoning is based on an ancient formula called *Kòng Xián Dān,*[207] in which *bái jiè zǐ* is used.

小陥胸湯之方
Xiǎo Xiàn Xiōng Tāng

黄連（五分半）・半夏（二戔七分）・括蔞仁（八分）。

huáng lián	黄連	5.5 fēn
bàn xià	半夏	2 qián and 7 fēn
guā lóu rén	瓜蔞仁	8 fēn

右、水一盞八分を以て、括蔞仁を煮て九分に取り、滓を去て、二味を入れ、六分に取り、一度に服す。

206. The source for this is unclear. Furthermore, because no MHLW-approved Kampō drug contains *gān suì*, *tíng lì*, or *bái jiè zǐ*, there has been little research in Japan concerning the application of said ingredients.

207. There are several ancient formulae with the name *Kòng Xián Dān* 控涎丹 (Jp: *Kōzen-Tan*; drool-controlling elixir). Because all of these formulae include *bái jiè zǐ* 白芥子, it is difficult to know which formula the author is refers to. Perhaps the most famous is the version (containing equal quantities of *dà jǐ*, *gān suì*, and *bái jiè zǐ*) found in *Sān Yīn Jí Yī Bìng Zhèng Fāng Lùn*《三因極一病症方論》(Jp: *San'in-Kyokuitsu-Byōshō-Ron*; A Unified Treatise on Diseases, Patterns, and Remedies According to the Three Causes). At present, no version of *Kòng Xián Dān* is covered by the Japanese National Health Insurance program or is commonly used in Japan.

First boil *guā lóu rén* in one cup and eight *fēn* of water to make nine *fēn* of the decoction. Remove the dregs and add the other two ingredients to make six *fēn* of the decoction; take in a single dose.

芍藥甘草湯之方
Sháo Yào Gān Cǎo Tāng

芍藥・甘草（ 各一戔八分 ）。

sháo yào	芍藥	1 qián and 8 fēn
gān cǎo	甘草	1 qián and 8 fēn

右 、水一盞二分を以て 、六分に煮とり 、一度に服す 。

Boil the above [ingredients] in one cup and two *fēn* of water to make six *fēn* of the decoction; take in a single dose.

葛根湯之方
Gé Gēn Tāng

葛根（ 一戔 ）・麻黄・大棗・生姜（ 各七分半 ）・桂枝・芍藥・甘草（ 各五分半 ）。

gé gēn	葛根	1 qián
má huáng	麻黄	7.5 fēn
dà zǎo	大棗	7.5 fēn
shēng jiāng	生薑	7.5 fēn
guì zhī	桂枝	5.5 fēn
sháo yào	芍藥	5.5 fēn
gān cǎo	甘草	5.5 fēn

右 、水二盞を以て 、六分に煮取り 、一度に服す 。

Boil the above ingredients in two cups of water to make six *fēn* of the decoction; take in a single dose.

黄連湯之方
Huáng Lián Tāng

桂枝・甘草・黄連・乾姜・人参・大棗（ 各五分半 ）・半夏（ 一戔一分 ）。

guì zhī	桂枝	5.5 fēn
gān cǎo	甘草	5.5 fēn
huáng lián	黄連	5.5 fēn
gān jiāng	乾薑	5.5 fēn
rén shēn	人參	5.5 fēn
dà zǎo	大棗	5.5 fēn
bàn xià	半夏	1 qián and 1 fēn

右、水二盞を以て、一盞二分に取り、滓を去て、再煎し、六分に取り、日に三服、夜に二服す。

Boil the above [ingredients] in two cups of water to make one cup and two *fēn* of the decoction. Remove the dregs and boil again to make six *fēn* of the decoction. Take three times during the day and twice at night.

甘遂半夏湯之方
Gān Suì Bàn Xià Tāng

甘遂（ 二分 ）・半夏（ 一戔二分 ）・芍藥・甘草（ 各八分 ）。

gān suì	甘遂	2 fēn
bàn xià	半夏	1 qián and 2 fēn
sháo yào	芍藥	8 fēn
gān cǎo	甘草	8 fēn

右、水一盞六分を以て、四分に取り、蜜四分を入れ煎じて、六分にとり、一度に服す。

Boil the above ingredients in one cup and six *fēn* of water to make four *fēn* of the decoction. Add four *fēn* of honey and boil again to make six *fēn* of the decoction; take in a single dose.

大黄甘草湯之方
Dà Huáng Gān Cǎo Tāng

大黄（ 一戔四分 ）・甘草（ 四分半 ）。

dà huáng	大黄	1 qián and 4 fēn
gān cǎo	甘草	4.5 fēn

右 、水一盞二分を以て四分に煮取り 、一度に服す 。

Boil the above [ingredients] in one cup and two *fēn* of water to make four *fēn* of the decoction; take in a single dose.

厚朴三物湯之方
Hòu Pò Sān Wù Tāng

厚朴（ 一戔六分 ）・大黄（ 八分 ）・枳實（ 一戔 ）。

hòu pò	厚朴	1 qián and 6 fēn
dà huáng	大黄	8 fēn
zhǐ shí	枳實	1 qián

右 、水二盞四分を以て 、二味を煮て一盞に取り 、大黄を入れ 、六分に取り 、一度に服す 。

Boil the above two ingredients in two cups and four *fēn* of water to make one cup of the decoction. Add *dà huáng* to make six *fēn*; take in a single dose.

乾姜附子湯之方
Gān Jiāng Fù Zǐ Tāng

乾姜・附子（ 各一戔 ）。

gān jiāng	乾薑	1 qián
fù zǐ	附子	1 qián

右、水一盞八分を以て、六分に煮とり、一度に服す。

Boil the above [ingredients] in one cup and eight *fēn* of water to make six *fēn* of the decoction; take in a single dose.

芎歸膠艾湯之方
Xiōng Guī Jiāo Ài Tāng

川芎・阿膠・甘草（各四分半）・芍藥（八分半）・艾葉・當歸（各六分）・乾地黄（一戔二分）。

chuān xiōng	川芎	4.5 fēn
ē jiāo	阿膠	4.5 fēn
gān cǎo	甘草	4.5 fēn
sháo yào	芍藥	8.5 fēn
ài yè	艾葉	6 fēn
dāng guī	當歸	6 fēn
gān dì huáng	干地黃	1 qián and 2 fēn

右、水一盞と清酒とを以て、六分に煮取り、滓を去て消へしめて、一度に服す。

Boil the above [ingredients] in one cup of water and sake to make six *fēn* of the decoction. Remove the dregs and [mix until all ingredients] are dissolved; take in a single dose.

豬苓湯之方
Zhū Líng Tāng

豬苓・茯苓・阿膠・滑石・澤瀉（各八分半）。

zhū líng	豬苓	5.5 fēn
fú líng	茯苓	5.5 fēn
ē jiāo	阿膠	5.5 fēn
huá shí	滑石	5.5 fēn
zé xiè	澤瀉	5.5 fēn

右、水一盞二分を以て六分に煮とり、阿膠を入れ消へしめて、一度に服す。

Boil the above [ingredients] in one cup and two *fēn* of water to make six *fēn* of the decoction. Add *ē jiāo* and dissolve [into the decoction]; take in a single dose.

苓桂朮甘湯之方
Líng Guì Zhú Gān Tāng

茯苓(一戔二分)・桂枝(一戔半)・甘草(各七分半)。

fú líng	茯苓	1 qián and 2 fēn
guì zhī	桂枝	1.5 qián
gān cǎo	甘草	7 fēn

右、水一盞二分を以て、六分に煮とり、一度に服す。

Boil the above [ingredients] in one cup and two *fēn* of water to make six *fēn* of the decoction; take in a single dose.

大黄牡丹皮湯之方
Dà Huáng Mǔ Dān Pí Tāng

大黄(一戔二分)・牡丹皮(九分)・芒硝・桃仁(各六分)・瓜子(一戔五分、かも瓜の子、可なり)。

dà huáng	大黄	1 qián and 2 fēn	
mǔ dān pí	牡丹皮	9 fēn	
máng xiāo	芒硝	6 fēn	
táo rén	桃仁	6 fēn	
guā zǐ	瓜子	1 qián and 5 fēn	the seed of a *kamouri* may be used*

* Kamouri is the colloquial Japanese name of *dōng guā* 冬瓜 (Jp: *tōgan*; wax gourd).

右、水三盞六分を以て、六分に煮とり、滓を去て、芒硝を入れ消へしめて、一度に服す。

Boil the above [ingredients] in three cups and six *fēn* of water to make six *fēn* of the decoction. Remove the dregs, add *máng xiāo,* and dissolve [into the decoction]; take in a single dose.

癥痼圓之方
Chōko-En

茯苓・大黄（ 各二十戔 ）・牡丹皮・桃仁・芍藥・桂枝・當歸（ 伊吹可なり 、各十戔 ）。

fú líng	茯苓	12 qián	
dà huáng	大黄	12 qián	
mǔ dān pí	牡丹皮	10 qián	
táo rén	桃仁	10 qián	
sháo yào	芍藥	10 qián	
guì zhī	桂枝	10 qián	
dāng guī	當歸	10 qián	the Ibuki variety

右 、末とし 、練蜜を以て丹となす 。

Grind the above ingredients into a powder and mix with *liàn mì* to make an elixir.

薏苡附子敗漿散之方
Yì Yǐ Fù Zǐ Bài Jiàng Sǎn

薏苡（ 二戔 ）・附子（ 四分 ）・敗漿（ 一戔 、女郎花の根なり 。花白し 。黄花を「 男めし 」と云ふ 。もしこの物なくば 、かりやすをかへ用ひて効あり ）。

yì yǐ	薏苡	2 qián	
fù zǐ	附子	4 fēn	
bài jiàng	敗漿	1 qián	This refers to the root of [the plant that is referred to in Japan as] *ominaeshi* 女郎花, which has white flowers. The type that has yellow flowers is [commonly] called *otokoeshi* 男郎花 [in Japan].* If this ingredient is not available, [the root of the plant known in Japan as] *kariyasu* 刈安 may be substituted.†

* *Bài jiàng* 敗漿 (Jp: *haishō*; herba patriniae), normally written as 敗醬, refers to the entire plants of Patrinia scabiosaefolia Fisch. and Patrinia villose Juss. of the family Valerianaceae. There are several varieties of patrinia that are used in China and Japan: as the mentioned in the text, the most popular is what is commonly called *ominaeshi* 女郎花 (i.e., Patrinia scabiosaefolia Fisch.), followed by *otokoeshi* 男郎花 (i.e., Patrinia villosa Juss.).
† *Kariyasu* 刈安 generally refers to Miscanthus tinctorius, a plant endemic to Japan. In China, the root of Miscanthus sinensis (Ch: *máng gēn* 芒根; Jp: *bōkon*) is used.

右、散となし、一戔を水一盞二分を以て、煮て半を減らして、頻りに服す。

Grind the above [ingredients] into a powder. Boil one *qián* of the powder in one cup and two *fēn* of water until half remains; take repeatedly.

四逆湯之方
Sì Nì Tāng

甘草（八分）・乾姜・附子（各六分）。

gān cǎo	甘草	8 fēn
gān jiāng	乾薑	6 fēn
fù zǐ	附子	6 fēn

右、水一盞を以て、四分に煮とり、一度に服す。

Boil the above [ingredients] in one cup of water to make four *fēn* of the decoction; take in a single dose.

抵當湯之方
Dǐ Dāng Tāng

水蛭・虻蟲・桃仁（各七分）・大黄（二戔）。

shuǐ zhì	水蛭	7 fēn
méng chóng	虻蟲	7 fēn
táo rén	桃仁	7 fēn
dà huáng	大黄	2 qián

右、末となし、水一盞を以て、六分に煮とり、一度に服す。

Make the above [ingredients] into a powder and boil in one cup of water to make six *fēn* of the decoction; take in a single dose.

抵當丸之方
Dǐ Dāng Wán

水蛭（二戔五分）・虻蟲・桃仁（各二戔）・大黄（六戔）。

shuǐ zhì	水蛭	2 qián and 5 fēn
méng chóng	虻蟲	2 qián
táo rén	桃仁	2 qián
dà huáng	大黄	6 fēn

右、末となし、糊丸す。六分、或るひは一戔を溫酒を以て送下す。

Grind the above [ingredients] into a powder to make flour and water paste pills. Take six *fēn* or up to one *qián* with warm sake.

梔子豉湯之方
Zhī Zǐ Chǐ Tāng

山梔子（六分）・香豉（一戔九分）。

shān zhī zǐ	山梔子	6 fēn
xiāng chǐ	香豉	1 qián and 9 fēn

右、水一盞一分を以て、先づ山梔子を煮て七分に取り、滓を去て、香豉を入れ、煮て四分にとり、一度に服す。

First boil *shān zhī zǐ* in one cup and one *fēn* of water to make seven *fēn* of the decoction. Remove the dregs and add *xiāng chǐ* to make four *fēn* of the decoction; take in a single dose.

克曰く、此の書は世の沈痾・痼疾と稱して、醫藥の治すること能はざる者を療する爲に著す所なり。醫藥も治すること能はざるは、是れその病毒あつく積むを以ての故なり。因りて其の藥を投ずるも、尋常の規矩に拘はらずして其の毒に應じて藥湯の分量を增加せざれば効なきことを知るべし。故にその藥力、病毒に敵せざれば治せず。敵する時は必ず瞑眩す。いはゆる「藥、瞑眩せざれば、厥の病ひ瘳へざる者」なり。

I, Katsu, wrote this book in order to treat those diseases that are commonly referred to as heavy or intractable diseases and cannot be cured by [conventional] medicinals. The reason why [these] medicinals are unable to cure [such intractable diseases] is because a pathotoxin has accumulated [in the body of the patient]. Thus, when administering drugs, [the physician] should not adhere to conventional rules and understand that unless the quantity of the decoction is increased according to the [size of the] toxin, [the treatment] will be ineffective. For this reason, unless the power of the drug contends against the pathotoxin as one contends against an enemy, the [disease] will not be cured. When [the drug] contends against [the toxin, the patient] will undoubtedly experience dizziness. This is what is meant by [the famous proverb], "unless the medicinal causes dizziness, the disease will not be cured."[208]

又た世に某々の藥を與へて、病者拒むを以て受けずと云ふ者あり。是れ則ち方症相敵するを以て、病毒、之れを拒むなり。たとへ藥を與へ、直に嘔する者といへども、強ひて用ゆべし。良藥は口に苦くして、病に利あるを知るべし。五雜組に「江左の商人左膊上に人面瘡あり、物を食らふ。醫者、藥石を試むることを教ゆ、皆苦しむことなし。ただ貝母に至りては口を閉ぢたり。口を抉りて之れを灌げば、遂に痂結んで癒ゆ」と。是れ其の藥、病毒に的中する故に之れを拒むの証なり。

Moreover, there are cases in which [the physician] administers various types of medicinals to the patient, but the patient refuses to take them. This is a case of the formula and pattern being [perfectly] matched to one another; [in such cases] the pathotoxin refuses [the medicinals]. Even if the patient begins to retch soon after the medicinal is admin-

208. As explained in the section for *Xiǎo Chái Hú Tāng* 小柴胡湯, this is a quote from the "Charge to Yue, Part I (Ch: *Yuè Mìng Shàng* 說命上; Jp: *Etsu-Mei-Jō*)" of *Shū Jīng*《書經》(Jp: *Shokyō*; Book of History). The original text is as follows: "若藥弗瞑眩、厥疾弗瘳" (Unless the medicinal causes distress [i.e., dizziness] in the patient, his disease will not be cured by it).

istered, [the physician] should force [the patient] to use [i.e., take] it. We can [thus] understand [the meaning of the phrase] "good medicinals that are effective in [curing] diseases have a bitter taste."[209] In the *Wŭ Zá Zŭ* 《五雜組》,[210] it is written that "there was a merchant of Jiāng Zuǒ who had sores [similar to sores] of the face on his left upper arm.[211] Physicians attempted various treatments, and none of them caused any suffering [to the patient]. The mouth [of the patient] shut only when administration of *bèi mŭ* was attempted. When [the patient's] mouth was forced open and the drug was poured down [his throat], the scabs [on his arm] eventually crusted over and he was cured." This [retching] is a sign that [the pattern] refused the drug because it was perfectly matched to [attack] the pathotoxin.

予、衆病者を療するに、此くの如きこと甚だ多きを以て、定極することあり。故に嘔して飲まず、拒んで受けずといへども、醫人、必ず方症相對するの藥を用ひ、病者に阿りて妄りに分量を増減せず。よく告げさとし、用ひ得て、其の効を奏すべし。

I have treated a multitude of patients, and have made a thorough investigation [into this principle] during my experience [treating] a great number of cases similar to this [case found in *Wŭ Zá Zŭ* 《五雜組》]. For this reason, even if the patient experiences retching and is unable to drink [the decoction] or refuses to take [the prescribed medicinal], the physician must, without fail, coax the patient to use the [correct] medicinal that was elucidated through [the process] formula-pattern matching, without carelessly changing the quantity of [ingredients]. If [the physician] succeeds in persuading [the patient] to use the drug, he will be able to achieve an effective result.[212]

209. This is a famous quote from *Kŏng Zĭ Jiā Yŭ* 《孔子家語》(Jp: *Kōshi-Ke-Go*; The Family Sayings of Confucius), collected in the third century CE. The original quote is as follows: 「良藥苦於口而利於病。」

210. *Wŭ Zá Zŭ* 《五雜組》(Jp: *Go-Zakko*; Five Miscellaneous Groups) is a *Míng* dynasty book of miscellaneous jottings by Xiè Zhàozhì 謝肇淛 (Jp: Sha Chōsei; 1567–1624 CE). It appears to have been widely read in Japan during the Edo period as a sort of encyclopedia.

211. Jiāng Zuǒ 江左 (Jp: Kōsa) refers to the southern region of modern-day Jiāngsū 江蘇 Province.

212. This is the end of the first half of the work.

後編序

Preface for the Latter Half [of the Work]

Ch: 古曰、三折臂而成良醫、稻葉意仲翁、嘗爲初學著診腹之書、已行于世、今玆又欲刻其後編、因屬序於予、予雖不文、於翁者義不可辭者、予夙有賴翁之治而免二豎之難焉、於是深奇其技、迺問其所以爲醫、

Jp: 古に曰く、「三たび臂を折りて、良醫と成る」と。稻葉意仲翁は嘗て初學のために診腹の書を著し、すでに世に行はる。今ここに又た其の後編を刻せんと欲す、因りて序を予に屬す。予、不文なりと雖も、翁に於いては義として辭すべからざる者あり。予、夙に翁の治に賴りて二豎の難を免るる者あり。ここに於いて深く其の技を奇とし、すなはち其の醫を爲す所以を問ふ。

The ancients had a saying: "One must break his arm three times before he can become a good physician."[208] The venerable Inaba Ichū previously authored a primer on abdominal examination, which has been put into practice across the land.[209] I desired to record the follow-up volume [of the previous work, and having completed this,] I therefore have written a preface for it here.[210] As I am no [scholar of] letters, I could not well express [the details of the art of] my venerable [sensei] in words, although I have relied on his treatment [in the past] and managed to avoid the two demons of deathly illnesses [because of him].[211] Being deeply [impressed], I regarded his techniques as extraordi-

208. The original phrase (Ch: *sān zhé gōng wéi liáng yī* 三折肱知爲良醫; Jp: *mitabi hiji wo orite ryōi taru koto wo shiru*) can be found in "Book XI, Duke Ding (Ch: *Dìng Gōng* 定公; Jp: *Teikō*)" of *Chūn Qiū Zuǒ Shì Zhuàn*《春秋左氏傳》(Jp: *Shunjū-Sashi-Den*; Commentary of Zuǒ of the Spring and Autumn Annals). This proverb has come to mean that experience is the best teacher.

209. Ichū was the nickname of the author.

210. This volume was written a couple of years after the first volume was published. In this preface, the pupil who recorded this volume explains his experience studying under the author.

211. Although *èr shù* 二豎 (Jp: *niju*) literally means "two children," it is an allusion to the following story found in "Book VIII, Duke Chéng (Ch: *Chéng Gōng* 成公; Jp: *Seikō*)" of *Chūn Qiū Zuǒ Shì Zhuàn*: "Duke Chéng dreamt that his disease turned into two boys, who said, 'That is a skillful physician. It is to be feared he will hurt us; how shall we get out of his way?' One of them then said, 'If we take our place above the heart and below the throat, what can he do to us?' When the physician arrived, he said, 'Nothing can be done for this disease. Its seat is above the heart

nary, and thus inquired of him concerning [the details of] his medical treatments.

Ch:翁曰、予之所爲、大異於今之醫、予見世醫、論巧而術拙、實徒誦而已、所謂以書爲御者、不盡馬之情、以古制今者、不達事之變者也、予有觀于斯、深信先師之教、直遡其本源、憤然努力、確然精研、故雖古人之言、無効于治病者、舍而不取、雖今人之方、有功於面生者、擇而用之、壹是徵之病者而已以故海隅山陬、無所不趾、樵人漁郎、莫疾不療、其間頗有得起死肉骨之驗、或有噬臍銘心者、毎有其奏効者、輒文以記其治圖以明其病無以不視于諸弟子者、是予之梓此書、而欲使救天下後世之微意也、

Jp:翁曰く、「予の爲す所、大いに今の醫に異なるなり。予、世の醫を見るに、論巧なるも術拙し。實に徒誦するのみ。所謂書を以て御を爲す者は、馬の情を盡さず。古を以て今を制する者、事の變に達せざる者なり。予、斯に觀ること有り、深く先師の教を信じ、直に其の本源に遡り、憤然として努力し、確然として精研す。故に古人の言と雖も、治病に効無き者は舍てて取らず。今人の方と雖も、回生に功有る者は擇びて之れを用ゆ。壹是に之れを病者に徵するのみ。故を以て海隅山陬も、所として趾せざるは無く、樵人漁郎、疾として療せざるは莫し。其の間、死せるを起し、骨ばるを肉づくるの驗を得ること、頗る有り。或るひは臍を噬み、心に銘せる者有り。其の効を奏するもの有る毎に、輒ち文し以て其の治を記し、圖し以て其の病を明らかにし、以て諸弟子に視さざる者無し。是れ予の此の書を梓にして、天下後世を救はしめんと欲するの微意なり」と。

He responded, "My [medical] practice is much different from other contemporary physicians. I regard the physicians of the world as being skilled in [the art of] debate but having poor [clinical] skills. Indeed, they are only [capable of] empty recitation! As [the famous proverb] says, 'Those who have [only] studied how to drive a horse [carriage] through books cannot fully understand the feelings of horses. Those who use ancient [laws] to govern the present are unable to understand the changes that take

---

and below the throat. If I assail it [with medicine], it will be of no use; if I attempt to puncture it, it cannot be reached. Nothing can be done for it.'" The original text is as follows:「公夢疾爲二豎子曰、彼良醫也、懼傷我、焉逃之、其一曰、居肓之上、膏之下、若我何、醫至、曰、疾不可爲也、在肓之上、膏之下、攻之不可、達之不及、藥不至焉、不可爲也。」

place in things.'[212] I have seen this [in my own experience], and thus I deeply believed the teachings of my sensei and went back directly to the source [of those teachings]. I have since ardently applied myself in order to achieve concrete results from my training and research. For this reason, I reject the sayings that are not useful in curing diseases, even if they have been handed down from the ancients. I select and use [formulae] that are successful in resuscitating patients, even if the formulae were developed by a modern person. In all [formulae], I look for evidence [of efficacy] in my patients. Consequently, [in my search,] I have traveled to every nook and cranny of the mountains and seas [across Japan], treating woodcutters and fishermen; there is no disease that I have not yet experienced treating. During that period, I experienced raising patients [who were near] death and fattening patients who were bony [and emaciated. However,] some [of the cases that I have experienced] made me full of regret [due to my inability to save them] and I have engraved [such cases] on the tablet of my heart. Each time [a formula] was successful, I wrote down an explanation of the treatment and drew an illustration in order to elucidate the disease. There is nothing that I have not shown to my pupils. This was my reasoning for having this book published, as I wanted to save future generations [from intractable diseases]."

Ch: 予嘆曰、嗚乎、翁之所爲、真良醫之志也、夫張長沙之醫古猿孫真人之救青蛙、於翁不足深奇扁鵲之鑒五臟之癥結丹溪之治一女之情病、亦於翁不多讓也、

Jp: 予、嘆じて曰く、「ああ、翁の爲す所は、真に良醫の志なり。夫れ張、長沙の古猿を醫し、孫真人の青蛙を救へるも、翁に於いては深く奇とするに足らず。扁鵲が五臟の癥結に鑒み、丹溪が一女の情病を治せるも亦た翁に於いては多くは譲らざるなり」と。

I was moved [by his words] and exclaimed, "Oh, venerable sir, the work that you are attempting truly comes from the will of a good physician. Zhāng Zhòngjǐng treating the old monkey of Cháng Shā[213] and Sūn Zhēnrén[214] saving a frog cannot be called extraor-

212. This proverb was originally found in the "Strategies of Zhào (Ch: *Zhào Cè* 趙策; Jp: *Chō-Saku*) Chapter" of *Zhàn Guó Cè*《戦國策》(Jp: *Sengoku-Saku*; Strategies of the Warring States). The original text is as follows:「以書爲御者、不盡於馬之情、以古制今者、不達於事之變。」

213. Zhāng Zhòngjǐng 張仲景 (Jp: Chō Chūkei; 150-219 CE) was an eminent physician who was renowned for his skill in pulse diagnosis. He is said to have been able to correctly diagnose disease in an old monkey who pretended to be human and came to him asking for treatment.

214. Sūn Zhēnrén 孫真人 (Jp: Son Shijin) is the pseudonym of Sūn Sīmiǎo 孫思邈 (Jp: Son Shibaku; ca. 581–682 CE), an eminent physician who authored voluminous formularies that have

dinary in comparison [with you]. Biǎn Què[215] [could treat diseases by] examining the concretions and binds of the five viscera, and Dān Xī[216] could treat the emotional condition of a woman [without the use of medicinals], but they are no greater than you."

Ch: 三折之醫、於翁初見之耳、且此書、在於翁蓋不過爲九牛之一毛、然大益于初學、則不可措也乎、因不辭、遂爲記其言以爲序、翁名克、字文禮、僦居於浪華、父名文内、字武次、其先出于河野七郎、世住于江州菩提寺邨云、

Jp: 三折の醫、翁に於いて初て之れを見るのみ。且つ此の書、翁に在りては、蓋し九牛の一毛爲るに過ぎず。然れども大いに初學に益あれば、則ち措くべからざらんか。因りて辭せず、遂に爲に其の言を記して、以て序と爲す。翁の名は「克」、字は「文禮」。浪華に僦居す。父の名は「文内」、字は「武次」、其の先は河野七郎より出づ。世は江州の菩提寺邨に住すと云ふ。

He is the first physician that I have met who exemplifies the meaning of "a physician who has broken his arm three times." Moreover, this book is but a drop in the bucket of [his knowledge].[217] Even so, if it is a great help to beginners, how could I not write down [what he knows]?" Therefore, I have not refused to write anything down, and hereby conclude my introduction [to the book]. My sensei's name is Katsu, and his style name is Bunrei. He is [currently] residing in Naniwa. His father's name was Bundai, and his style name was Takeji, coming from [the lineage of] Kōno Shichirō.[218] For generations, [the family] is said to have resided in Bodaiji Village in Gōshū.[219]

---

been influential in China and Japan. He is said to have had the skill to cure even frogs.

215. Biǎn Què 扁鵲 (Jp: Hen Jaku, ca. 401-310 BCE) was a legendary physician of ancient China. *Shǐ Jì*《史記》(Jp: *Shiki*; The Records of the Grand Historian) states that he had the ability to completely see the abdominal concretions and binds causing diseases in the five viscera (Ch: *jǐn jiàn wǔ zàng zhēng jié* 盡見五臟癥結; Jp: *jin-ken-gozō-chōketsu*).

216. Dān Xī 丹溪 (Jp: Tankei) was the pseudonym of Zhū Zhènhēng 朱震亨 (Jp: Shu Shinkō; 1281–1358 CE), one of the four great expert physicians of the *Jīn* and *Yuán* periods (Ch: *Jīn Yuán sì dà jiā* 金元四大家; Jp: *Kin-Gen-Shidaika*).

217. Literally, "a single hair out of nine ox (hides)," a famous Chinese idiom (Ch: *jiǔ niú yī máo* 九牛一毛; Jp: *kyūgyū-ichimō*).

218. There is no available information concerning the members of the author's family. Kōno Shichirō may refer to Kōno Shichirōzaemon 河野七郎左衛門 (1383-1442 CE), an ancient warrior.

219. Gōshū 江州 is the abbreviated name of Ōmi Province (Jp: *Ōmi-No-Kuni* 近江國), which today comprises Shiga Prefecture (Jp: *Shiga-Ken* 滋賀縣).

Ch:時享和紀元龍次辛酉上巳後三日

Jp:時に享和紀元、龍次辛酉、上巳の後三日

[Written in] the first year of the Kyōwa era [i.e., 1801],[220] on the third day after the Jōshi Festival [i.e., the sixth day of the third lunar month],[221]

Ch:布衣後學南阿荒井公廉題於浪華蠖屈軒

Jp:布衣、後學・南阿・荒井公廉浪華蠖屈軒に於いて題す

in a humble abode in Naniwa by the pupil Arai Kōren[222] of Nan-A.[223]

220. The Kyōwa 享和 era spanned the period from 1801 to 1804.
221. The Shangsi Festival (Ch: *shàng sì jié* 上巳節; Jp: *jōshi-setsu*), also known as the Double Third Festival, is an ancient Chinese and Japanese spring festival celebrated on the third day of the third month of the traditional lunisolar calendar. In Japan, it is currently celebrated on March third of the Western calendar, and is usually called (*momo-no-sekku* 桃の節句 [the peach festival] or more popularly *hina-matsuri* 雛祭り [the doll festival]).
222. This may refer to Arai Kōren 荒井公廉, also known as Arai Meimon 荒井鳴門 (1775–1853), a famous Confucian scholar of the Edo period.
223. Nan-A 南阿 refers to southern Awa Province (Jp: *Awa-No-Kuni* 阿波國), which currently comprises part of Tokushima Prefecture (Jp: *Tokushima-Ken* 德島縣).

腹證奇覽後編巻之上

First half of the Second Volume of Fukushō-Kiran
《腹證奇覽》
(Extraordinary Views of Abdominal Patterns)

湖南稲葉克文禮父著
Written by Master "Konan" Inaba (Katsu) Bunrei

余つらつら腹證の診察を以て難治と稱するを考ふるに、凡そ腹底より動氣する者多し。或るひは臍底臍下臍の兩邊、或るひは小腹、或るひは心下・心上・胸膈に動氣を發し、又たは奔豚氣、腹底より起りて、甚しき者は死せんとす。此くの如き類あげて數ふべからず。

Through my detailed study of abdominal pattern diagnosis, I have found that most cases of what are known as intractable diseases are actually due to [the presence of] stirring qì in the depths of the abdomen.[224] In some cases, the stirring qì may emerge in the depths of the umbilical region, subumbilical region, or both sides of the umbilicus. In other cases, it may emerge from the region below the heart, the region above the heart, or the chest and diaphragm. Moreover, running piglet qì may also arise in the depths of the abdomen, leading to death in severe cases. It would be impossible to count the number of such [cases that I have experienced].

余、諸州に奔走し、之れを患ふるものを治療して以て按ずるに、凡そ世に癪と號する者、或るひは小兒の驚風と稱する者、かくの如き症を發する者多し。此れに因りて之れをみるに、諸病みな一毒にして諸患をなすことを知れり。皆、状に因りて其の名を命ずる也。

I have roamed the various provinces [of Japan], busily engaged in treating these [intrac-

224. Although short, this preface by the author is important in outlining his rejection of traditional Chinese medical theory and establishment of a theoretical framework of abdominal examination.

table cases]. Based on [my experience], I believe that many patients [with diseases] that are popularly known as "*shaku*" or pediatric fright wind present with symptoms similar [to the ones mentioned above].[225] For this reason, it can be known that the various symptoms of any of the multitude of diseases [that patients may present with] are caused by a single toxin.[226] [Diseases] all [simply] differ in name based on the symptoms [that they cause].

しかるに是れ等を治するの方、天然自然の術有りて治すべきことなり。然るを今世醫家者流の治療する所を見るに、速やかに之れを治する者甚だまれなり。たとひ治すといへども、四、五日にして復た發し、他日にして又た發す。是こに於いてみな云ふ、「癪は治すべからざる者なり」と。

However, the formulae to cure these [diseases] are in line with nature and can thus [naturally] cure [patients], unlike the treatment methods performed by modern physicians that [I have] witnessed. There are few [current physicians] who can quickly cure [diseases]. Even if [a physician] can [temporarily] cure [an intractable disease], it will recur four or five days later, and eventually recur once again in the future. [Such physicians] all say, "Cases of '*shaku*' are incurable."

たまたま諸州中に名家ありて、その治効を奏すると云ふを聞くごとに、余、敬んでが行いて教へをこひ、之れを得て療ぜんとするに、皆脈を主とし、或るひは五行の論を以て教へをなす。余、謹んで此の教へを奉じて治を施すに、彼れ治して此れは治せざる者多し。

During my travels across various provinces, each time I heard that a famous physician had been successful in treating [the aforementioned cases], I would go to that physician

225. This is explained in greater detail the section for *Xiǎo Pǐn Bēn Tún Tāng* 小品奔豚湯.
226. Based on this, it can be seen that similar to other members of the Ancient School (Jp: *Kohō-Ha* 古方派), the author was heavily influenced by the theory of the "myriad diseases arising from one toxin" (Jp: *manbyō-ichidoku-setsu* 萬病一毒說; Ch: *wàn bìng yī dú shuō*) developed by Yoshimasu Tōdō 吉益東洞. Yoshimasu is famously recorded as having said, 「萬病一毒，衆藥皆毒物、以毒攻毒、毒去體佳、初無益損於元氣也、何補云乎哉」(The myriad diseases [arise from] a single toxin. The multitude of medicinals are all toxins [in themselves]. It is splendid to use an [external] toxin to attack the [patho]toxin [in the body] and make the [patho]toxin leave the body. [In the] first [place], there are no [such things as] reducing or boosting [what is known as] original qì. [Therefore,] what need is there to speak of supplementing [original qì when diagnosing diseases]).

and respectfully ask for instruction. However, they all principally relied on pulse [examination] or five-phase theory to treat [patients. Although] I humbly dedicated myself to these teachings, I found that while some patients were cured, in many cases, the patients were not cured.

是こに於いて診脈・五行の論はみな空論にして、病を治するの實用たらざることを悟れり。故に余、腹診の術を以て方法を考へて、その規模を立つ。實に十に八、九中らざることなし。然りといへども、是れ余が自ら知る所に非ず。天然自然の治法にして、なま険しき邪智の私ならざること、諸君子つとめて以て知るべし。

I therefore realized that pulse examination and five-phase theory are nothing more than empty theories and are [therefore] useless in curing diseases. For this reason, I have researched the technique of abdominal examination and established its scope [in clinical practice]. It is indeed effective in eight or nine out of every ten cases. This [method] is not something that I learned out of my own [wisdom]. Esteemed gentlemen [i.e., readers], I ask you to understand that this is an all-natural method of treatment,[227] and is by no means a cunning [trick to deceive you] for my own profit.

227. In the present work, the author repeatedly combines the two words in Japanese/Chinese for "natural," i.e., *tiān rán* 天然 (Jp: *tennen*; literally, "in line with heaven"), and *zì rán* 自然 (Jp: *shizen*; literally, "in line with itself"), to emphasize the naturalness of abdominal treatment in contrast with the perceived contrivances of traditional Chinese diagnostic theory.

當歸芍藥散之圖

Illustration for the Dāng Guī Sháo Yào Sǎn [Pattern][228] 當歸芍藥散

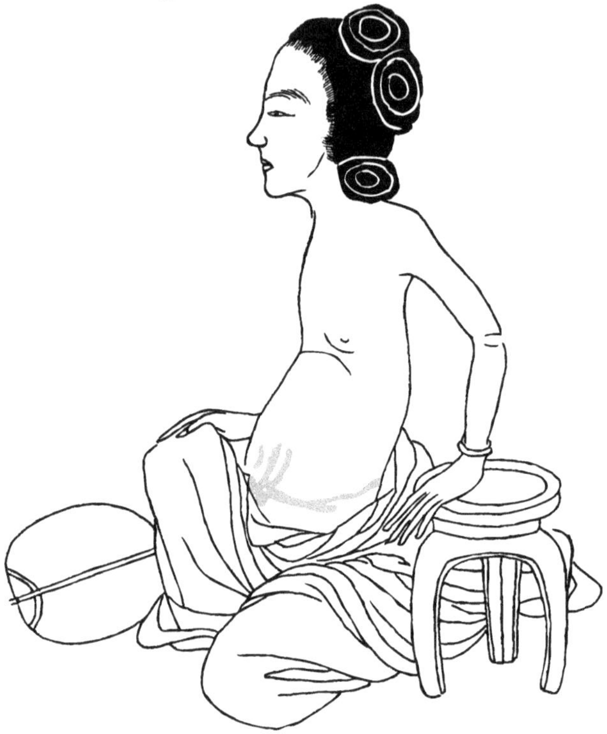

Fig. 43

圖の如く、臍傍に拘攣するものあり。指頭にささへ、之れを按して痛腰背に徹する者、或るひは心下悸し、或るひは小腹強痛、或

228. The formula for *Dāng Guī Sháo Yào Sǎn* 當歸芍藥散 (Jp: *Tōki-Shakuyaku-San*; Chinese angelica and peony powder) was originally found in *Jīn Guì Yào Lüè*. The extract preparation of the formula is covered by the Japanese National Health Insurance program as a prescription drug, and is also commonly sold in Japanese drug stores as an over-the-counter drug. It is currently indicated by the MHLW for: irregular menstruation, menstrual disorder, menstrual pain, menopause, prepartum, postpartum, or miscarriage-related symptoms (anemia, fatigue, dizziness, edema), dizziness or lightheadedness when standing up quickly, dull headache, stiff shoulders, low back pain, poor circulation in legs, frostbite, edema, skin spots, and tinnitus in persons with weak physical strength who have cold extremities and anemic tendency and are easily fatigued and present with occasional symptoms such as lower abdominal pain, dull headache, dizziness, stiff shoulders, tinnitus, or palpitations（體力虚弱で、冷え症で貧血の傾向があり疲労しやすく、ときに下腹部痛、頭重、めまい、肩こり、耳鳴り、動悸などを訴えるものの次の諸症：月經不順、月經異常、月經痛、更年期障害、產前產後あるいは流產による障害（貧血、疲労倦怠、めまい、むくみ）、めまい・立ちくらみ、頭重、肩こり、腰痛、足腰の冷え症、しもやけ、むくみ、しみ、耳鳴り）.

るひは冒して渇し、小便小不利の者、此の方の正証なり。男女老若をとはず、何の病ひをとはず、此の方を用ひて、病患治せざることなし。

As shown in the illustration, [there is] hypertonicity in [the regions] lateral to the umbilicus. The patient presents with pain that stretches through to the back and lumbus upon pressing [the abdomen] with the fingertips. In some cases, the patient has palpitations in the region below the heart, strong pain in the smaller abdomen, or veiling accompanied by thirst and inhibited urination; [these are] the true pattern[s] for this formula. Regardless of whether the patient is a man or a woman, and regardless of the disease presented, there is no disease that this formula cannot cure when used [correctly according to formula-pattern matching theory].

然れども毒の淺深厚薄に因りて、敢へて瞑眩せざる者あり。又たその毒厚深にして瞑眩甚しく、若しくは腹痛忍ぶべからざる者あり。或るひは志氣、冒して樂しまざる者間々あり。必ずしも驚くべからず。ますます服藥をかさね進めて可なり。

However, depending on the depth and thickness of the toxin, the patient may not necessarily experience dizziness [when the drug is administered]. When the toxin is thick and deep, some patients experience severe dizziness or insufferable abdominal pain [upon administration]. In some cases, the mind-qì of the patient is veiled and the patient feels depressed. There is no need to be frightened. The drug may be continued to be administered all the more.

則ち當歸芍藥散之方
Dāng Guī Sháo Yào Săn

當歸（一戔、伊吹可也）・芍藥（真の生干）・茯苓（各八分）・澤瀉・唐蒼朮（各四分）。

dāng guī	當歸	1 qián	the Ibuki variety may be used*
sháo yào	芍藥	8 fēn	crude, dried
fú líng	茯苓	8 fēn	
zé xiè	澤瀉	4 fēn	
cāng zhú	蒼朮	4 fēn	Chinese†

* There is still some confusion between the varieties of *dāng guī* (Jp: *tōki*) that are used in China and Japan. *Dāng guī* generally refers to Angelica sinensis in China (referred to as

kara-tōki 唐當歸 [literally, "Chinese *dāng guī*"] in Japan). However, *dāng guī* usually refers to Angelica acutiloba in Japan (which is called *dōng dāng guī* 東當歸 [literally, "eastern *dāng guī*"] in China). There are several varieties of Angelica acutiloba endemic to Japan. The Ibuki 伊吹 variety, (also known as *miyama-tōki* 深山當歸), is Angelica acutiloba Kitagawa (subsp. iwatensis Hikino), which grows north of Mt. Ibuki (Jp: *Ibuki-San* 伊吹山) in Shiga Prefecture (Jp: *Shiga-Ken* 滋賀縣). Perhaps due to a lack of knowledge concerning pharmacognosy, the varieties of *dāng guī* are often not strictly differentiated in ancient and modern Japanese Kampō formularies and medical texts.

† In Japan, *cāng zhú* (Jp: *sōjutsu*; atractylodes rhizome) and *bái zhú* (Jp: *byakujutsu*; white atractylodes rhizome) were and continue to be confused. In China as well, early texts concerning herbology such as *Shén Nóng Běn Cǎo Jīng* 《神農本草經》(Jp: *Shinnō-Honzō-Kyō*; The Divine Husbandman's Herbal Foundation Canon; compiled some time between 200 BCE and 300 CE, however the complete original text is nonextant) did not seem to differentiate between the two ingredients, and listed only *zhú* 朮 in formulae. By the *Sòng* (宋) dynasty (960–1279 CE), a firm distinction between the two was largely established. The *Tài Píng Huì Mín Hé Jì Jú Fāng* 《太平惠民和劑局方》(Jp: *Taihei-Keimin-Wazai-Kyoku-Hō*; Tài Píng Imperial Grace Pharmacy Formulas; published from 1107 to 1110), the first state-supported medical formula compilation in China, lists *bái zhú* in the formula for *Dāng Guī Sháo Yào Sǎn* 當歸芍藥散, which has become standard in traditional Chinese medicine (TCM) currently used in China. Nevertheless, Tsumura & Co., the largest seller of extract Kampō medicines in Japan, uses *cāng zhú* in this formula and most others, whereas Kracie Pharma, Ltd., the second largest seller, uses *bái zhú*.

右、五味散となし、清酒を以て一戔を送下す。日三たび、夜二たび。又た煎方、水一盞と酒半盞を以て六分に煮取り、一度に服す。

The powder made from these five ingredients is to be drunk with one *qián* of clear [rice] liquor [i.e., sake] three times during the daytime and twice at night. The method to decoct the formula is to boil the ingredients in [a mixture of] one cup of water and a half-cup of sake and then administer the ingredients together in a single dose.

又た此の証にして便閉の者、三黄丸、毎夜一戔を兼用して可なり。又た傳に云ふ、婦人妊身便閉、或るひは便遠の者、必ず產重し。此の方を用ひて可なり、亦た三黄丸兼用をかくべからず。

Moreover, patients [who match] this pattern and present with a fecal block may be simultaneously given one *qián* of *Sān Huáng Wán* 三黄丸 each night.[229] One text states

229. There are several different formulae with the name *Sān Huáng Wán* 三黄丸. The formula for this version of *Sān Huáng Wán* (Jp: *San'Ō-Gan*; three yellows pill) is the same as the formu-

that pregnant women who have a fecal block or difficulty in passing stools will definitely have a difficult delivery. This formula may be used [in such cases]. Moreover, [it could be said that] the simultaneous use of *Sān Huáng Wán* is essential [in these cases].

則ち三黄丸の方
Sān Huáng Wán

唐大黄（ 三戔 。古渡・重實の者可也 ）・黄連・黄芩（ 各一戔 。五分 ）。

Chinese dà huáng*	大黄	3 qián	the kowatari variety;† the heavy variety may be used
huáng lián	黄連	1 qián and 5 fēn	
huáng qín	黄芩	1 qián and 5 fēn	

* There are several varieties of *dà huáng*. In Japan, the crude drug referred to as Chinese *dà huáng* (Jp: *kara-daiō* 唐大黄) is Rheum undulatum, which is considered to have a weaker effect than the more commonly used Rheum palmatum or Rheum officinale.

† During the Edo period, foreign goods that entered Japan during or before the Muromachi 室町 period (1336–1573) were referred to as *kowatari* 古渡り (literally, "ancient migration.")

右 、三味末となし丸す 。

Grind the three above ingredients into a powder to make pills.

---

lae for *Sān Huáng Sǎn* 三黄散 (Jp: *San'Ō-San*; three yellows powder) and *Sān Huáng Xiè Xīn Tāng* 三黄瀉心湯 (Jp: *San'Ō-Shashin-Tō*; three yellows heart-draining decoction), which were originally found in *Shāng Hán Lùn*. The extract preparations of the formulae for *Sān Huáng Sǎn* and *Sān Huáng Xiè Xīn Tāng* are covered by the Japanese National Health Insurance program as prescription drugs, and are also commonly sold in Japanese drug stores as over-the-counter drugs. They are currently indicated by the MHLW for: various symptoms associated with hypertension (i.e., hot flashes, stiff shoulders, tinnitus, dull headache, insomnia, anxiety), nosebleed, bleeding hemorrhoid, constipation, menopause, and [what is known in Japan as] "blood path disease" in persons with moderate or strong physical strength who have slight hot flashes, facial flushing, anxiety, feeling of a knot in the solar plexus, or tend to experience constipation. Note: Blood path disease (Jp: *chi-no-michi-shō* 血の道症) refers to neuropsychiatric and physical symptoms such as anxiety and irritation that occur [in women] due to hormonal fluctuations associated with menstruation, pregnancy, childbirth, postpartum period, menopause, etc. (體力中等度以上で 、のぼせ氣味で顔面紅潮し 、精神不安 、みぞおちのつかえ 、便祕傾向などのあるものの次の諸症：高血壓の隨伴症狀「 のぼせ 、肩こり 、耳なり 、頭重 、不眠 、不安 」、鼻血 、痔出血 、便祕 、更年期障害 、血の道症 。血の道症とは 、月經 、妊娠 、出產 、產後 、更年期など女性のホルモンの變動に伴って現れる精神不安やいらだちなどの精神神經症狀および身體症狀のことである).

人参去朮加桂湯之圖
Illustration for the Rén Shēn Qù Zhú Jiā Guì Tāng[230] [Pattern]
人参去朮加桂湯

圖の如く、本動氣臍底に在りて、時々臍上をつくもの、是れ腎氣動ずる也。心下痞鞕・胸中痺、或るひは胸膈痞塞、或るひは心を衝くもの奔豚氣に似たり。みな血証にして腎間の氣動くなり。

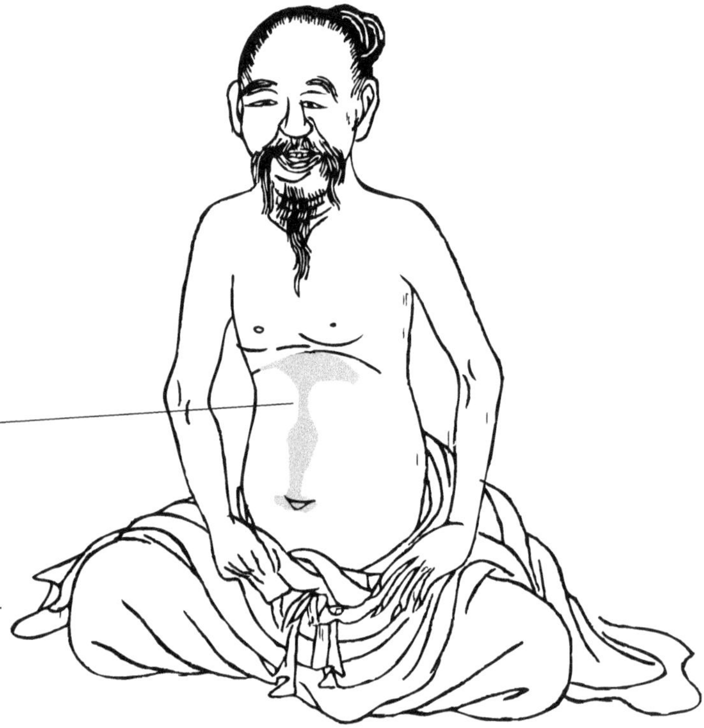

臍上をつく者
A case of a [toxin] surging into the supraumbilical region

Fig. 44

As shown in the illustration, the patient presents with a stirring qì in the depths of the umbilicus that occasionally surges into the supraumbilical region; this is the kidney qì stirring. [The patient may present with] glomus and hardness in the region below the heart, chest impediment, glomus blockage in the chest and diaphragm, or surging into the heart similar to a case of running piglet qì. These are all cases of a blood pattern in which there is a stirring qì in the kidney region.

230. The original source of *Rén Shēn Qù Zhú Jiā Guì Tāng* 人参去朮加桂湯 (Jp: *Ninjin-Kyo-Jutsu-Ka-Kei-Tō*; ginseng decoction minus [white] atractylodes plus cinnamon twig) is unclear. At present, the formula is not covered by the Japanese National Health Insurance program and is not commonly used in Japan.

古人云ふ、「腎間の動氣は十二經の根本なり。その動變じて百患をなす。則ち百証をあらはす」。乃ち百患・百証、一藥一方を以て、先後の取捨樞機たがはざる時は、百患・百証治せざることなし。

An ancient [physician] said that "stirring qì in the kidney region is the root of the twelve channels. The transmutations of the stirring cause the hundred afflictions [to arise] and the hundred patterns to manifest."[231] Thus, when the essential points concerning the order and additions and subtractions for each drug and each formula are correct, none of the hundred afflictions and hundred patterns will remain uncured.

則ち人參去朮加桂湯の方
Rén Shēn Qù Zhú Jiā Guì Tāng

人參（竹節）・甘草・乾姜（各二戔）・桂枝（二戔七分）。

zhú jié rén shēn*	竹節人參	2 qián
gān cǎo	甘草	2 qián
gān jiāng	乾薑	2 qián
guì zhī	桂枝	2 qián and 7 fēn

* Several varieties of ginseng are used in traditional Chinese and Japanese medicine. *Zhú jié rén shēn* 竹節人參 (Jp: *chikusetsu-ninjin,* more commonly called *tochiba-ninjin* 栃葉人參) refers to Panax japonicus.

右、末となし、密丸・雞子黄の大きさの如く、熱湯六分を以て研き砕き、溫めて服す。日三たび、夜二たび。

Grind the above ingredients into a powder, then tightly pack the powder into a pill the size of a yolk of a chicken egg. Break the pill into six *fēn* of boiling water and take [the decoction] while it is still warm. [The decoction should be administered] three times during the day and twice at night.

231. This is found in *Nàn Jīng*《難經》(Jp: *Nan-kyō*; The Classic of Difficult Issues), which is thought to have been written or compiled near the end of the Eastern Hàn (Ch: *Dōng Hàn* 東漢; Jp: *Tō-Kan*) dynasty (25–220 CE). The original text as found in the "Bowel and Visceral Well and Transport Points" Chapter (Ch: *Zàng Fǔ Jǐng Shū* 藏府井俞; Jp: *Zōfu-Seishu*) is as follows: "臍下腎間動氣者、人之生命也、十二經之根本也、故名曰原..." (The stirring qì in the kidney region is the life of humans and the root of the twelve channels, thus [the transport points] are named "the origin[s]...").

小品奔豚湯之圖
Illustration for the Xiǎo Pǐn [Fāng] Bēn Tún Tāng[232] [Pattern]
小品奔豚湯

圖の如く、其の人胸滿して氣急速迫、俗に云ふ「息だはしく」、時々息ぎれして、起居安からず、心細く、時々臍の左右より奔豚氣發こり、欝冒して項背強急し、或るひは手足逆冷する者。此の方の正証なり。腹診を審らかにして、此の方を與へて其の効を知るべし。余、此の方を數々用ひて、其の効驗あるを知る。

As shown in the illustration, the person [i.e., the patient] presents with fullness in the chest, a condition colloquially called "strenuous breathing." The patient sometimes experiences shortness of breath, is disquieted in daily living, feels helpless, sometimes feels running piglet qì in the left and right sides of the umbilicus, has veiling depression, stiffness of the nape and back, or counterflow cold of the extremities. [These are] the true patterns [matching] this formula. [The physician] should make [the pattern] clear through abdominal examination, and administer this formula. Having done so, he will understand the efficacy [of the formula]. I have often used this formula and understand its effectiveness [from experience].

232. There are several different formulae with the name *Bēn Tún Tāng* 奔豚湯 (Jp: *Honton-Tō*; running piglet decoction). Of these, three are listed in this work. As seen from the title of this section, this version was copied from *Xiǎo Pǐn Fāng*《小品方》(Jp: *Shōhin-Hō*; Formulary of Trifles), a text written by Chén Yánzhī 陳延之 (dates of birth and death unknown) in the mid-fourth century CE. The formulary was designated as a compulsory text for Japanese medical students during the eighth century, but was lost in Japan and China by the Northern *Sòng* (Ch: *Běi Sòng* 北宋; Jp: *Hoku-Sō*) dynasty (960–1127 CE) until it was found in a private Japanese library in 1985. Although the text remained lost during the Edo period, large sections of the work were quoted in Chinese texts such as *Wài Tái Mì Yào*《外臺秘要》(Jp: *Gedai-Hiyō*; Essential Secrets from Outside the Metropolis; compiled by Wáng Tāo 王燾 [dates of birth and death unknown] in 752 CE) and Japanese texts such as *Ishin-Pō*《醫心方》(Ch: *Yī Xīn Fāng*; (Formulary from the Heart of Medicine; published by Tamba No Yasunori 丹波康頼 [912–995 CE] in 984 CE). Thus, it appears that many Japanese physicians had some knowledge of the contents of the work. At present, this formula and the other two formulae for *Bēn Tún Tāng* listed in this work are not covered by the Japanese National Health Insurance program and are not commonly used in Japan. However, the versions from *Jīn Guì Yào Lüè* and *Zhǒu Hòu Bèi Jí Fāng*《肘後備急方》(Jp: *Chūgo-Bikyū-Hō*; Emergency Prescriptions Ready at Hand), not discussed in this work, are approved by the MHLW to be sold in Japanese drug stores as over-the-counter drugs. The details of these two formulae are explained in the section for "*Guǎng Jì* [*Fāng*]" *Bēn Tún Tāng*「廣濟[方]」奔豚湯.

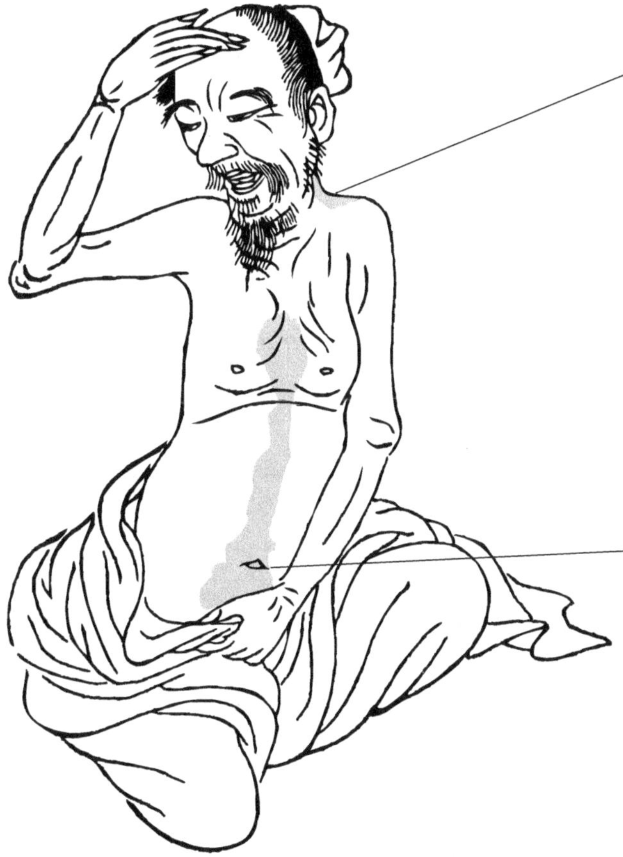
項背強急の毒
A toxin causing stiffness of the nape and back
奔豚氣發こるの毒
A toxin causing running piglet qì

Fig. 45

桂枝湯の証に似て、急迫甚だしく痞滿項背にこはり、頗る血証をかす。所謂癪聚家に間々此の証あり。甚だしき者は小兒驚風の如く、人事を知らず。此くの如き者に、大いに此の方效あり。此れに因りて之れを考ふるに、小兒驚風と號する者も、大人奔豚氣つき上がり、項背強急して死せんとする者も、其の名を命ずるところ異なりといへども、其の証をつまびらかにするに至つては、大いに異ならず。

[This pattern] is similar to the pattern for *Guì Zhī Tāng,* [in which the patient presents with] severe distress and glomus and fullness [that cause] hypertonicity in the nape and back and a severe blood pattern develops. Patients who present with a gathering of what is known [in Japan] as "*shaku*" have this pattern.[233] In severe cases, the patient presents

233. The character *shaku* 癪 was invented in Japan and cannot be found in the Chinese language. It is a combination of the disease radical (疒; Ch: *nè*; Jp: *yamai-dare*) and the character for accumulation (Ch: *jī* 積; Jp: *seki*). In traditional Japanese Kampō medicine, it may refer to mounting qì (Ch: *shàn qì* 疝氣; Jp: *senki*), or lower abdominal colic (severe colicky pain in the

with [symptoms] similar to those of pediatric fright wind, such as loss of consciousness.[234] This formula is extremely effective for these types of patients. Thus, when these [facts] are considered, although the names [of the afflictions experienced by] pediatric patients who present with fright wind and adult patients on the verge of death (who present with running piglet qì that surges upward, causing stiffness of the nape and back) are different, when their [abdominal] patterns are elucidated, there is in fact very little that differs [between the two conditions].

後世、狀に因つて其の命ずること異なるを以て、其の方も亦た異にして、治せざる者多し。只だ腹症に因らば多岐の惑ひを去るべし。亦た常に癇症間々あり。考ふべし。

Later generations [of physicians] incorrectly diagnose [these conditions] on the basis of the outward appearance [of patients]; because the formulae [that these physicians] prescribe are also different [from the true formulae that match the patterns], there are many patients who are not cured. If [the physician] relies only on abdominal patterns, then he will be able to remove all confusion [from his mind. This formula] generally [matches] patients who present with an epilepsy pattern. [In such cases, the formula] may be considered [for use].

則ち小品奔豚湯の方
Xiǎo Pǐn [Fāng] Bēn Tún Tāng

炙甘草（八分）・李根皮・葛根（各一錢五分）・黄芩・桂心・瓜蔞仁・人參（各四分。竹節）・川芎（五分）。

zhì gān cǎo	炙甘草	8 fēn
lǐ gēn pí	李根皮	1 qián and 5 fēn

lower abdomen usually accompanied by constipation and ischuria), accompanied by psychiatric conditions such as hysteria. According to the *Ishin-Pō*《醫心方》(Formulary from the Heart of Medicine), the oldest extant medical work in Japan, qì can accumulate in an organ to form a lump, causing severe pain and a variety of afflictions. The concept of *shaku* is thought to have corresponded to a variety of modern conditions that cause spasms of pain, such as stomach cancer, appendicitis, peritonitis, etc. In modern Japan, *shaku* commonly refers to general vexation or irritability.

234. Pediatric fright wind (Ch: *jīng fēng* 驚風; Jp: *kyōfū*), also known as "infantile convulsion," refers to infantile diseases marked by convulsions and loss of consciousness.

gé gēn	葛根	1 qián and 5 fēn
huáng qín	黄芩	4 fēn
guì xīn	桂心	4 fēn
guā lóu rén	栝蔞仁	4 fēn
zhú jié rén shēn	竹節人參	4 fēn
chuān xiōng	川芎	5 fēn

右五味、水一盞八分を以て、六分に煮取り、一度に服す。

Boil the above five ingredients in one cup and eight *fēn* of water to make six *fēn* of the decoction, and administer to the patient in a single dose.

廣濟奔豚湯之圖

Illustration for the Guǎng Jì [Fāng] Bēn Tún Tāng[235] [Pattern]

廣濟[方]奔豚湯

圖の如く、臍底の動氣築々として豚の奔るごとく上りて心胸に在りて下らず。吸々として氣急速迫、人語をきくことを欲せず。或るひは心下煩亂して安からず。發作時あり、或るひは四支煩疼、手足厥冷。其の脉、沈・遲若しくは微・濇冷氣を兼ぬるもの。此の症、世に癇氣と號する者に甚だ多し。諸藥投ずるに效なし。此の方に非ざれば、治せざるなり。

As shown in the illustration, there is a tingling feeling in the depths of the umbilicus (similar to a piglet running around) that surges up into the heart and chest without descending. [Moreover, the patient presents with] hasty rapid breathing and has no desire to listen to human speech. In some cases, the patient presents with recurrent vexation and derangement in the region below the heart and is disquieted. In some cases, the patient presents with vexing pain in the limbs and reversal cold of the extremities.

235. This is the second version of *Bēn Tún Tāng* 奔豚湯 (running piglet decoction) found in this work. This version was found in *Guǎng Jì Fāng*《廣濟方》(Jp: *Kōsai-Hō*; Broad Salvation Formulary). The text is no longer extant, but it was extensively quoted in *Wài Tái Mì Yào*《外臺秘要》(Jp: *Gedai-Hiyō*; Essential Secrets from Outside the Metropolis). Hence, many Japanese physicians in the Edo period appeared to have some knowledge of the contents of the work. At present, this formula is not covered by the Japanese National Health Insurance program and is not commonly used in Japan.

The pulse is sunken and slow or faint and rough, and a cold qì is present. This pattern is common in patients who present with what is commonly referred to as "*shaku*" qì. The administration of other drugs will be ineffective. Unless this formula is used, [the disease] will not be cured.

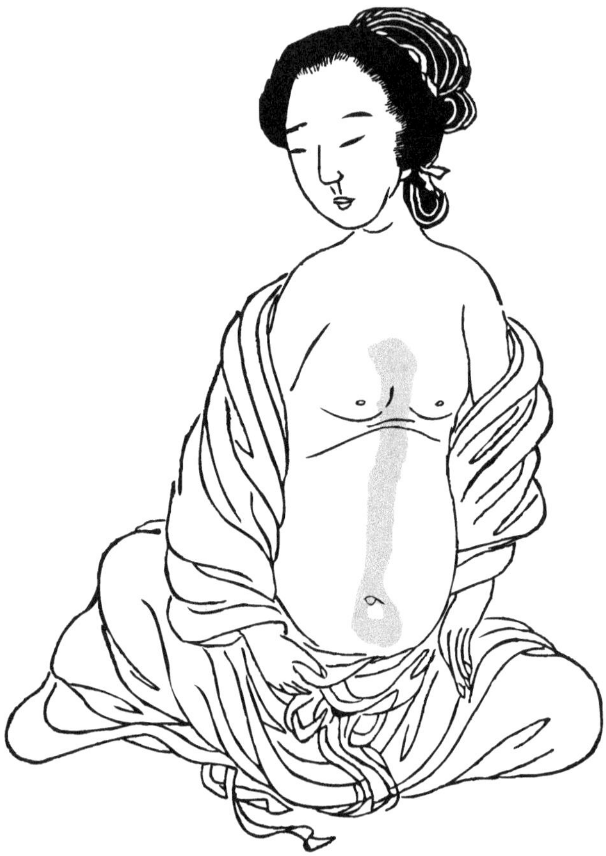

Fig. 46

則ち廣濟奔豚湯の方
Guǎng Jì [Fāng] Bēn Tún Tāng[236]

李根皮（一戔六分）・半夏（一戔四分）・乾姜・桂心（各八分）・茯苓（六分）・炙甘草・竹節人参（各四分）・炮附子（二分）。

lǐ gēn pí	李根皮	1 qián and 6 fēn	
bàn xià	半夏	1 qián and 4 fēn	
gān jiāng	乾姜	8 fēn	
guì xīn	桂心	8 fēn	
fú líng	茯苓	6 fēn	
zhì gān cǎo	炙甘草	4 fēn	
zhú jié rén shēn	竹節人参	4 fēn	
fù zǐ	炮附子	2 fēn	blast-fried

右八味、水一盞八分を以て、六分に煮とる。

Decoct the above eight ingredients in one cup and eight *fēn* of water to make six *fēn* of the decoction.

236. The formula for *Bēn Tún Tāng* which is found in Chapter 3, Section 23 of the *Zhǒu Hòu Bèi Jí Fāng*《肘後備急方》is as follows: "甘草（二兩），人參（二兩），桂心（二兩），茱萸（一升），生薑（一斤），半夏（一升）。以水一斗，煮取三升，分三服。此藥宜預蓄，得病便急合之。*gān cǎo* (2 *liǎng*), *rén shēn* (2 *liǎng*), *guì xīn* (2 *liǎng*), *wú zhū yú* (1 *shēng*), *shēng jiāng* (1 *jīn*), *bàn xià* (1 *shēng*). [Add the medicinals to] one *dòu* of water and reduce down to to three *shēng*. Separate into three doses and take. It is appropriate to store these medicinals beforehand, [so that when one] contracts disease [they can be] quickly and easily combined to [make the formula]." The *Zhǒu Hòu Bèi Jí Fāng* version of the formula and the version from *Jīn Guì Yào Lüè*《金匱要略》are approved by the MHLW for sale as over-the-counter drugs, but both are not well known in Japan at present. Both formulae are currently indicated by the MHLW for: paroxysmal palpitations and anxiety neurosis in persons with moderate or strong physical strength who have a feeling of palpitations being pushed up to the chest or throat (體力中等度以下で、下腹部から動悸が胸やのどに突き上げる感じがするものの次の諸症：發作性の動悸、不安神經症).

防風茯苓湯之圖

Illustration for the Fáng Fēng Fú Líng Tāng[237] [Pattern] 防風茯苓湯

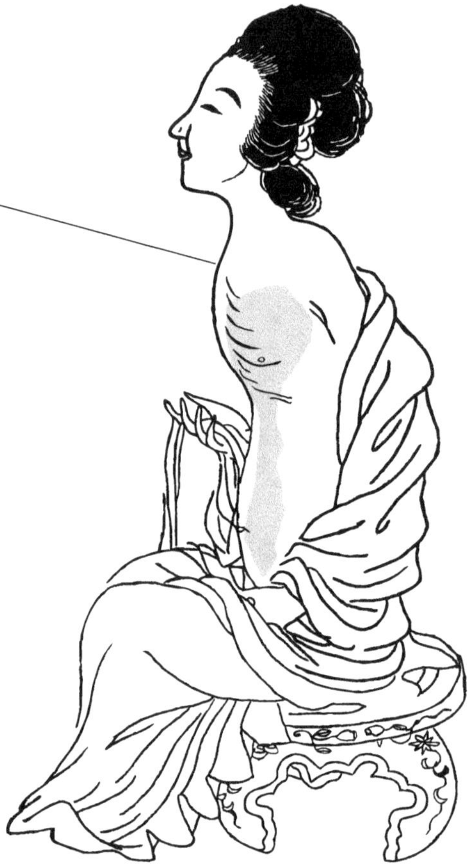

臍上動氣心を衝して痛胸滿短氣冷涎を吐するもの

A case in which supraumbilical stirring qì surges into the heart, causing pain and fullness in the chest, shortness of breath, and ejection of cold drool [from the mouth].

圖の如く、臍底の動氣衝して、胸滿、氣急速迫、心痛して涎を吐し、痰飲・冷涎ある者、此の方を用ひて效あり。

As shown in the illustration, the patient presents with a stirring qì in the depths of the umbilicus that surges [upward], causing fullness in the chest, distressed rapid [breathing], heart pain, and ejection of drool, phlegm-rheum, or cold drool. This formula is effective when used [in such cases].

Fig. 47

237. There are at least two versions of the formula for *Fáng Fēng Fú Líng Tāng* 防風茯苓湯 (*Bōfū-Bukryō-Tō*; saposhnikovia and poria decoction); this version appears to have been copied from *Wài Tái Mì Yào* (Jp: *Gedai-Hiyō*; Essential Secrets from Outside the Metropolis), albeit with some changes made to the quantities of ingredients. At present, no version of the formula is covered by the Japanese National Health Insurance program and none is commonly used in Japan.

則ち防風茯苓湯の方
Fáng Fēng Fú Líng Tāng

桂枝（ 一戔二分 ）・半夏・乾姜（ 各八分 ）・竹節人參（ 六分 ）・甘草・茯苓・防風（ 各四分 ）。

guì zhī	桂枝	1 qián and 2 fēn
bàn xià	半夏	8 fēn
gān jiāng	乾姜	8 fēn
zhú jié rén shēn	竹節人參	6 fēn
gān cǎo	甘草	4 fēn
fú líng	茯苓	4 fēn
fáng fēng	防風	4 fēn

右七味 、水一盞半を以て 、六分に煮取る 。

Boil the above seven ingredients in one and one-half cups of water to make six *fēn* of the decoction.

小品牡蠣奔豚湯之圖
Illustration for the Xiǎo Pǐn [Fāng] Mǔ Lì Bēn Tún Tāng [Pattern]
小品[方]牡蠣奔豚湯

圖の如く 、臍底に動氣ありて 、時々奔豚氣 、小腹より起りて 、胸を撞き 、上逆或るひは心痛 、手足逆冷の者 。この方 、此れを治す 。

As shown in the illustration, the patient presents with a stirring qì in the depths of the umbilicus and occasionally experiences running piglet qì and counterflow that arises from the smaller abdomen and surges into the chest, in some cases [causing] heart pain or counterflow cold of the extremities. This formula cures these [conditions].

則ち小品牡蠣奔豚湯の方
Xiǎo Pǐn [Fāng] Mǔ Lì Bēn Tún Tāng[238]

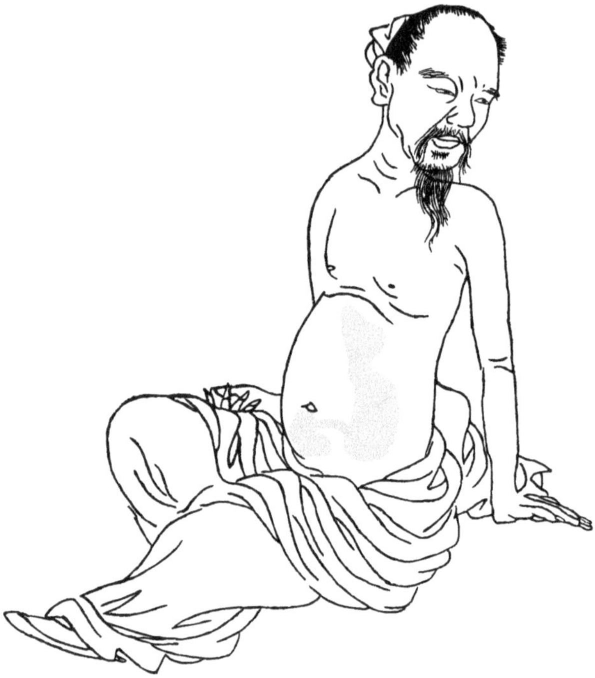

Fig. 48

238. As previously mentioned, this formula and the other two formulae for *Bēn Tún Tāng* 奔豚湯 noted in this work are not covered by the Japanese National Health Insurance program and are not commonly used in Japan. The formula for the MHLW-*approved Bēn Tún Tāng* as found in *Zhǒu Hòu Bèi Jí Fāng*《肘後備急方》(Jp: *Chūgo-Bikyū-Hō*; Emergency Prescriptions Ready at Hand), also known as *Zhǒu Hòu Jiù Zú Fāng*《肘後救卒方》(Jp: *Chūgo-Kyūsotsu-Hō*; Prescriptions Ready at Hand for Rescuing the Dying), which was written by the prolific scholar Gé Hóng 葛洪 (283–343 CE), is as follows: *gān cǎo* 甘草 (2g), *rén shēn* 人參 (2g), *guì pí* 桂皮 (4g), *wú zhū yú* 呉茱萸 (2g), *shēng jiāng* 生薑 (1g), *bàn xià* 半夏 (4g). It is indicated for paroxysmal palpitations and anxiety neurosis in persons with moderate or weak physical strength who experience the feeling of palpitations from the hypogastric region heaving upward to the chest or throat (體力中等度以下で、下腹部から動悸が胸やのどに突き上げる感じがするものの次の諸症：發作性の動悸、不安神經症).
Furthermore, the formula for *Bēn Tún Tāng* as found in *Jīn Guì Yào Lüè*《金匱要略》, which is also approved by the MHLW, is as follows: *gān cǎo* 甘草 (2g), *chuān xiōng* 川芎 (2g), *dāng guī* 當歸 (2g), *bàn xià* 半夏 (4g), *huáng qín* 黄芩 (2g), *gé gēn* 葛根 (5g), *sháo yào* 芍藥 (2g), *shēng jiāng* 生薑 (1–1.5g), [*gān*] *lǐ gēn bái pí* [甘]李根白皮 (5–8g; *sāng bái pí* 桑白皮 may be substituted). It is indicated for paroxysmal palpitations and anxiety neurosis in persons with moderate physical strength who experience the feeling of palpitations from the hypogastric region heaving upward to the chest or throat (體力中等度で、下腹部から動悸が胸やのどに突き上げる感じがするものの次の諸症：發作性の動悸、不安神經症).

牡蠣（ 六分 ）・桂心（ 一戔六分 ）・李根皮（ 一戔五分 ）・炙甘草（ 六分 ）。

mǔ lì	牡蠣	6 fēn
guì xīn	桂心	1 qián and 6 fēn
lǐ gēn pí	李根皮	1 qián and 5 fēn
zhì gān cǎo	炙甘草	6 fēn

右四味 、水一盞半を以て 、六分に煮とる 。

Decoct the above four ingredients in one and one-half cups of water to make six *fēn* of the decoction.

當歸建中湯之圖

Illustration for the Dāng Guī Jiàn Zhōng Tāng[239] [Pattern]

當歸建中湯

圖の如く 、腹中拘攣急迫して 、數縄を引つぱるが如くにして 、小腹腰背より引き痛むもの 。或るひは手足疼痛して浮腫する者 。或るひは卒かに手足攣痛し 、俗に「 筋戻 」と云ふもの 。或るひは血症にして虚羸 、氣息吸々としてまさに絶せんとする者 。みな 、此の方用ひて 、其の效いちじるし 。

As shown in the illustration, the patient presents with hypertonicity and distress in the abdomen, as well as a pulling pain (similar to the feeling of being pulled by several ropes) induced from the smaller abdomen, lumbus, and back. In some cases, the patient presents with pain and puffy swelling in the extremities. In some cases, the patient presents with a sudden hypertonic pain in the extremities, something that is colloquially called

239. The formula for *Dāng Guī Jiàn Zhōng Tāng* 當歸建中湯 (Jp: *Tōki-Kenchū-Tō*; Chinese angelica center-fortifying decoction) was originally found in *Jīn Guì Yào Lüè*. The extract preparation of the formula is covered by the Japanese National Health Insurance program as a prescription drug, and may be sold in Japanese drug stores as an over-the-counter drug. It is currently indicated by the MHLW for: menstrual pain, dysmenorrhea, irregular menstruation, abdominal pain, lower abdominal pain, low back pain, hemorrhoids, pain associated with prolapse, and decreased physical strength after childbirth or sickness in persons with weak physical strength who are easily fatigued and have poor complexion (體力虛弱で 、疲勞しやすく血色のすぐれないものの次の諸症 : 月經痛 、月經困難症 、月經不順 、腹痛 、下腹部痛 、腰痛 、痔 、脱肛の痛み 、病後・術後の體力低下).

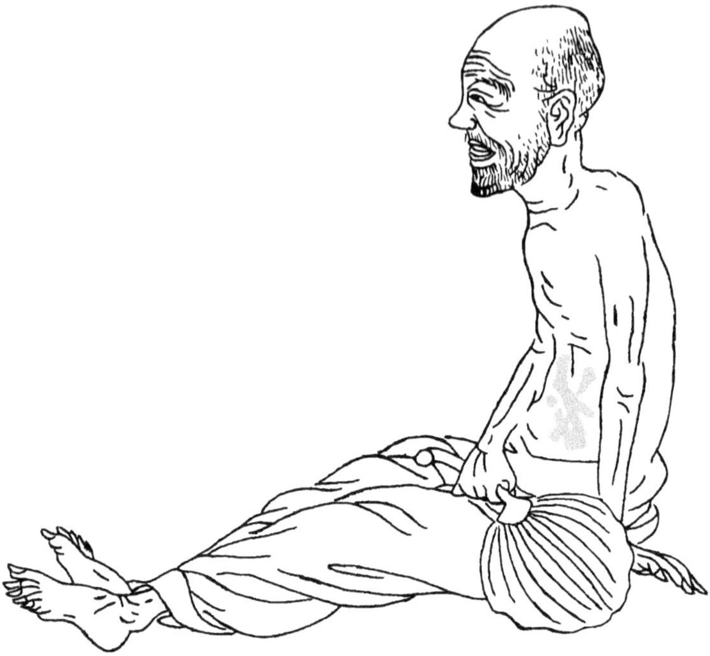

Fig. 49

"*suji-chigai.*"[240] In some cases the patient presents with a blood pathocondition, vacuous marked emaciation and weakness, and heavy breathing that verges on expiration. This formula is remarkably effective when used [to treat] all [of these patterns].

余按ずるに、凡そ重病にして、世醫その療を失ふもの、或るひは大承氣湯、或るひは桃仁承氣、或るひは大黄牡丹皮などの症、全く備はりて、久しく攻むる者、時として其の毒瞑眩してうごき諸症を發す。其の發する症を詳らかにして、ゆるさず攻め追ひ去りて、又た本の備はりたる症をせめて、月日をへて全く治すべし。

I believe that in all cases of severe diseases for which the physicians of the world mistake treatment, [the formulae corresponding to] patterns such as [the patterns for] *Dà Chéng Qì Tāng, Táo Rén Chéng Qì* [*Tāng*], or *Dà Huáng Mǔ Dān Pí* [*Tāng*] are complete and sufficient [to treat the patterns]; when [such medicinals are] used over long periods of time to attack [a pattern], the toxin [causing the disease] is stirred, often causing dizziness and various other symptoms.[241]

240. Although *suji-chigai* 筋戾 literally means "sinew perversion," it commonly refers to muscle strain or sprain in Japan.

241. As mentioned in the section for *Guì Zhī Tāng* 桂枝湯, in both Japan and China, it was often considered that unpleasant side effects such as dizziness are signs that the toxin is leaving the body and the treatment is successful.

凡そ下劑を以て攻め下す時は、忽ち上衝拘攣し、或るひは急迫などして、桂枝加桂湯。或るひは面浮腫し、手足攣痛などする者は、當歸建中湯。或るひは上衝・頭眩、小便不利をなして、苓桂朮甘湯。或るひは上衝・胸脇苦滿するは柴胡桂枝湯等の諸症を發すること、舉げてかぞふべからず。就中、血証家、虚脱のもの、又た血動ひて和せざるもの、當歸建中湯の症多し。學者、つつしんで考へ用ゆべし。或る傳に云ふ、「當歸建中湯の症にして、脫血・崩漏のもの、此の方内に於ひて、劉寄奴を大いに加へて可なり」。

If [the physician] elucidates the pattern that the patient presents with and attacks it unrelentingly in order to drive [the toxin] out [of the patient] while attacking the original pattern that the patient presents with, the patient will be completely cured within a matter of days or months.

Generally speaking, when a laxative is used to attack and precipitate [the toxin], and the patient suddenly experiences [symptoms such as] upward surging and hypertonicity [in some cases,] or distress in other cases; [these symptoms are signs of the pattern for] *Guì Zhī Jiā Guì Tāng.*[242] When the patient presents with puffy swelling of the face and hypertonic pain in the extremities, [it is the pattern for] *Dāng Guī Jiàn Zhōng Tāng.* When the patient presents with upward surging, a dizzy head, and inhibited urination, [it is the pattern for] *Líng Guì Zhú Gān Tāng.*

There are a countless number of patterns such as *Chái Hú Guì Zhī Tāng* in which the patient presents with upward surging and bitter fullness in the chest and rib-sides. In many cases when the patient especially presents with a blood pattern [i.e., pathocondition], vacuity desertion, or stirring blood that is not harmonized, it is the pattern for *Dāng Guī Jiàn Zhōng Tāng.* The student [of abdominal patterns] should carefully consider [these indications] when using [the drugs]. One text states that "when the patient presents with the pattern for *Dāng Guī Jiàn Zhōng Tāng* and has blood desertion or flooding and spotting,[243] a large quantity of *liú jì nú*[244] may be added to this formula."

242. The formula for *Guì Zhī Jiā Guì Tāng* 桂枝加桂湯 (Jp: *Keishi-Ka-Kei-Tō*; cinnamon twig decoction with extra cinnamon) was originally found in *Shāng Hán Lùn* and *Jīn Guì Yào Lüè*. At present, this formula is not covered by the Japanese National Health Insurance program and is not widely used in Japan.

243. Flooding and spotting (Ch: *bēng lòu* 崩漏; Jp: *bōrō*) generally refers to bleeding or dribbling blood from the vagina which is not due to normal menses. It may be seen in menstrual diseases, metrostaxis and metrorrhagia, stony uterine mass, vaginal bleeding during pregnancy, ectopic pregnancy, postpartum profuse vaginal bleeding, postpartum lochiorrhea, epidemic hemorrhagic fever, purpura and blood extravasation.

244. The author glossed *liú jì nú* 劉寄奴 (Jp: *ryūkido*; anomalous artemisia) as *otogirisō* 弟切

則ち當歸建中湯の方
Dāng Guī Jiàn Zhōng Tāng

當歸（ 一戔四分 。伊吹可也 ）・芍藥（ 一戔二分 ）・桂枝・生姜・（ 各六分 ）・甘草（ 四分 ）。

dāng guī	當歸	1 qián and 4 fēn	the Ibuki variety is acceptable.
sháo yào	芍藥	6 fēn	
guì zhī	桂枝	6 fēn	
shēng jiāng	生姜	6 fēn	
gān cǎo	甘草	4 fēn	

右五味 、水一盞半を以て 、六分に煮とる 。

Boil the five ingredients in one and one-half cups of water to make six *fēn* of the decoction.

若しくは大虛の者には 、飴糖三戔を加ふ 。或るひは 、血を去ること過多の者 、或るひは崩症（ くずれるごとく血出る ）にして止まざる者には 、地黄（ 一戔二分 ）・阿膠（ 八分 ）を加へて可なり 。傳に云ふ 、「 この症 、廣東人參二戔を濃煎にして 、時々用ひて可なり 」。

If the patient presents with major vacuity, add three *qián* of (hard) *yí tāng*. In cases when the patient presents with excessive blood loss or a persistent [blood] flooding pattern (in which the hemorrhage is similar to a flood), *dì huáng* (one *qián* and two *fēn*) and *ē jiāo* (eight *fēn*) may be added [to the formula]. According to [one] tradition (i.e., text), "a concentrated decoction of *guǎng dōng rén shēn*[245] (two *qián*) may be occasionally used for this pattern."

草, the Japanese name of *xiǎo lián qiào* 小連翹 (Jp: *shō-rengyō*; erect hypericum). Because both have antihemorrhagic properties, it is unclear which ingredient the author refers to. It is possible that the gloss may be a mistake of the author, but it is also possible that *liú jì nú* and *xiǎo lián qiào* were regarded as intersubstitutable: Japanese physicians during the Edo period often substituted local Japanese crude herbs when the indicated Chinese herbs could not be found.

245. There are several varieties of *rén shēn* 人參 (Jp: *ninjin*; ginseng). *Guǎng dōng rén shēn* 廣東人參 (Jp: *Kanton-ninjin*; literally, "Cantonese ginseng") generally refers to American ginseng i.e., Panax quinquefolius). However, considering that Japan was under a policy of isolation (Jp: *sakoku* 鎖國) during the Edo period, it is unlikely that American ginseng was meant here. In *Kokun-Iden* 《 古訓醫傳 》 (Chronicles of the Ancient Instruction of Physicians), written by the renown physician Utsuki Kondai 宇津木昆臺 (1779–1848 CE), it is noted that *guǎng dōng rén shēn* refers to Panax notoginseng, which is normally called *tián qī* 田七 (Jp: *denshichi*) or *sān qī* 三七 (Jp: *sanshichi*).

黄土湯之圖

Illustration for the Huáng Tǔ Tāng[246] [Pattern] 黄土湯

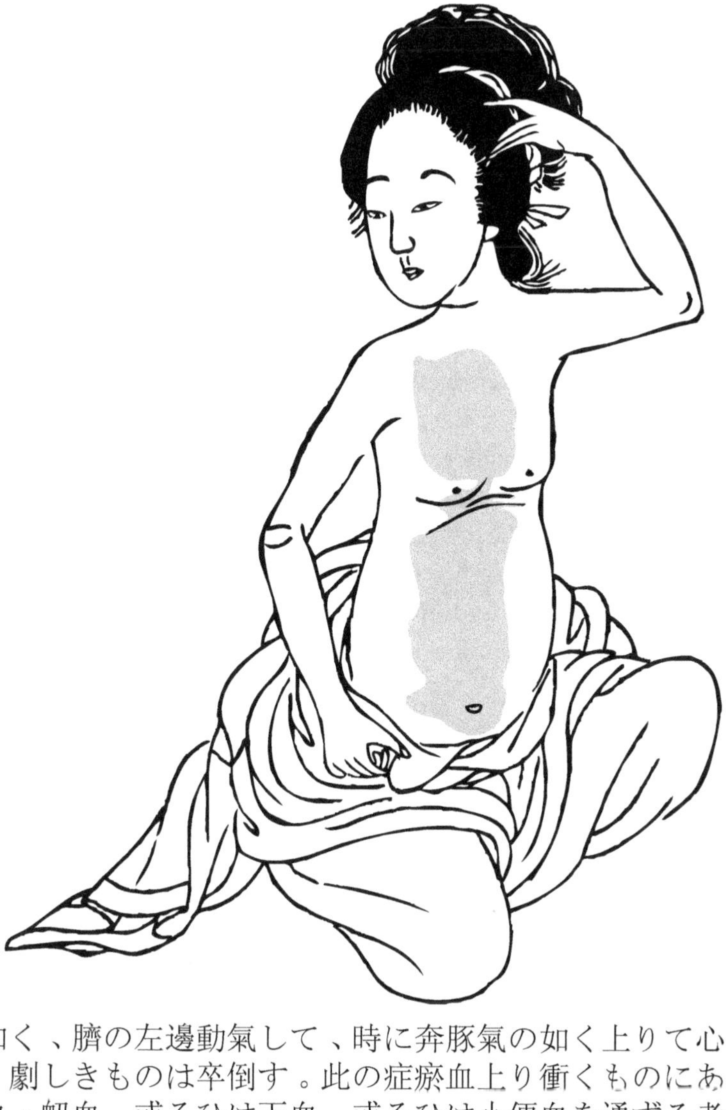

Fig. 50

圖の如く、臍の左邊動氣して、時に奔豚氣の如く上りて心胸にせまり、劇しきものは卒倒す。此の症瘀血上り衝くものにあり。故に吐血・衄血、或るひは下血、或るひは小便血を通ずる者、みな、此の方を用ひて大效あり。

246. The formula for *Huáng Tǔ Tāng* 黄土湯 (Jp: *Ōdo-Tō*; yellow earth decoction) was originally found in *Jīn Guì Yào Lüè*. At present, this formula is not covered by the Japanese National Health Insurance program and is not well known in Japan.

As shown in the illustration, in the region to the left of the umbilicus, the patient presents with a stirring qì that often surges upward to the heart [region] and chest; it is similar to a case of running piglet qì. In severe cases, [the patient may] suddenly collapse. This pattern involves the upward surging of static blood. Thus, this formula is extremely effective in patients who present with blood ejection, nosebleed, blood descent, or hematuria.[247]

余、此の方を數用數效するに、墮胎後に此の症甚だ多し。或るひは產後惡露不盡して、上りて心を攻むるもの、此の症多し。その腹診の分かち右に記するの方劑、みな、動氣奔豚を以て眼とす。此の方のごときは、瘀血上りて心を衝ものゆへ奔氣に似て實は奔豚にあらず。謹んで診察を違ふことなかれ。

I have often used this formula and experienced its efficacy. This pattern is extremely common [in women] after miscarriage. When a [female] patient presents with a postpartum persistent flow of lochia that ascends and attacks the heart, it is often a case of this pattern. The previously mentioned formulae, which are listed by abdominal [symptoms as revealed by] examination, are all indicated for [cases of] stirring qì [or] running piglet [qì]. In cases similar to [the pattern for] this formula, [the patient presents with] static blood that surges up into the heart. Thus, although [such cases] appear similar to a running [piglet] qì [pattern], they are in fact not cases of running piglet [qì]. Carefully perform the [abdominal] examination and do not make any mistakes [in diagnosing the pattern]!

則ち黄土湯の方
Huáng Tǔ Tāng

黄土(二錢六分)・炙甘草・干地黄・唐蒼朮・附子・阿膠・黄芩(各一錢)。

huáng tǔ	黄土	2 qián and 6 fēn
zhì gān cǎo	炙甘草	1 qián
gān dì huáng	干地黄	1 qián
cāng zhú	蒼朮	1 qián

247. Nosebleed or epistaxis (Ch: *nǜ xuè* 衄血; Jp: *jikuketsu*) generally refers to non-traumatic external bleeding, including bleeding from the ear, nose, gingiva, and tongue, and subcutaneous hemorrhage.

fù zǐ	附子	1 qián
ē jiāo	阿膠	1 qián
huáng qín	黄芩	1 qián

右七味、水二盞を以て七分に煮とる。

Boil the seven ingredients in two cups of water to make seven *fēn*.

黄土の眞物を得るの傳あり。山野僻地の民家、他土をまじへず。生土を以て竈を作り、毎日たくこと、土をまじへず。生土、年をへて凡そ廿年餘にして、其の色紫になる者可也。此れを水干すること七度。砂石灰を去りよく清らかにほして用ゆべし。

There is a text explaining how to obtain authentic *huáng tǔ*.[248] [According to the text,] there are homes located in remote fields and mountains where the soil is not mixed with other types. The virgin soil is used to make ovens; the ovens are used for cooking everyday, and no mixing of the soil takes place. Over a period of approximately twenty or more years, the virgin soil becomes purple in color; this soil is acceptable [for use]. It may be used after washing in water and drying seven times and subsequently removing the sand-lime in order to achieve a pure product.

右、黄土一味を龍肝散と云ふ。その功能、左に記す。龍肝散の功能、心痛・反胃・中悪に可なり。腋臭に頻りに塗り付けて可也。小児臍瘡にも亦た可也。小児の重舌に酢に和してぬる。又た産後に悪血・心を攻めて痛む者、酒を以て二戔を服す。崩漏・帯下・吐血・欬血及び催生胞衣を下すの大効あり。

When *huáng tǔ* is used individually, it is called *Lóng Gān Sǎn*.[249] The effects of [the drug] are written below. *Lóng Gān Sǎn* is indicated for heart pain, stomach reflux, and malignity

248. As explained later in the text, although the author uses the term *huáng tǔ* 黄土 (Jp: *ōdo*; loess), he is actually referring to *fú lóng gān* 伏龍肝 (Jp: *fukuryūkan*; oven earth; terra flava usta), also known as *zào xīn huáng tǔ* 灶心黄土 (Jp: *sōshin-ōdo*). Because *fú lóng gān* was not always easily available in Japan during the Edo period, Yoshimasu Tōdō 吉益東洞 and other physicians were known to substitute earthenware bricks for *fú lóng gān*.
249. At present, the formula for *Lóng Gān Sǎn* 龍肝散 (Jp: *Ryūkan-San*; oven earth powder) is not covered by the Japanese National Health Insurance program and is not commonly used in Japan.

stroke. It may be frequently smeared [on the armpits to prevent] armpit odor. It may also be used [to treat] pediatric umbilical sores. It may be mixed with vinegar and directly applied to treat double tongue in children. Moreover, when the patient presents with postpartum malign blood that attacks the heart and causes pain, [the formula] should be taken with two *qián* of sake. [The formula] is extremely effective in [treating cases of] flooding and spotting, vaginal discharge,[250] blood ejection, or coughing of blood,[251] hastening delivery, and causing the placenta to descend.

桂枝加附子湯之圖

Illustration for the Guì Zhī Jiā Fù Zǐ Tāng[252] [Pattern]

桂枝加附子湯

圖の如く、假令へば身體或るひは手足毒あつて痛み、事にふれて疼痛甚しく、或るひは動搖して疼み忍び難きもの、或るひは疝氣と號するもの、疼み上りて心下に充塞し、疼痛甚しきもの、此の方を用ひて效あり。

As shown in the illustration, this formula is effective when used in patients who present with conditions such as the following: generalized pain or pain in the extremities associated with a toxin, severe pain upon being touched, shaking and trembling of the body accompanied by insufferable pain, the condition that is referred to as "mounting qì," ascendant pain that fills and blocks the region below the heart, or excruciating pain.

250. Vaginal discharge or leukorrhea (Ch: *dài xià* 帶下; Jp: *taige*) refers to increased vaginal discharge with abnormal color, texture and smell. It can be seen in vulva infection or uterine disease, especially in leukorrhagia.

251. Coughing of blood, normally written as 咳血 (Ch: *ké xuè*; Jp: *kakketsu*), refers to the expectoration of blood or blood-stained sputum.

252. The formula for *Guì Zhī Jiā Fù Zǐ Tāng* 桂枝加附子湯 (Jp: *Keishi-Ka-Bushi-Tō*; cinnamon twig decoction plus aconite) was originally found in *Jīn Guì Yào Lüè*. At present, this formula is not covered by the Japanese National Health Insurance program and is not commonly used in Japan. However, several variations of *Guì Zhī Tāng* 桂枝湯 with additions are covered by the Japanese National Health Insurance program as prescription drugs. The most similar of these is *Guì Zhī Jiā Zhú Fù Tāng* 桂枝加朮附湯 (Jp: *Keishi-Ka-Jutsu-Bu-Tō*; cinnamon twig decoction plus [white] atractylodes and aconite). It is currently indicated by the MHLW for: arthralgia and neuralgia in persons with weak physical strength who experience sweating, have cold extremities that feel stiff or occasional oliguria (體力虛弱で、汗が出、手足が冷えてこわばり、ときに尿量が少ないものの次の諸症：關節痛、神經痛).

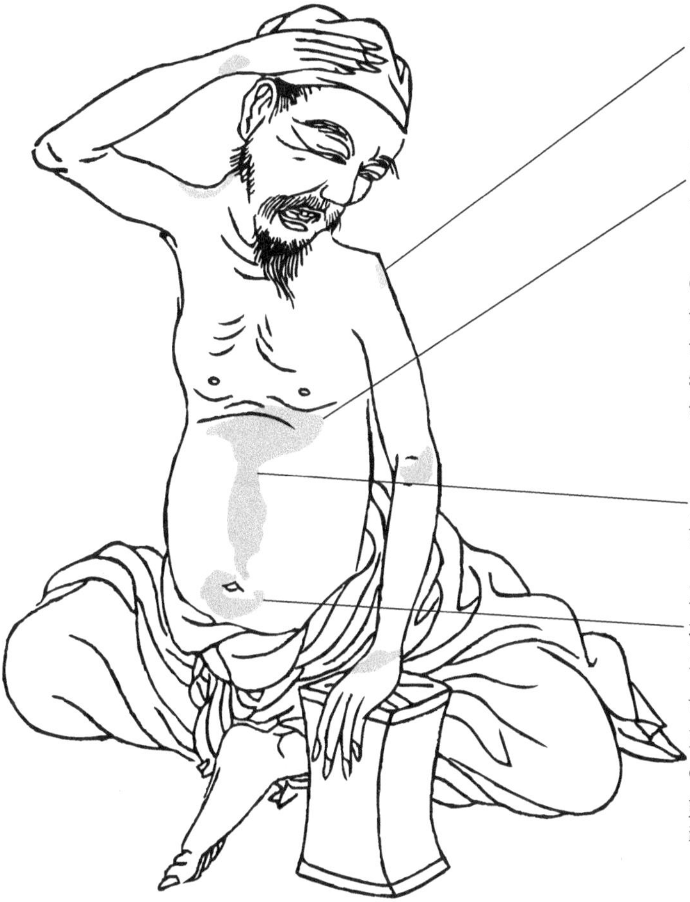
骨節疼痛
Joint pain
心下に結聚の
毒。その餘、文
面を以て考ふべ
し
Gathering and binding toxin in the region below the heart. The text [of this section] should be referred to in other [similar] cases.
氣上衝
Upward surging of qì
右の臍傍下結し
接して痛もの附
子の症なり
When the region to the lower right of the umbilicus is bound and pain is present upon palpation, it is the pattern for *fù zǐ*.

Fig. 51

又た云ふ、心腹、痞満・疼痛し飲食せず、日々水數升を吐き、骨立倦怠の者。まづ茯苓湯、或るひは大半夏湯、或るひは小半夏加茯苓湯、或るひは茯苓澤瀉湯、或るひは半夏瀉心湯、或るひは茯苓飲等。その正症を審らかにして之れを用ひ、吐やんで桂枝加附子湯、之れを主る。その效、神なり。

Furthermore, [this formula is also indicated for] patients who have glomus and fullness [or] pain in the heart [region] and abdomen and no [thought of] food or drink, eject several *sheng*[253] of water everyday, appear bony [due to emaciation], and have fatigue. [In such cases,] formulae such as *Fú Líng Tāng, Dà Bàn Xià Tāng, Xiǎo Bàn Xià Jiā Fú Líng Tāng, Fú Líng Zé Xiè Tāng, Bàn Xià Xiè Xīn Tāng,* or *Fú Líng Yǐn* [should be used] first.[254]

253. A *shēng* 升 (Jp: *shō*) was a traditional unit of measurement of volume used in East Asia. The exact volume varied depending on the time period and region it was used, but it was standardized as approximately 1.8 liters during the Meiji period in Japan.

254. Of the above-mentioned formulae, only *Bàn Xià Xiè Xīn Tāng* 半夏瀉心湯 is explained in

[Only] after [the physician] has elucidated the true pattern and used these [formulae], and [the patient] has ceased to vomit, *Guì Zhī Jiā Fù Zǐ Tāng* [may] govern this [pattern]. The efficacy [of the drug] is divine [when used in this way].

又た云ふ、惡寒・發熱・頭痛・煩騒して、心下に結聚ありて、之れを按して暗然として冷氣ありて時々鳴動する者、桂枝加附子湯の正症なり。

Furthermore, [when] the patient presents with chills, heat [effusion], headache, vexation, gathering and binding in the region below the heart, a cold qì that can be subtly felt when pressing [the region], and occasional rumbling movements [in the abdomen], [this] is the true pattern for *Guì Zhī Jiā Fù Zǐ Tāng.*

又た云ふ、時々五心煩熱、心氣樂しまず。羸痩倦怠し、或るひは心下に現然として塊あり。之れを按せば、冷氣ありて鳴動する者。まづ大黄附子湯を與へ、毒を下して後、桂枝加附子湯を用ひて可なり。

---

a separate section. There are many different versions of *Fú Líng Tāng* 茯苓湯 (Jp: *Bukuryō-Tō*; poria decoction). Hence, it is unclear which formula the author refers to. The extract preparations of *Dà Bàn Xià Tāng* 大半夏湯 (Jp: *Dai-Hange-Tō*; major pinellia decoction), *Xiǎo Bàn Xià Jiā Fú Líng Tāng* 小半夏加茯苓湯 (Jp: *Shō-Hange-Ka-Bukuryō-Tō*; minor pinellia decoction plus poria), *Fú Líng Zé Xiè Tāng* 茯苓澤瀉湯 (Jp: *Bukuryō-Takusha-Tō*; poria and alisma decoction) and *Fú Líng Yǐn* 茯苓飲 (Jp: *Bukryō-In*; poria beverage) are covered by the Japanese National Health Insurance program as prescription drugs and may be sold in Japanese drug stores as over-the-counter drugs. *Dà Bàn Xià Tāng* is currently indicated by the MHLW for the following symptoms: vomiting, dry heaving, nausea, and queasiness in persons with moderate or weak physical strength who have a feeling of a knot in the solar plexus (體力中等度以下で、みぞおちがつかえた感じがあるものの次の諸症：嘔吐、むかつき、はきけ、惡心). *Xiǎo Bàn Xià Jiā Fú Líng Tāng* is currently indicated by the MHLW for the following symptoms: morning sickness, vomiting, nausea, and gastritis in persons who feel queasy and occasionally vomit. This drug may be used regardless of physical strength (體力に關わらず使用でき、惡心があり、ときに嘔吐するものの次の諸症：つわり、嘔吐、惡心、胃炎). *Fú Líng Zé Xiè Tāng* is currently indicated by the MHLW for the following symptoms: gastritis and gastrointestinal weakness in persons with moderate or weak physical strength who have either an upset stomach, nausea, or vomiting and have thirst (體力中等度以下で、胃のもたれ、惡心、嘔吐のいずれかがあり、渇きを覺えるものの次の諸症：胃炎、胃腸虛弱). *Fú Líng Yǐn* is currently indicated by the MHLW for the following symptoms: gastritis, neurotic gastritis, gastrointestinal weakness, and heartburn in persons with moderate or weak physical strength who have nausea, heartburn, upper abdominal distension, or oliguria (體力中等度以下で、はきけや胸やけ、上腹部膨滿感があり尿量減少するものの次の諸症：胃炎、神經性胃炎、胃腸虛弱、胸やけ).

Furthermore, the patient [may] present with occasional heat vexation in the five hearts and depressed heart qì.[255] In some cases, the patient may present with marked emaciation and fatigue or an apparent lump in the region below the heart. Upon palpation, the patient may experience cold qì and rumbling and stirring [in the abdomen]. *Dà Huáng Fù Zǐ Tāng*[256] should be first administered [to the patient], and after precipitating the toxin, *Guì Zhī Jiā Fù Zǐ Tāng* may be used.

又た云ふ、心痛久しく止まず。心下痞鞕、毒、心・脾に客し上衝して、心をせめ痛む者に用ひて大いに效あり。然れども腹底に冷氣あるを眼として用ゆべし。

Furthermore, [the patient may] also present with enduring heart pain that does not cease. [In cases when the patient presents with] glomus and hardness in the region below the heart and a toxin that has settled in the heart and spleen and surges upward, attacking the heart and causing pain, [this formula] is extremely effective. However, [the medicinal] should be used on the basis of the presence of a cold qì in the depths of the abdomen.

又た云ふ、寒疝、心腹疼痛、手足逆冷して身體拘攣の者、みな此の方を用ひてしるしあり。

Furthermore, all patients who present with cold mounting,[257] pain in the heart [region or] abdomen, or counterflow cold of the extremities accompanied by generalized hypertonicity are indicated for the use of this formula.

則ち桂枝加附子湯の方
Guì Zhī Jiā Fù Zǐ Tāng

桂枝・芍藥・附子・大棗（各七分半）・生姜・甘草（各五分）。

255. The five hearts (Ch: *wǔ xīn fán rè* 五心煩熱; *goshin-hannetsu*) refers to the feeling of heat in the palms of hands, soles of feet and in the chest, accompanied by uneasiness or restlessness.
256. *Dà Huáng Fù Zǐ Tāng* 大黄附子湯 (Jp: *Daiō-Bushi-Tō*; rhubarb and aconite decoction) is discussed in its own section in this book.
257. Cold mounting (Ch: *hán shàn* 寒疝; Jp: *kansen*) refers to acute abdominal pain due to cold, also called cold-induced colic or cold abdominal colic.

guì zhī	桂枝	7.5 fēn
sháo yào	芍藥	7.5 fēn
fù zǐ	附子	7.5 fēn
dà zǎo	大棗	7.5 fēn
shēng jiāng	生姜	5 fēn
gān cǎo	甘草	5 fēn

右六味、水一盞八分を以て、六分に煮とる。

Boil the above six ingredients in one cup and eight *fēn* of water to make six *fēn* of the decoction.

附子湯之圖

Illustration for the Fù Zǐ Tāng[258] [Pattern] 附子湯

圖の如く、心下悸して痞鞕、腹拘攣、小便不利、或るひは腹痛、或るひは身攣痛の者。余、此の方を數しば用ひ、數しば效有りて、その傳に云ふ、「この『痞鞕』と云ふ者、敢へて痞鞕するに非ず」。然れども心下の邊に結聚する處ありて、之れを按せば、暗然として冷氣あり。是れ則ち附子の與る所なり。謹んで腹診を審らかにせざれば、方症相對することを得べからず。

As shown in the illustration, the patient presents with palpitations in the region below the heart, glomus and hardness, abdominal hypertonicity, inhibited urination, and in some cases abdominal or generalized hypertonic pain. I have often used this formula and obtained an effective result. According to one text, "This 'glomus and hardness' does not necessarily mean [severe] glomus and hardness." However, there is gathering and binding present in the sides of the region below the heart, in which a cold qì can be subtly felt when pressed [during the abdominal examination]. This is [the pattern] for *fù zǐ*. If the abdominal pattern is not carefully elucidated, [the physician] will be unable to [correctly] perform formula-pattern matching.

258. The formula for *Fù Zǐ Tāng* 附子湯 (Jp: *Bushi-Tō*; aconite decoction) was originally found in *Jīn Guì Yào Lüè* and *Shāng Hán Lùn*. At present, this formula is not covered by the Japanese National Health Insurance program and is not commonly used in Japan.

又た云ふ、心下悸し且つ痞鞕、胸下の兩傍に結聚する者。此れを診察するに、よく心氣を定靜し、之れを按して自づから暗然として腹底に冷氣あるを覺ふ。或るひは腹拘攣、小便不利、或るひは時々腹痛する者、これ全き附子湯の正症なり。學ぶ者、もちひて以て其の奇功をしるべし。

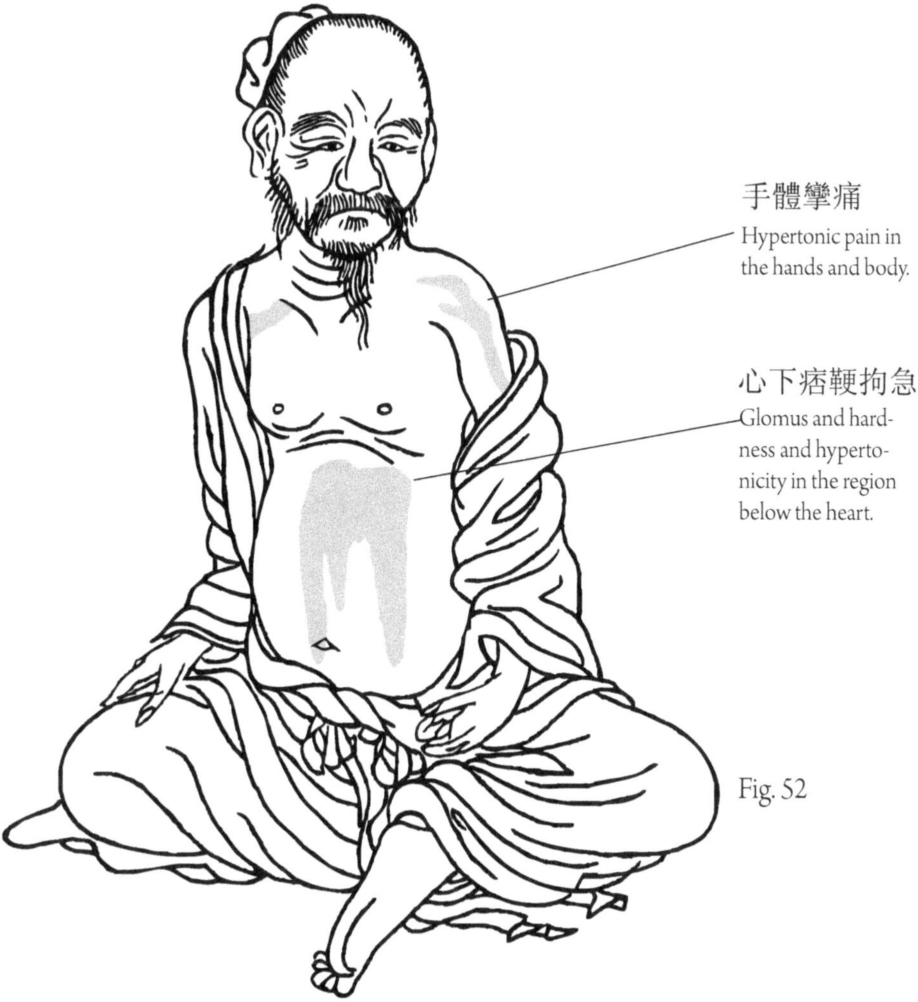

Fig. 52

Furthermore, [the patient may present with] palpitations in the region below the heart, glomus and hardness, and bilateral gathering and binding in the rib-sides below the chest. When examining this [type of patient, the physician should] quiet his heart qì and press [the abdomen]; a subtle cold qì can be naturally felt in the depths of the abdomen. When the patient presents with abdominal hypertonicity, inhibited urination, or in some cases occasional abdominal pain, this is truly the right pattern for *Fù Zǐ Tāng*. [If] the student [of abdominal patterns] uses the formula [correctly], he will understand its extraordinary efficacy.

又た一症。或る人云ふ、病人、舌上赤くただれ、皮を剥ぐが如く、食鹽の味に痛みを覺へ、食ふこと能はず。食する時は津を吐く。或るひは口中ねばり、或るひは涸渴する者。產後に此の症多し。男子も亦たあり。附子湯の方内においひて、當歸八分を加ふ(但し伊吹に非ざれば、効なし)。又た鹿胎子の霜一錢を兼用すべし。

Here is another pattern [that matches the formula]. According to one person, patients [who present with this pattern] have ulceration of the tongue, and the skin appears as if it is being peeled off. The patient feels pain when eating and thus is unable to eat; he ejects liquid when eating. Some patients present with a sticky feeling inside the mouth and others present with desiccation and thirst.[259] This pattern is common in postpartum women. [However,] men also present with [this pattern]. Add eight *fēn* of *dāng guī* to the formula for *Fù Zǐ Tāng*. (However, unless the Ibuki [variety] is used, it will be ineffective). Furthermore, one *qián* of charred *lù tāi* may be used simultaneously.

則ち附子湯の方
Fù Zǐ Tāng

茯苓・芍藥・附子(各六分)・朮(八分)・人參(四分)。

fú líng	茯苓	6 fēn
sháo yào	芍藥	6 fēn
fù zǐ	附子	6 fēn
[bái] zhú	[白]朮	8 fēn
rén shēn	人參	4 fēn

五味、水一盞六分を以て、六分に煮とる。

Boil the above five ingredients in one cup and six *fēn* of water to make six *fēn* of the decoction.

259. Desiccation and thirst (Ch: *hé kě* 涸渴; Jp: *kokatsu*) refers to a feeling of dryness of the mouth with a desire to drink.

又た云ふ、茯苓は赤。芍藥は眞の生干。附子は大にして十戔の物。朮は唐。人參は竹節を用ゆべし。但し自然に生じやせたる者可なり。凡そ諸藥、近世糞汁を用つて作りたるは効なし。

Moreover, the red [variety of] *fú líng* [should be used]. *Sháo yào* that has been correctly half dried [should be used]. Large *fù zǐ* of ten *qián* in size [should be used]. *Zhú* refers to the Chinese variety [i.e., *cāng zhú*]. *Zhú jié rén shēn* should be used for *rén shēn*. However, [only herbs] that are grown in nature are acceptable. Any medicinal [ingredient] that is grown in manure, as is done in recent generations, will be ineffective.

理中加附子湯之圖

Illustration of Lǐ Zhōng Jiā Fù Zǐ Tāng[260] 理中加附子湯

圖の如く、心下痞鞕・小便不利・胸中痹、或るひは急痛・急迫・上衝して、手足厥冷、惡寒の者。

As shown in the illustration, the patient presents with glomus and hardness in the region below the heart, inhibited urination, and chest impediment. In some cases, the patient presents with acute pain, distress, upward surging, reversal cold of the extremities, or chills.

260. The formula for *Lǐ Zhōng Jiā Fù Zǐ Tāng* 理中加附子湯 (Jp: *Richū-Ka-Bushi-Tō*; center-rectifying decoction plus aconite) appears to have been copied from *Sān Yīn Jí Yī Bìng Zhèng Fāng Lùn*《三因極一病症方論》(Jp: *San'in-Kyokuitsu-Byōshō-Ron*; A Unified Treatise on Diseases, Patterns, and Remedies According to the Three Causes) published by Chén Yán 陳言 (Jp: Chin Gen; 1131–1189) in 1174, although many Japanese sources claim it was taken from *Tài Píng Huì Mín Hé Jì Jú Fāng*《太平惠民和劑局方》(Jp: *Taihei-Keimin-Wazai-Kyokuh Ō*; Tài Píng Imperial Grace Pharmacy Formulas. It is also known as *Fù Zǐ Lǐ Zhōng Tāng* 附子理中湯 (Jp: *Bushi-Richū-Tō*; aconite center-rectifying decoction) or *Fù Zǐ Rén Shēn Tāng* 附子人參湯 (Jp: *Bushi-Ninjin-Tō*; aconite and ginseng decoction). In Japan, it is commonly known as *Bushi-Richū-Tō* 附子理中湯. The extract preparation of the formula is covered by the Japanese National Health Insurance program as a prescription drug and is also commonly sold in Japanese drug stores as an over-the-counter drug. It is currently indicated by the MHLW for: gastrointestinal weakness, diarrhea, vomiting, stomach pain, abdominal pain, and acute or chronic gastritis in persons with weak physical strength who have a severe cold feeling in the extremities and are easily fatigued (體力虛弱で、手足の冷えが強く、疲れやすいものの次の諸症：胃腸虛弱、下痢、嘔吐、胃痛、腹痛、急・慢性胃炎).

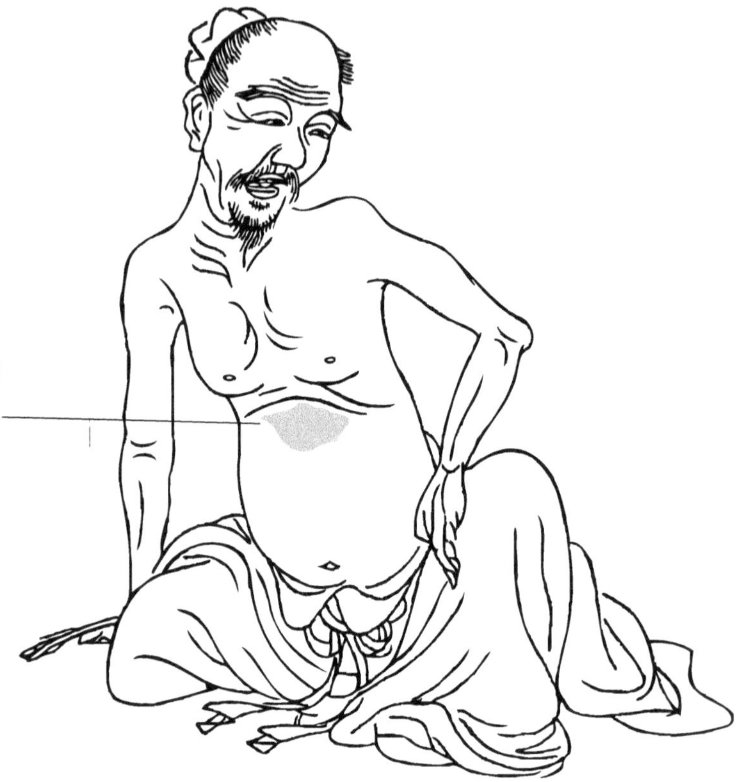

Fig. 53

又た云ふ、心腹痛、嘔吐して下痢、或るひは煩熱・悪寒、或るひは噎逆の者、この方に効あり。

Furthermore, this formula is effective in patients who present with gripping pain in the heart [region] and abdomen, vomiting and retching, heat vexation, chills, or counterflow dysphagia.[261]

則ち理中加附子湯の方
Lǐ Zhōng Jiā Fù Zǐ Tāng

261. In traditional Chinese medical theory, a distinction was made between vomiting and retching: vomiting (Ch: *tù* 吐; Jp: *to*) referred to the forcible expulsion of gastric contents through the mouth, and retching (Ch: *ǒu* 嘔; Jp: *ō*) referred to making the sounds and movements of vomiting bringing up little or nothing from the stomach. However, many Japanese physicians, including the author, do not differentiate the two, and often use the expression *ǒu tù* 嘔吐 as a general word for vomiting.

桂枝・甘草(各八分)・竹節人参・唐蒼朮・乾姜(各六分)・附子(一戔)。

guì zhī	桂枝	8 fēn
gān cǎo	甘草	8 fēn
zhú jié rén shēn	竹節人参	6 fēn
cāng zhú	蒼朮	6 fēn
gān jiāng	乾姜	6 fēn
fù zǐ	附子	1 qián

右六味、水二盞を以て、六分に煮とる。

Boil the above six ingredients in two cups of water to make six *fēn* of the decoction.

余、此の方、身體厥冷、大便自利の者に、數しば用ひて數しば効を奏す。然れども何れも皆、心下に痞満するを以て此の証の眼的とすべし。

I have often used this formula [to treat] patients who present with generalized reversal cold and uninhibited defecation.[262] However, in all cases, glomus and fullness in the region below the heart should be used as the [primary] indication for this pattern.

眞武湯之圖

Illustration of Zhēn Wǔ Tāng[263] 眞武湯

262. Uninhibited defecation (Ch: *dà biàn zì lì* 大便自利; Jp: *daiben-jiri*) refers to spontaneous diarrhea, that is, diarrhea not attributable to purgation.

263. The formula for *Zhēn Wǔ Tāng* 眞武湯 (Jp: *Shinbu-Tō*; true warrior decoction) was originally found in *Shāng Hán Lùn*. The formula was originally called black turtle decoction (Ch: *Xuán Wǔ Tāng* 玄武湯; Jp: *Genbu-Tō*) in reference to Xuán Wǔ 玄武, the Chinese mythological creature/spirit of the North; in traditional Chinese five-phase (Ch: *wǔ xíng* 五行; Jp: *go-gyō*) theory, the North was associated with the kidneys. The name of the formula was apparently later changed during the reign of Emperor Zhēnzōng 真宗 (Jp: *Shinsō*; 968–1022 CE) of the *Sòng* (宋) dynasty (Jp: *Sō*; 960–1279 CE) to avoid using the character 玄, which had been decreed to be a taboo character used in the personal name of the emperor. The extract preparation of the formula is covered by the Japanese National Health Insurance program as a prescription drug, and is also commonly sold in Japanese drug stores as an over-the-counter drug. It is currently indicated by the MHLW for: diarrhea, acute or chronic gastroenteritis, gastrointestinal weakness, dizziness, palpitations, common cold, edema, eczema, dermatitis, and itchy skin in persons with weak physical strength who have cold extremities, fatigue, occasional diarrhea, abdominal pain, or

圖の如く、腹滿これを按せば軟にして拘攣し、あるひは心下悸して、時々目眩し、身瞤動し、或るひは腹痛惡寒し、小便不利、或るひは嘔する者。又た云ふ、此の症、四支疼重、或るひは沈重疼痛する者間々あり。其の餘、何病ひをとはず、前に云ふ如く腹診

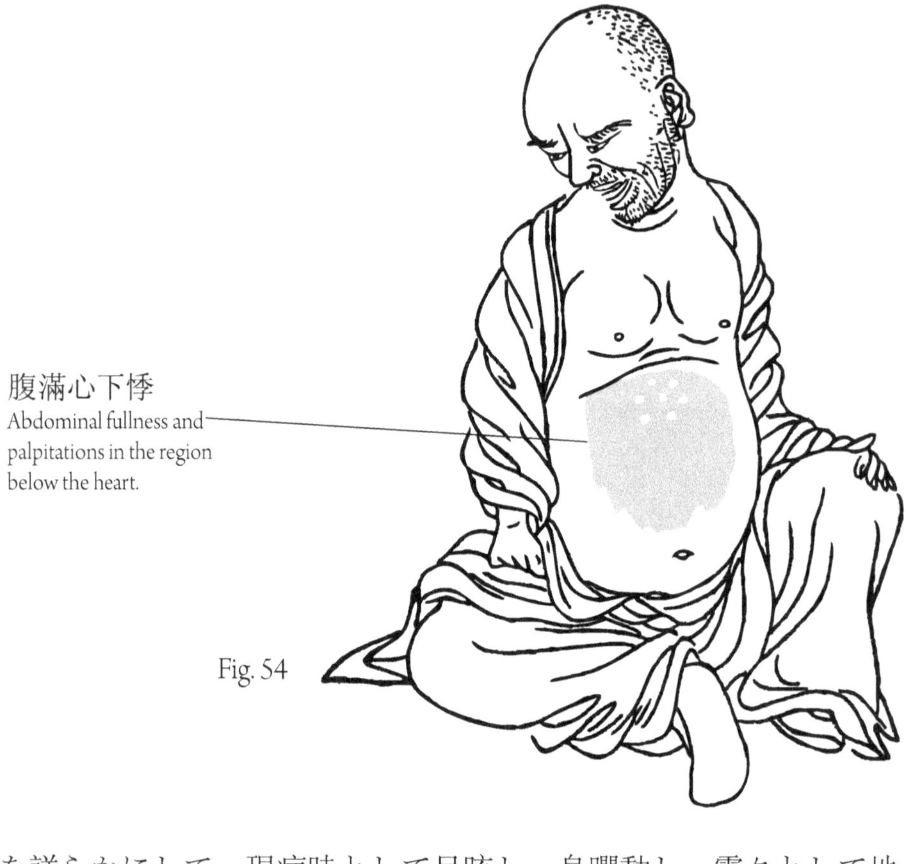

Fig. 54

を詳らかにして、現症時として目眩し、身瞤動し、震々として地に擗たんと欲する者を眼として、之れを用ひて其の効有らざることなし。

As shown in the illustration, the patient presents with abdominal fullness; the abdomen is soft when pressed, and hypertonicity [can be felt]. In some cases, the patient may present with palpitations in the region below the heart, occasional dizzy vision, or generalized twitching. In other cases, the patient may present with abdominal pain, chills, inhibited urination, or retching. Furthermore, in this pattern, the patient presents

---

dizziness (體力虛弱で、冷えがあって、疲勞倦怠感があり、ときに下痢、腹痛、めまいがあるものの次の諸症：下痢、急・慢性胃腸炎、胃腸虛弱、めまい、動悸、感冒、むくみ、濕疹・皮膚炎、皮膚のかゆみ).

with heavy aching limbs or [generalized] heaviness accompanied by pain.[264] In addition, regardless of [the name of] the disease [that the patient presents with], if [the physician] elucidates [the pattern] through the aforementioned [method of] abdominal examination and finds that the patient has dizzy vision, generalized twitching, and [violent] shaking as if [the body is] being thrown to the ground, there are no cases [in which the medicinal] is not effective.

又た云ふ、此の症にして、腹底に寒冷を覺ゆる者大ひにあり。附子の分量、或るひはは一倍、或るひは二倍、三倍に加ふるの多少。みな、腹底の冷、或るひは寒の現然たるか、暗然たるか。その厚薄淺深を以て、附子の多少を考ふべし。すべて附子を隊伍するの法、此の言を以てかんがふべし。

Furthermore, patients who present with this pattern feel great coldness in the depths of the abdomen. With regard to the quantity of *fù zǐ* [to be used], in some cases, the quantity [as written in the formula listed here] should be used, and in other cases, two or three times that quantity should be used. In all cases, [the quantity depends on] if coldness is present in the depths of the abdomen, and if that coldness is [readily] apparent or hidden [i.e., can only be subtly felt on palpation]. The quantity of *fù zǐ* [to be used] should be determined on the basis of the thickness and depth [of the toxin]. This saying [applies] when considering any formula that includes *fù zǐ*.

則ち眞武湯の方
Zhēn Wǔ Tāng

茯苓・芍藥・生姜（各七分半）・唐蒼朮（五分）・附子（四分）。

fú líng	茯苓	7.5 fēn
sháo yào	芍藥	7.5 fēn
shēng jiāng	生姜	7.5 fēn
cāng zhú	蒼朮	5 fēn
fù zǐ	附子	4 fēn

264. Heavy pain (normally written as Ch: *zhòng tòng* 重痛; Jp: *jūtsū*) refers to a pain accompanied by a sensation of heaviness.

右五味、水一盞六分を以て、六分に煮とる。

Boil the above five ingredients in one cup and six *fēn* of water to make six *fēn* of the decoction.

余、此の方を數しば用ひて効を得ること有るを云ふ。たとへば半身不遂の者、此の症にして、其の腹底寒冷、且つ項背強急、痰喘ありて、時々發熱・頭痛、腹中塊物あり。之れを按して痛む者、則ち此の方に附子を益すこと三倍して、葛根湯を合して本劑大劑を以て與へ、『德本十九方』中の順氣丸を兼用すること毎夜一錢二分。此くの如くかさね進めて、その治を奏すること多し。

I have often used this formula and obtained successful results. For example, some patients who present with hemiplegia have cold in the depths of the abdomen, stiffness of the nape and back, phlegm panting, occasional heat effusion [accompanied by] headache, and a lump [or lumps] in the abdomen.[265] When the [abdomen] is pressed and pain is present, increase [the quantity of] *fù zǐ* in this formula threefold and mix this formula with *Gé Gēn Tāng* and administer [the formulas together as a] great [i.e., combined] formula. According to *Tokuhon-Ō-Jūku-Hō*, one *qián* and two *fēn* of *Junki-Gan*,[266] may [also] be simultaneously administered each night. When [these formulae are] repeatedly [administered in] this way, the treatment is usually effective.

眞武葛根湯の合方
Zhēn Wǔ Gé Gēn Tāng[267]

265. Phlegm panting (Ch: *tán chuǎn* 痰喘; Jp: *tanzen*) refers to difficulty in breathing due to the presence of phlegm.

266. As explained in the text, *Junki-Gan* 順氣丸 (Ch: *Shùn Qì Wán*; qì-normalizing pill) is an original formula by Nagata Tokuhon 永田德本. As such, this formula is not covered by the Japanese National Health Insurance program and was probably never commonly used in Japan.

267. *Zhēn Wǔ Gé Gēn Tāng* 眞武葛根湯 (Jp: *Shinbu-Kakkon-Tō*; true warrior pueraria decoction) is more commonly known in Japan as *Kakkon-Ka-Jutsu-Bu-Tō* 葛根加朮附湯 (Ch: *Gé Gēn Jiā Zhú Fù Tāng*; pueraria decoction plus atractylodes and aconite). It appears to be an original formula of Yoshimasu Tōdō and originally published in *Hōki*《方機》(Formula Mechanisms; 1811 CE). Although the formula is not currently well known in Japan, the extract preparation of the formula is approved by the MHLW to be sold in Japanese drug stores as an over-the-counter drug. It is currently indicated by the MHLW for: stiff shoulders, scapular neuralgia, and rheumatoid arthritis of the upper body in persons with aversion to cold with fever, headache, and tension in the neck or scapular region (惡寒發熱して、頭痛があり、項部・肩背部に緊張感あるものの次の諸症：肩こり、肩甲部の神經痛、上半身の關節リウマチ).

葛根(七分)・麻黄(五分)・芍藥・大棗・生姜・茯苓(各六分)・桂枝・甘草・附子(各四分)・唐蒼朮(五分)。

gé gēn	葛根	7 fēn	
má huáng	麻黄	5 fēn	
sháo yào	芍藥	6 fēn	
dà zǎo	大棗	6 fēn	
shēng jiāng	生姜	6 fēn	
fú líng	茯苓	6 fēn	
guì zhī	桂枝	4 fēn	
gān cǎo	甘草	4 fēn	
fù zǐ	附子	4 fēn	
cāng zhú	蒼朮	5 fēn	Chinese

右十味、水二盞を以て、六分に煮とる。前に云ふ如く、腹底の寒冷・厚薄淺深に因りて、謹んで附子の多少を考ふべし。

Boil the above ten ingredients in two cups of water to make six *fēn* of the decoction. As previously mentioned, the quantity of *fù zǐ* [in the formula] should be carefully considered based on the presence of cold in the abdomen and the thickness and depth of the toxin.

徳本翁順氣丸の方
Venerable Tokuhon's Junki-Gan

大黄・芒硝(各等分)。

dà huáng	大黄	equal amounts
máng xiāo	芒硝	

右二味、末と爲して丸す(丸する時に臨みて、蜜を少し入りて丸と爲べし)。右順氣丸の主治、血症にして塊物有りて、之れを按していたむ者、何病ひをとはず毎夜一匁を白湯にて送下す。久しく用ひて治せざることなし。

Grind the above two ingredients into a powder to make pills (when making the pills, [the powder] should be mixed with a little honey). The aforementioned *Junki-Gan* is primarily indicated for blood pathoconditions in which a lump is present; regardless of the [name of] the disease [that was diagnosed], if the patient presents with pain when [the abdomen] is pressed, one *qián* [of the drug] should be taken with hot water each night. If used for a long period of time, there will be no [patient with the pattern] who is uncured.

古人、附子を用ひて効ある症を記す。古人某云ふ、「寒疝にして心腹脇皆痛み、諸藥効なきに、蜜製の烏頭丸を用ひて神妙也」云々。余、按ずるに、此の症、惡寒・厥冷、手足厥逆して、腰足引痛し、或るひは腹痛、或るひは體痛み、時として上衝し、惡風煩燥、或るひは絞痛しのびがたき者に、之れを用ひてしばしば効あり。

The ancients wrote about the patterns for which *fù zǐ* is effective. A certain ancient [physician] once said that "honey-processed *Wū Tóu Wán*[268] is divinely effective in all cases of cold mounting in which pain (that cannot be treated by other drugs) is present in the heart [region], abdomen, and rib-sides." I believe that this formula is often successful for patterns in which the patient presents with aversion to cold, reversal cold in the extremities, or for cases of taut pain in the lumbus and legs, cases of abdominal pain, cases of a generalized pain that often surges upward and is accompanied by aversion to wind and vexation and agitation,[269] or cases of unbearable gripping pain.[270]

則ち蜜製烏頭丸の方
Honey-Processed Wū Tóu Wán

268. There are many different versions of *Wū Tóu Wán* 烏頭丸 (Jp: *Uzu-Gan*; aconite pill). This version, which contains only honey-processed *wū tóu* 烏頭, seems to have been taken from *Pǔ Jì Fāng*《普濟方》(Jp: *Fusai-Hō*; Universal Salvation Formulary), published by Zhū Sù 朱橚 (Jp: Shu Shuku; ca. 1361–1425 CE) et al. in 1406 CE. At present, this formula is not covered by the Japanese National Health Insurance program and is not commonly used in Japan.
269. Aversion to wind (Ch: *wù fēng* 惡風; Jp: *ōfū*) refers to a strong dislike of wind, also known as wind intolerance in traditional Chinese medical theory. Although physicians of the Ancient School (Jp: *Kohō-Ha* 古方派) of Kampō medicine, including the author of this book, generally focused on clinical symptoms in performing diagnosis and eschewed the complexities of traditional Chinese medical theory, they occasionally used concepts such as aversion to cold, wind, or heat as indications for treatment.
270. Gripping pain (Ch: *jiǎo tòng* 絞痛; Jp: *kōtsū*) refers to an acute pain in the chest or abdomen, often caused by spasm, obstruction or twisting, also called spasm and pain.

大烏頭角を去りて四つに破り、白蜜一合を以て煎じ盡して、之れをとる。よく焙り干し末となし、別に熟蜜を以て丸とす。毎日之れを服するに、冷へたる鹽湯を以て送下す。余、之れを用ゆるの傳に云ふ、初め五分を用ひて瞑眩せず、まして七分に至る。尚瞑眩せず。又たまして一戔、或るひは一戔五分、二戔に至るべし。

Remove the skin of a large *wū tóu,* break into four pieces, completely boil in one gě of *bái mì,* and collect the [residue of the decoction].[271] Mix-fry, dry, and grind [the ingredients] into powder. Add processed honey separately to make pills. [The pills are] to be taken every day with chilled salt water. According to a text that I have referred to, when five *fēn* is used at first, the patient will not experience dizziness [i.e., side effects]. Even when the dose is increased to seven *fēn,* the patient will still not experience dizziness. [The quantity] may be increased up to one *qián,* or in some cases up to one *qián* and five *fēn* or two *qián.*

又た姜附湯の方法
The Method [to Make] Jiāng Fù Tāng

大附子（四つにわり、一枚）・生姜（十枚）。右二味、水一盞を以て、七分に煎じ、溫服す。

[Use a] large *fù zǐ* (broken into four pieces, use one piece), *shēng jiāng* (ten pieces). Boil the above two ingredients in water to make seven *fēn* of the decoction; drink [while still] warm.[272]

冷瘴・寒熱往來、頭痛・身疼、痰を吐し、或るひは汗多くして渇し、或るひは自利して煩燥する者、之れを用ひて妙効あり。余、此の方を用ひて按ずるに、其の人痰喘甚だしく、手足厥冷・下

271. *Gě* 合 (Jp: *gō*) is a traditional unit of volume that was used in East Asia. The exact volume differed depending on the region and period in which it was used, but during the Meiji period in Japan, it was calculated as one-tenth of a *shēng* 升 (Jp: *shō*), that is, 180.4ml.
272. There are several formulas with the name *Jiāng Fù Tāng* 薑附湯 (Jp: *Kyō-Bu-Tō*; ginger and aconite decoction). This version appears to have been taken from *Bèi Jí Qiān Jīn Yào Fāng* (Jp: *Bikyū-Senkin-Yōhō*), albeit with different quantities of ingredients. At present, this formula is not covered by the Japanese National Health Insurance program and is not commonly used in Japan.

利・身體厥逆、或るひは自利する者、死に向はんと欲する者に、數しば用ひて數しば効を得たり。學者、用ひて効をしるべし。

[This formula] is wondrously effective for patients who present with cold miasmic diseases, alternating heat [effusion] and [aversion to] cold, headache, generalized pain, or ejection of phlegm, or for patients present with copious sweating and thirst, or for patients who present with uninhibited vexation and agitation. I have often used this formula and experienced its efficacy in [treating] patients who present with: severe phlegm panting, reversal cold of the extremities, diarrhea, generalized reverse flow, patients who have spontaneous [diarrhea], or patients who are facing [i.e., on the verge of] death. The student [of abdominal patterns] will [also] come to understand the efficacy of the formula when it is used [in clinical practice].

又た大渇引飲の者に、附子の症あり、石膏の症あり。其の分別の密傳有つて云ふ、「たとへば病人大ひに熱し大渇引飲の者に、身屈(かが)まり縮む者、その腹底を按じて寒冷なる者は、附子の症也。又た身體厥冷し、手足厥逆すといへども、身を伸ばし衾の中をのり出づる者、其の腹底を按ずるに少しく熱するは石膏の症也」。

Moreover, of the patients who present with great thirst with fluid intake, some have the pattern for *fù zǐ*, and others have the pattern for *shí gāo*. Concerning the differentiation [of patterns], there is a secret text that explains, "If the patient has a high fever and great thirst with fluid intake, a back that is curved and contracted, and cold that can be felt in the depths of the abdomen upon palpation, it is the [right] pattern for *fù zǐ*. [By contrast,] in the pattern for *shí gāo*, although the patient presents with generalized reversal cold and reverse flow in the extremities, [the patient] stretches out his body and pops out of the bedding. Upon palpation of the depths of the abdomen, a slight heat [can be felt]."

朮防己去石膏加茯苓芒硝湯之圖[273]

Illustration of [the Pattern for] Jutsu-Bōi-Kyo-Sekkō-Ka-Bukuryō-Bōshō-Tō[274] 朮防己去石膏加茯苓芒硝湯

273. In Japan, the character *jǐ* 己 in [*mù*] *fáng jǐ* [木]防己 is always written with the character *yǐ* 已, thus the Japanese pronunciation of the herb is [*moku*]*bōi* [木]防已 (Ch: [*mù*] *fáng yǐ*) and never [*moku*]*bōko* (Ch: [*mù*] *fáng jǐ*). Although the names slightly differ in Japan, the herbs themselves are generally the same as those used in China.

274. As later explained in the text, *Jutsu-Bōi-Kyo-Sekkō-Ka-Bukuryō-Bōshō-Tō* 朮防已去石膏

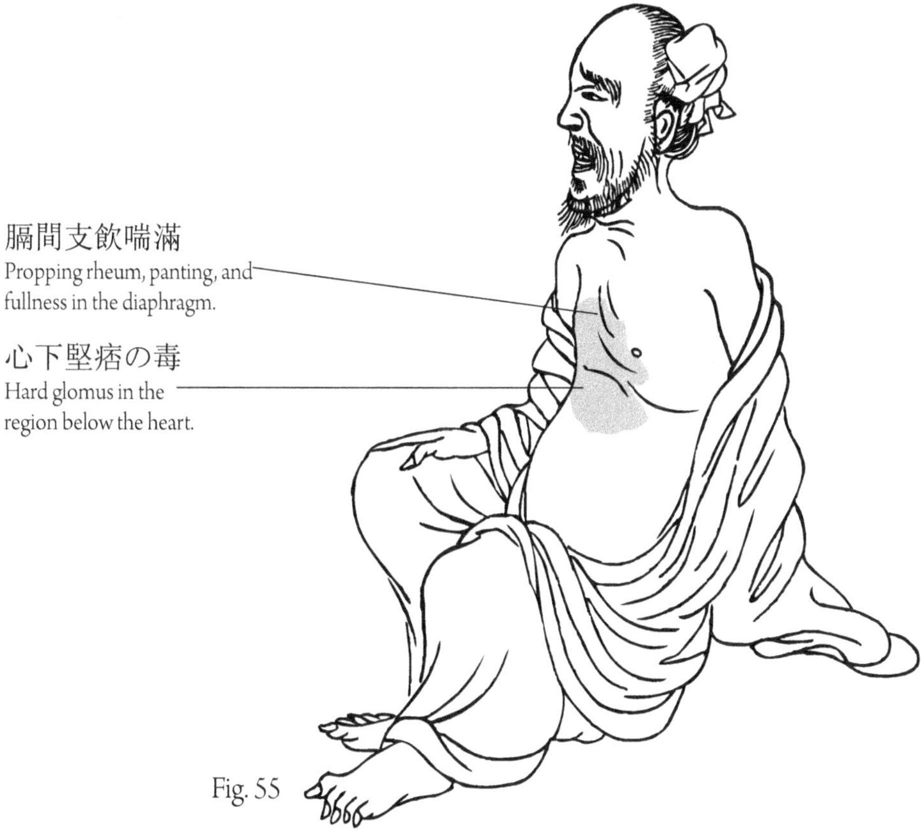

Fig. 55

圖の如く、心下堅痞し、膈間に支飲ありて喘滿し、面色黧黑。其の形腫るが如く水氣あるもの、此の方の正症なり。余、腹診の術を以て藥劑を投ずることを定極するに、凡そ心下の毒動かずして患ふる者多し。たとへば腹中の毒に中りて方症相對して、治方を定極すると云へども、心下の毒さらざる時は食すること能はず。

加茯苓芒硝湯 (Ch: *Zhú Fáng Jǐ Qù Shí Gāo Jiā Fú Líng Máng Xiāo Tāng*; atractylodes and fangji decoction minus gypsum plus poria and mirabilite) is an original formula of the author based on his particular interpretation of the formula for *Mù Fáng Jǐ Qù Shí Gāo Jiā Fú Líng Máng Xiāo Tāng* 木防已去石膏加茯苓芒硝湯 (Jp: *Mokubōi-Kyo-Sekkō-Ka-Bukuryō-Bōshō-Tō*; woody fangji decoction minus gypsum plus poria and mirabilite), which was originally found in *Jīn Guì Yào Lüè*. At present, both formulae are not covered by the Japanese National Health Insurance program and are not commonly used in Japan. However, the extract preparation of the base formula of *Mù Fáng Jǐ Tāng* 木防已湯 (Jp: *mokubōi-tō*; woody fangji decoction) is covered by the Japanese National Health Insurance program as a prescription drug, and may be sold in Japanese drug stores as an over-the-counter drug. It is currently indicated by the MHLW for: palpitations, shortness of breath, bronchial asthma, and edema in persons with moderate or strong physical strength who have a feeling of a knot in the solar plexus and poor complexion (體力中等度以上で、みぞおちがつかえ、血色すぐれないものの次の諸症：動悸、息切れ、氣管支ぜんそく、むくみ).

故に先づ心下の毒を去らんと欲すとも、方症相對せざる時は動かず、治せざるなり。余、之れを苦しむこと久し。近ごろ少しく分別することあるを以て左に記す。

As shown in the illustration, the patient presents with hard glomus in the region below the heart, propping rheum[275] in the diaphragm, panting and fullness, and a soot-black facial complexion. When the patient presents with water qì that causes swelling [i.e., edema], it is the right pattern for this formula. During my thorough investigations concerning the administration of drugs in accordance with abdominal [findings discovered during] examination, I have found that many patients suffer [from a pattern in which] there is an unmoving toxin in the region below the heart. Even in cases in which [the physician] matches the formula according to the pattern and thoroughly investigates the [appropriate] method of treatment to attack the toxin present the abdomen, unless the toxin leaves region below the heart, [the patient] will remain unable to eat. For this reason, although [the physician may] first desire to remove the toxin from the region below the heart, unless the formula and pattern are [correctly] matched, [the toxin] will not be moved and [the patient] will not be cured. I struggled [to understand this pattern] for a long period of time. As I have recently become somewhat able to differentiate [patterns], I shall write my [recent] findings below.

凡そ上衝急迫して心下痞鞕する者、桂枝人參湯の症なり。或るひは只だ心下痞鞕、胸中痹にして時々急痛、小便不利の者、人參湯の症なり。或るひは胸下實滿して、心下痞鞕、四逆散の症なり。或るひは胸下結聚して、心下痞鞕、之れを按して底に冷氣を覺ゆる者、附子湯の症なり。或るひは大便閉、心下痞鞕、且つ心下臍上の問實して、之れを按して痛むこと甚だし、調胃承氣湯の症なり。或るひは心煩・吐下して、心下痞鞕の者、乾姜黄芩黄連人參湯の證なり。或るひは腹中雷鳴して、心下痞鞕の者、半夏瀉心湯の症なり。或るひは便閉、浮腫して心下痞鞕、雷鳴する者、桃花人參湯の症なり。或るひは心胸張出・便閉し、心下痞して鞕滿の者、大陷胸丸の症なり。或るひは腹拘攣・急迫して、心下痞鞕・實滿する者、甘遂半夏湯の症なり。前編の甘遂半夏湯の條下に於いて、つぶさに論ず。其の餘の方、みな之れに倣へ。

Generally speaking, when the patient presents with upward surging, distress, and glomus and hardness in the region below the heart, it is the pattern for *Guì Zhī Rén Shēn*

275. Propping rheum (Ch: *zhī yǐn* 支飲; Jp: *shi-in*) refers to water in the region below the heart with cough and copious phlegm, leading to the inability to lie down and swelling (i.e., edema) and distention of the body.

Tāng. When the patient presents with only glomus and hardness in the region below the heart, chest impediment with occasional acute pain, and inhibited urination, it is the pattern for *Rén Shēn Tāng.* When the patient presents with replete fullness in the region below the chest and glomus and hardness in the region below the heart, it is the pattern for *Sì Nì Sǎn.*[276] When the patient presents with gathering and binding in the region below the chest, glomus and hardness in the region below the heart, and the feeling of a cold qì in the depths [of the abdomen] upon palpation, it is the pattern for *Fù Zǐ Tāng.* When the patient presents with a fecal block, glomus and hardness in the region below the heart, and repletion in the region that is below the heart and above the umbilicus that causes severe pain when pressed, it is the pattern for *Tiáo Wèi Chéng Qì Tāng.* When the patient presents with heart vexation, vomiting and diarrhea, and glomus and hardness in the region below the heart, it is the pattern for *Gān Jiāng Huáng Qín Huáng Lián Rén Shēn Tāng.*[277] When the patient presents with thunderous rumbling in the abdomen and glomus and hardness in the region below the heart, it is the pattern for *Bàn Xià Xiè Xīn Tāng.* When the patient presents with a fecal block, puffy swelling, glomus and hardness in the region below the heart, and thunderous rumbling [in the abdomen], it is the pattern for *Táo Huā Rén Shēn Tāng.*[278] When the patient presents with distention in the heart and chest, fecal block, and glomus and hard fullness in the region below the heart, it is the pattern for *Dà Xiàn Xiōng Wán.* When the patient presents with abdominal hypertonicity and distress, glomus and hardness, and replete fullness in the region below the heart, it is the pattern for *Gān Suì Bàn Xià Tāng.* I have discussed the details [of the formula] in the section for *Gān Suì Bàn Xià Tāng* in the previous volume. Use [the information for] these [formulae] as a reference for all other [related] formulae.

且つ本文に、「朮・防己」とあるは恐らくは訛也。余考ふるに、「朮」の字の一點を落したるが故に、「蒼朮」を隊伍せざるか。今、「蒼朮」を加へて、「朮防己去石膏加茯苓芒硝湯」と爲て用ゆるに、その効いちじるし。或るひは心下痞鞕、飲食停滯して、大便せざる者、大簇丸を兼用して可なり。

276. *Sì Nì Sǎn* 四逆散 (Jp: *Shigyaku-San*; counterflow cold powder) is discussed separately in the next section.

277. The details of *Gān Jiāng Huáng Qín Huáng Lián Rén Shēn Tāng* 乾薑黃芩黃連人參湯 (Jp: *Kankyō-Ōgon-Ōren-Ninjin-Tō*; dried ginger, scutellaria, coptis, and ginseng decoction) are not discussed in this work. The formula was originally found in *Shāng Hán Lùn*. However, at present, this formula is not covered by the Japanese National Health Insurance program and is not commonly used in Japan.

278. The details of *Táo Huā Rén Shēn Tāng* 桃花人參湯 (Jp: *Tōka-Ninjin-Tō*; peach blossom and ginseng decoction) are not discussed in this work, and the source of the formula and its ingredients are unclear.

According to the main text [of *Shāng Hán Lùn*,[279] this formula] contains *zhú fáng jǐ*,[280] but this is likely a [typographical] error. The character *zhú* 朮 is missing a character [before it]; hence, I believe that [the correct word] should be *cāng zhú*. When *cāng zhú* is added to the formula to make *Jutsu-Bōi-Kyo-Sekkō-Ka-Bukuryō-Bōshō-Tō*, its efficacy is remarkable. If the patient presents with glomus and hardness in the region below the heart, collection and stagnation of food and drink, and the inability to defecate, the coadministration of *Taisō-Gan* is permissible.[281]

朮防己去石膏加茯苓亡硝湯の方
Jutsu-Bōi-Kyo-Sekkō-Ka-Bukuryō-Bōshō-Tō

唐蒼朮・防己（各七分半）・桂枝（五分）・茯苓・人參（各一戔）・芒硝（一戔五分）。

cāng zhú	蒼朮	7.5 fēn	Chinese
fáng jǐ	防己	7.5 fēn	
guì zhī	桂枝	5 fēn	
fú líng	茯苓	1 qián	
rén shēn	人參	1 qián	
máng xiāo	芒硝	1 qián and 5 fēn	

279. The author is referring to Chapter 12 of the *Jīn Guì Yào Lüè* (Ch: *Tán Yǐn Ké Sòu Bìng Mài Zhèng Bìng Zhì* 痰飲咳嗽病脈證并治 (Jp: *Tan'in-Gaisō-Byōmyakuō-Hei-Chi*) Pulse, Signs, and Treatment of Diseases Involving Phlegm-Rheum and Cough.
280. The author has interpreted the character *mù* 木 of the herb *mù fáng jǐ* 木防己 (Jp: *mokubōi*; woody fangji [radix cocculi]) as the character *zhú* 朮. That is, the author believes that the correct formula should list *zhú*/ *fáng jǐ* 朮/防己, i.e., a combination of *cāng zhú* 蒼朮 (Jp: *sōjutsu*; rhizoma atractylodes) and *fáng jǐ* 防己 (Jp: *bōi*; fangji [radix stephaniae tetrandrae]). However, at present, the name of the main herb used in this formula is generally considered to be *mù fáng jǐ* 木防己 in both China and Japan. Thus, this interpretation seems to have never received wide support in Japan, and *Mù Fáng Jǐ Tāng* 木防己湯 rather than *Zhú Fáng Jǐ Tāng* 朮防己湯 is currently covered by the Japanese medical insurance system.
281. The formula for *Taisō-Gan* 大簇丸 (Ch: *Tài Cù Wán*; tài cù pill) is an original formula found in *Tōdō-Sensei-Kajuku-Hō*《東洞先生家塾方》(Master Tōdō's Family Formulary). The name was taken from *tài cù* 大簇 (usually written as 太簇), the third note of the Chinese twelve-note musical scale (Ch: *shí èr lǜ* 十二律). At present, this formula is not covered by the Japanese National Health Insurance program and is not commonly used in Japan. However, it has the same ingredients as *Sān Huáng Wán* 三黃丸 and the MHLW-approved *Sān Huáng Xiè Xīn Tāng* 三黃瀉心湯 (Jp: *San'ō-Shashin-Tō*; three yellows heart-draining decoction), albeit with different quantities of the ingredients.

右六味、水一盞八分を以て、六分に煮とり、滓を去りて芒硝を入れ、一度に服す。

Boil the above six ingredients in one cup and eight *fēn* of water to make six *fēn* of the decoction, remove the residue, add *máng xiāo*, and administer together.

大簇丸の方
Taisō-Gan

大黄（十戔）・黄芩・黄連（各五戔）。

dà huáng	大黄	10 qián
huáng qín	黄芩	5 fēn
huáng lián	黄連	5 fēn

右三味、末丸となし、清酒を以て送下す、又た白湯にて送下するも可なり。

Grind the above three ingredients into a powder pill and take with clear sake. It may also be taken with hot water.

四逆散之圖
Illustration of [the Pattern for] Sì Nì Săn[282] 四逆散

圖の如く、臍下の左右、心下或るひは脇下の傍、みな實滿して、たとへば大柴胡湯の腹に似て、胸膈實滿・胸膈攣急する者、所謂積聚家に間々此の方のしやうあり。又た云ふ、凡そ衆病者、此の症、或るひは柴胡湯の症、傍らに有らざることなし。總べて難症・重病を療ずるに、一症の毒を攻むる時は、必ず變じて諸症を

282. The formula for *Sì Nì Săn* 四逆散 (Jp: *Shigyaku-San*; counterflow cold powder) was originally found in *Shāng Hán Lùn.* The extract preparation of the formula is covered by the Japanese National Health Insurance program as a prescription drug, and is also commonly sold in Japanese drug stores as an over-the-counter drug. It is currently indicated by the MHLW for: gastritis, stomach pain, abdominal pain, and neurosis in persons with moderate or strong physical strength who have symptoms such as a heavy painful feeling in the chest and abdomen, anxiety, or insomnia (體力中等度以上で、胸腹部に重苦しさがあり、ときに不安、不眠などがあるもののの次の諸症：胃炎、胃痛、腹痛、神經症).

現はす 。その方法 、みな具はれり 。故に古人の方法大ひに同じふして少しく異なる者多し 。

As shown in the illustration, this formula may be used in cases when replete fullness is present in the left and right sides of the subumbilical region and the regions below the heart or under the rib-sides. [The pattern] is similar to the abdominal [pattern] for *Dà Chái Hú Tāng*, as replete fullness and hypertonicity are present in the chest and diaphragm. This formula may be also used for patients who have what are known as "accumulations and gatherings."[283] Furthermore, patients with comorbid diseases generally also present with the pattern for [one of the variant formulae of] *Chái Hú Tāng*. When any type of intractable or severe disease is treated by attacking the toxin causing the pattern, [the said pattern] will undoubtedly transmutate and manifest into various other patterns. The [ancient] methods [of treatment] all possess [the efficacy to cure such intractable diseases]. Thus, there are many [physicians] now who use almost the same methods [i.e., formulae] of the ancients with only slight differences.

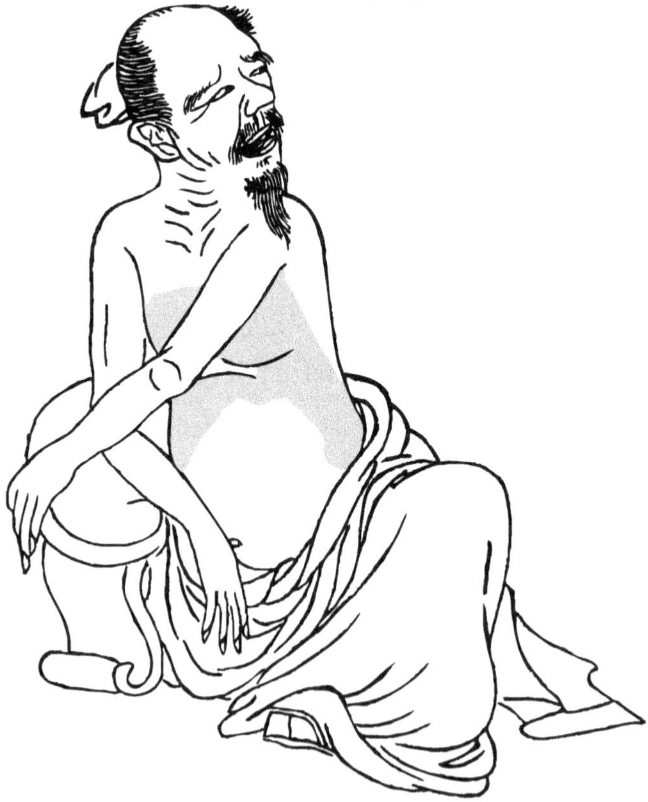

Fig. 56

283. Accumulations and gatherings (Ch: *jī ju* 積聚; Jp: *shakuju*), also known as aggregation-accumulation, is a general term referring to mass formation in the chest and abdomen, also called abdominal mass.

則ち四逆散の方

Sì Nì Săn

芍藥・柴胡・甘草・枳實(各一錢)。

sháo yào	芍藥	1 qián
chái hú	柴胡	1 qián
gān căo	甘草	1 qián
zhĭ shí	枳實	1 qián

右四味 、爲末每服二錢白湯にて送り下す 。

Grind the above four ingredients into a powder and take with two *qián* of hot water.

調胃承氣湯之圖

Illustration for the Tiáo Wèi Chéng Qì Tāng[284] [Pattern]

調胃承氣湯

圖の如く 、心下臍上の間 、實して堅く 、之れを按して病者痛みを覺ゆる者 、此の方の正症なり 。是れ乃ち胃實して大便 。

As shown in the illustration, when the region from below the heart to the supraumbilical region is replete and hard, and the patient feels pain upon palpation [of the abdomen], it is the right pattern for this formula. This is [a case of] stomach repletion and [difficult] defecation.

284. The formula for *Tiáo Wèi Chéng Qì Tāng* 調胃承氣湯 (Jp: *Chōi-Jōki-Tō*; stomach-regulating qì-infusing decoction) was originally found in *Shāng Hán Lùn*. The extract preparation of the formula is covered by the Japanese National Health Insurance program as a prescription drug, and may be sold Japanese drug stores as an over-the-counter drug. It is currently indicated by the MHLW for: constipation and dull headache, hot flashes, eczema, dermatitis, pimples (acne), anorexia (appetite loss), abdominal distension, abnormal intestinal fermentation, and hemorrhoids associated with constipation in persons with moderate physical strength (體力中等度なものの次の諸症：便祕 、便祕に伴う頭重・のぼせ・濕疹・皮膚炎・ふできもの「 にきび 」・食欲不振「 食欲減退 」・腹部膨滿 、腸内異常醗酵・痔などの症狀の緩和).

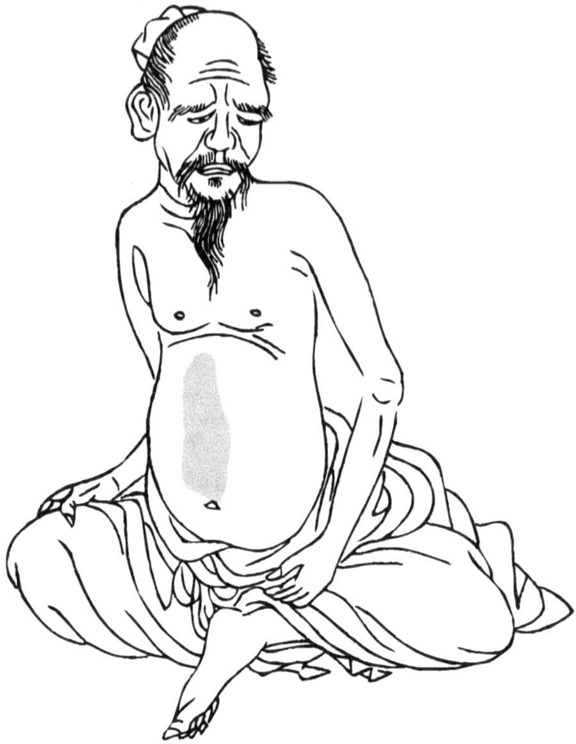

Fig. 57

則ち調胃承氣湯の方
Tiáo Wèi Chéng Qì Tāng

大黄（一戔二分）・甘草・芒硝（各六分）。

dà huáng	大黄	1 qián and 2 fēn
gān cǎo	甘草	6 fēn
máng xiāo	芒硝	6 fēn

右三味、水一盞一分を以て、四分に煮とり、滓を去りて、芒硝を入れ、一度に服す。日々二、三度服す。

Boil the three ingredients in one cup and one *fēn* of water to make six *fēn* of the decoction. After removing the residue, add *máng xiāo* and administer in a single dose. This formula should be administered two or three times daily.

鶴家甘遂桃花湯之圖

Illustration for the Kaku Family's Kanzui-Tōka-Tō[285]

鶴家甘遂桃花

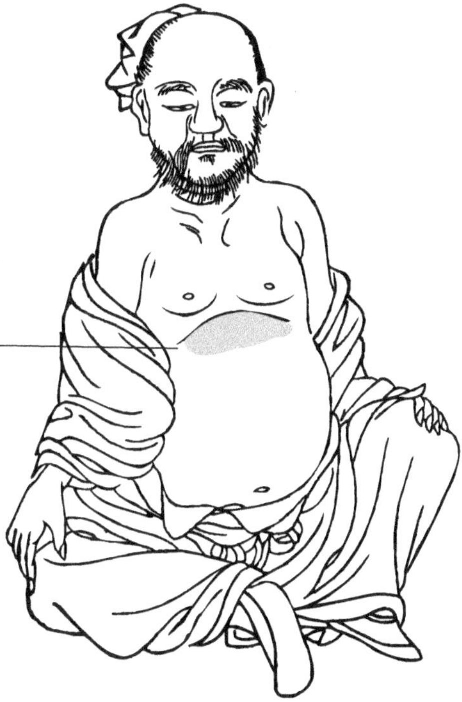

水毒、心下に結聚す
Water toxin binding to the region below the heart.

Fig. 58

圖の如く、四逆散の腹に似て苦滿せず。心下痞滿、之れを按して軟水鳴ずること瀝々として少しく聲あり。又た雷鳴する者もあり。たとへば人參湯、或るひは甘遂半夏湯、或るひは朮防己去石膏加茯苓芒硝湯、或るひは大陷胸丸などをあたへて効なき者、この方尤も効あり。

As shown in the illustration, [this pattern] resembles the abdominal [pattern for] *Sì Nì Săn,* in which bitter fullness is not present. The patient presents with glomus and fullness in the region below the heart. Upon palpation, the abdomen feels soft, and a slight gurgling sound of water [can be heard]. Furthermore, some patients present with thunderous rumbling [in the abdominal region]. This formula is exceptionally effective in cases

285. As implied by the name of the formula, the Kaku Family's *Kanzui-Tōka-Tō* 鶴家甘遂桃花 (Ch: *Hè Jiā Gān Suì Táo Huā Tāng*; the Kaku family's kansui and peach blossom decoction) is an original formula of Kaku Taiei 鶴泰榮. At present, this formula is not covered by the Japanese National Health Insurance program and was perhaps never well known in Japan.

which other formulae such as *Gān Suì Bàn Xià Tāng, Rén Shēn Tāng, Jutsu-Bōi-Kyo-Sekkō-Ka-Bukuryō-Bōshō-Tō*, or *Dà Xiàn Xiōng Wán* have not been effective.

且つ此の一腹症を考へ知る者は、播州二見の處士、室谷某の弟、茶人大口如翁の女直なり。彼、女子にして、古人未だ達せざる所を發明す。是れ醫を好むの厚き、實に斯の道の忠臣ともいふべし。古人の云ふ、「片玉も以て琦とすべし」とは、大口氏の女を謂ふなるべし。

One person who has studied and deeply understood this abdominal pattern was Nao, the wife of the famous tea ceremony master Ōguchi Joō,[286] and younger sister of a certain Mr. Muroya, who lived as a private citizen in the Futami area of Banshū.[287] [Although] she was a woman, she was able to discover levels [of medicine] that the ancients had not yet reached. Her love of medicine was so deep that she could be called a [true] faithful follower of this way [of medicine]. An ancient once said, "A broken shard of jade can also become a beautiful stone."[288] This phrase is most fitting to describe Mr. Ōguchi's wife.

則ち鶴家甘遂桃花湯の方
Kaku Family's Kanzui-Tōka-Tō

甘遂（一戔）・白桃花（一戔五分）・大黄（五分）。

gān suì	甘遂	1 qián
bái táo huā	白桃花	1 qián and 5 fēn
dà huáng	大黄	5 fēn

右三味、水一盞二分を以て六分に煮とり、滓を去りて甘遂の末を入れ、頓に服す。但し空心（すきはら）に服すべし。又た云ふ、

286. Ōguchi Joō 大口如翁 (year of birth unknown–1778 CE) was the son of Ōguchi Shōō 大口樵翁 (1689–1764 CE), who founded the Ōguchi tea school. There is no available information concerning his wife.

287. Banshū is the abbreviated name of Harima Province (Jp: *Harima-No-Kuni* 播磨國), which comprises the southwestern region of present-day Hyōgo Prefecture (Jp: *Hyōgo-Ken* 兵庫縣).

288. In a commentary of *Hòu Hàn Shū*《後漢書》(Jp: *Gokan-Jo*; History of the Later *Hàn* Dynasty) it states that「片玉可以琦、奚必俟盈尺」(...a broken shard of jade can also become a beautiful stone. What need is there for it to be over one cubit [in size?]). One cubit (Ch: *chǐ* 尺; Jp: *shaku*) ranged from approximately 23 to 35 centimeters in length.

前方の症に似て、心悸胸痛して水腫者、黄連桃花散を用ひて可なり。

Boil the three ingredients in one cup and two *fēn* of water to make six *fēn* of the decoction; remove the dregs, add *gān suì* powder, and take at once. However, [the medicinal] should be taken on an empty stomach.[289] Moreover, when the patient presents with [symptoms] similar to the aforementioned pattern [as well as] heart palpitations, chest pain, and water swelling [i.e., edema],[290] *Huáng Lián Táo Huā Sǎn*[291] may be used.

則ち黄連桃花散の方
Huáng Lián Táo Huā Sǎn

白桃花(四戔半)・黄連・大黄(各一戔)。

bái táo huā	白桃花	4.5 qián
huáng lián	黄連	1 qián
dà huáng	大黄	1 qián

右三味、末となし、白湯を以て一戔五分を送下す。瞑眩して大ひに効あり。

Grind the above three ingredients into a powder and take with one *qián* and five *fēn* of hot water. [The formula is] extremely effective [in treating] cases of dizziness.

大黄附子湯之圖
Illustration for the Dà Huáng Fù Zǐ Tāng[292] [Pattern] 大黄附子湯

289. Although the Chinese characters (Ch: *kōng xīn* 空心; Jp: *kūshin*) used literally mean *empty heart*, the author has glossed this term as *suki-hara*, the Japanese word for *empty stomach*.
290. Water swelling (Ch: *shuǐ zhǒng* 水腫; Jp: *suishu*) refers to edema (dropsy) of the eyelids, head, face, abdomen, back, or entire body.
291. The source of *Huáng Lián Táo Huā Sǎn* 黄連桃花散 (Jp: *Ōren-Tōka-Tō*; coptis and peach blossom powder) is unclear. At present, this formula is not covered by the Japanese National Health Insurance program and is not well known in Japan.
292. The formula for *Dà Huáng Fù Zǐ Tāng* 大黄附子湯 (Jp: *Daiō-Bushi-Tō*; rhubarb and aconite decoction) was originally found in *Jīn Guì Yào Lüè*. The extract preparation of the formula is covered by the Japanese National Health Insurance program as a prescription drug, and is also commonly sold in Japanese drug stores as an over-the-counter drug. It is currently indicated by the MHLW for: abdominal pain, neuralgia, and constipation in persons with moderate or weak

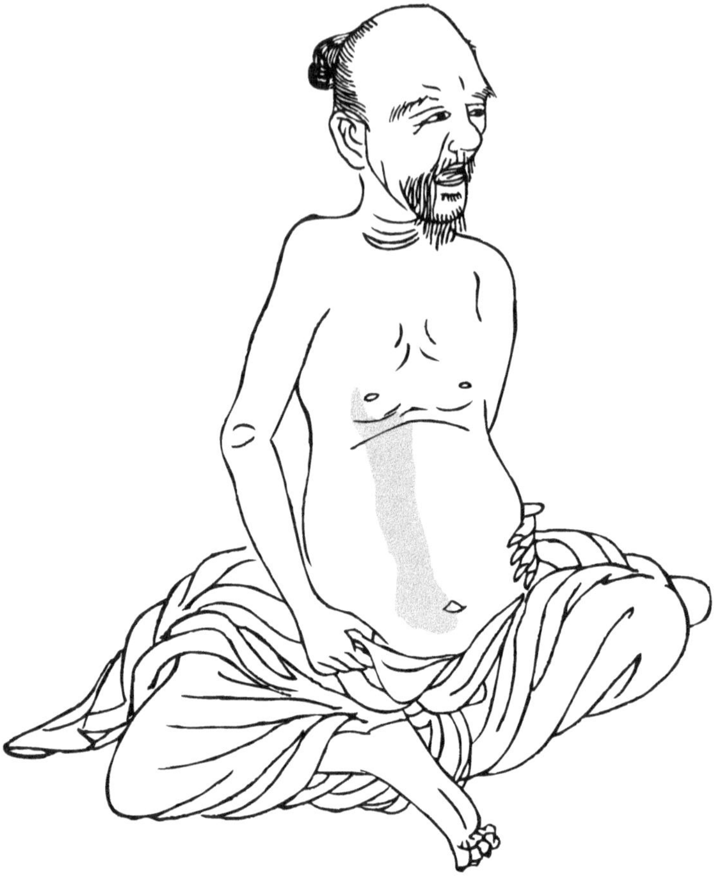

Fig. 59

圖の如く、臍の四邊に毒ありて絞痛忍びがたき者、或るひは腹底冷寒、或るひは身體惡寒するを以て、腹診の眼とすべし。或るひは脇下偏痛、或るひは身體冷へて惡寒するもの、若しくは臓寒の者。

As shown in the illustration, the abdominal indication [for the formula] is the presence of a toxin in the four sides of the umbilicus, causing insufferable gripping pain. In some cases the patient may present with cold in the depths of the abdomen, and in other cases the patient may present with generalized aversion to cold [i.e., shivering]. Some patients present with hemilateral pain under the rib-sides, and others present with cold in the body that causes aversion to cold or cold in the organs.

physical strength who feel cold and have occasional constipation (體力中等度以下で、冷えて、ときに便祕するものの次の諸症：腹痛、神經痛、便祕).

又た云ふ、小腹及び臍旁、或るひは臍下の拘攣急迫して絞痛の者、この方内に於いて芍藥・甘草各一戔を加へて大いに効あり。余、しばしば經驗するを以て此こに記せり。

Moreover, adding *sháo yào* and *gān cǎo* (one *qián* each) to the formula is extremely effective in cases when the patient presents with hypertonicity and distress, causing gripping pain in the smaller abdomen, [the regions] beside the umbilicus, or the subumbilical region. I have often experienced [the efficacy of this drug]; hence, I have listed [the formula] here.

則ち大黄附子湯の方
Dà Huáng Fù Zǐ Tāng

大黄（九分）・細辛（六分）・附子（一戔四分餘）。

dà huáng	大黄	9 fēn
xì xīn	細辛	6 fēn
fù zǐ	附子	a little more than 1 qián and 4 fēn

右三味、水一盞を以て、四分に煮とる。

Boil the three ingredients in one cup of water to make four *fēn* of the decoction.

大黄黄連瀉心湯之圖
Illustration for the Dà Huáng Huáng Lián Xiè Xīn Tāng[293] [Pattern] 大黄黄連瀉心湯

圖の如く、心下痞、之れを按して軟、心中煩悸衝逆するもの。余、此の方を數々用ひ、しばしば効有り。

As shown in the illustration, the patient presents with glomus in the region below the heart which feels soft upon palpation, [and there is also] heart vexation, palpitations, and

293. There are several different versions of *Dà Huáng Huáng Lián Xiè Xīn Tāng* 大黄黄連瀉心湯 (Jp: *Daiō-Ōren-Shashin-Tō*; rhubarb and coptis heart-draining decoction). This version was originally found in *Shāng Hán Lùn*. At present, this formula is not covered by the Japanese National Health Insurance program and is not commonly used in Japan.

surging counterflow. I have often used this formula and [seen that] it has been effective [in such cases].

『論』に云ふ、「心下痞、之れを按して軟。其の脉、關上浮なる者」と。案ずるに『金匱』云ふ、「關上積在臍傍、上關上積在心下」と云々。然らば則ち「關上」は臍傍より上中脘までの位を候ふものとす。之れを腹証に考ふるに、中脘、動氣浮かび高く病人自づから其の心下痞するをおぼへ、之れを按ずるに鞕實ならざるものは是れ血熱炎上の候なり。痞は病人自づから心下の痞を覺へるなり。軟鞕からざるの謂ひにして軟弱をいふにあらず。

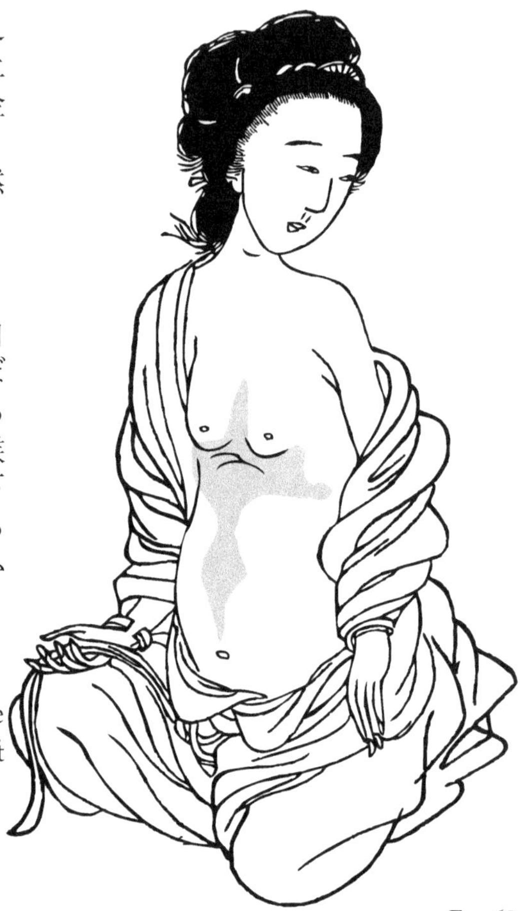

Fig. 60

In [Shāng Hán] Lùn,[294] it states that "... the patient presents with glomus in the region below the heart, which feels soft upon palpation, and [the patient] has a floating pulse in the *guān* [region of the radial-arterial pulse]..."[295] I believe that it states in the *Jīn Guì* [*Yào Lüè*][296]

294. The original text as found in the "On Identification of Pulse, Symptom Complex, and Treatment of Greater Yáng [Diseases], Chapter 7, Line 154 (Ch: *Biàn Tài Yáng Mài Zhèng Bìng Zhì Xià* 辨太陽脈證并治下; Jp: *Ben-Taiyō-Myakushō-Hei-Chi-Ka*)" is as follows:「心下痞、按之濡、其脈關上浮者、大黄黄連瀉心湯主之。」*Dà Huáng Huáng Lián Xiè Xīn Tāng* governs the pattern in which the patient presents with glomus in the region below the heart, which feels soggy upon palpation, and a floating pulse at the *guān* [position].
295. The *guān* refers to the middle region of the three radial-arterial regions used in traditional Chinese pulse diagnosis. The three regions of the pulse are as follows: 1) the distal or front *cùn* 寸 (Jp: *sun*; inch), located at the wrist crease, 2) the middle *guān* 關 (Jp: *kan*; bar), located medial to the radial styloid process, and 3) the proximal or rear *chǐ* 尺 (Jp: *shaku*; cubit).
296. The original text as found in Chapter 11, "On Pulse, Symptom Complex and Treatment of Accumulation and Gathering of Pathogenic Wind and Cold in the [Five] Viscera (Ch: *Zàng Fēng Hán Jī Jù Bìng Mài Zhèng Bìng Zhì* 臟風寒積聚病脈證并治; Jp: *Zō-Fūkan-Shakujubyō-*

that "...[when there is a feeling] in the *guān,* the accumulation is located to the sides of the umbilicus and when it is above the *guān,* [i.e. proximal to the *cùn kǒu*], the accumulation is in the region below the heart..." If this is true, then the *guān* corresponds to the [abdominal] region from the sides of the umbilicus to the upper center stomach duct.[297] Considering this [fact] in [the context of] abdominal patterns, when the patient presents with a stirring qì that floats high in the center stomach duct, naturally causing a feeling of glomus in the region below the heart, and palpatory findings do not reveal hard fullness, it is a case of blood heat flaming upward. The patient feels glomus in the region below the heart. [The region] is soft and not hard, but this does not mean that it is soft and weak.

又た三黄瀉心湯、心氣不定を治すと云ふ。此の証たる、俗に云ふ、よく物忘れして冒する者、甚だしきものは健忘と號する、是れあり。本方を用ひて治を奏すること擧げてかぞへがたし。一書に云ふ、「心下痞鞕・嘔吐吃逆、或るひは嚏する者、この方大ひに効あり」と。又た云ふ、心腹攪痛し、諸藥効なくして死せんと欲するものに即効あり。余、しばしば經驗す。

Furthermore, it is said that *Sān Huáng Xiè Xīn Tāng* can cure cases of fluctuating heart qì. [Persons with] this pattern are colloquially referred to as being forgetful, as if stupefied, and in severe cases, they are said to have amnesia. It is difficult to count all of the times that [I] have used this formula and obtained a successful result. One book states, "This formula is extremely effective for patients who have glomus and hardness in the region below the heart, retching and vomiting with counterflow, or sneezing." Furthermore, it also says that [the formula] has an immediate effect in patients in whom there is a churning pain present in the heart and abdomen, all medicinals have been ineffective, and are on the verge of dying. I have often experienced [the efficacy of this medicinal].

Myakushō-Hei-Chi)" is as follows:「脈來細而附骨者、乃積也。寸口積在胸中。微出寸口、積在喉中。關上積在臍傍。上關上、積在心下。微下關、積在少腹」(When the pulse is fine and attached to the bone, it is a case of accumulation. When [felt] in the *cùn kǒu,* the accumulation is in the chest. When it is faintly [felt] leaving the *cùn kǒu*, the accumulation is in the throat. When [felt] in the *guān*, the accumulation is located to the sides of the umbilicus and when [felt] above the *guān*, the accumulation is in the region below the heart. When it can be faintly [felt] below the *guān*, it is in the lesser abdomen....)

297. Although the meaning of the passage is disputed, it appears that the author of *Jīn Guì Yào Lüè* believed that the radial-arterial pulse regions constitute a microcosm of the abdomen, which itself can be considered to be a microcosm of the entire body, or at least an indicator of visceral health; this view is supported by the author of the present work.

則ち大黄黄連瀉心湯の方
Dà Huáng Huáng Lián Xiè Xīn Tāng

大黄（一戔二分）・黄連（六分）。（此の方、黄芩六分を加ふるときは即ち三黄瀉心湯なり）

dà huáng	大黄	1 qián and 2 fēn
huáng lián	黄連	6 fēn

When six *fēn* of *huáng qín* 黄芩 is added to this this formula, it becomes *Sān Huáng Xiè Xīn Tāng* 三黄瀉心湯.

右二味、水六分を以て、熱湯にして振り出だし用ゆ。

Boil the above two ingredients in six *fēn* of water, and administer after shaking in hot water.

大建中湯之圖
Illustration for the Dà Jiàn Zhōng Tāng[298] [Pattern] 大建中湯

圖の如く、腹の皮むくむくと起りて、頭足あるが如く。たとへば樹の枝を袋に包みて推してみるが如く。その病ひ發する時は大ひに寒痛。嘔して食すること能はず。上下いたむところ、手を近づくべからず。或るひは大便閉し、或るひは心胸、大寒・上衝の者。

As shown in the illustration, the abdominal skin rises up and becomes enlarged, [creating a pattern] as if a cephalopod[299] [were inside the abdomen]. The feeling can be compared to inserting the twigs of a tree into a bag and palpating [the outside of the bag].

298. The formula for *Dà Jiàn Zhōng Tāng* 大建中湯 (Jp: *Dai-Kenchū-Tō*; major center-fortifying decoction) was originally found in *Jīn Guì Yào Lüè*. The extract preparation of the formula is covered by the Japanese National Health Insurance program as a prescription drug, and may be sold in Japanese drug stores as an over-the-counter drug. It is currently indicated by the MHLW for: lower abdominal pain and abdominal distension in persons with weak physical strength who have a cold sensation in the abdomen accompanied by pain (體力虚弱で、腹が冷えて痛むものの次の諸症：下腹部痛、腹部膨満感). It is commonly prescribed by gastroenterologists in Japan for treatment of ileus, bowel obstruction, etc.

299. *Zusoku* 頭足, more commonly called *tōsokurui* 頭足類 (Ch: *tóu zú lèi*), refers to the molluscan class Cephalopoda, which includes animals such as squids and octopuses.

When the [symptoms of the] disease occur, severe cold pain [is present]. The patient experiences retching accompanied by the inability to eat. There is pain in upper and lower regions that is exacerbated by the slightest touch of the hand [during the abdominal examination]. In some cases, the patient presents with a fecal block, and in some cases, and great cold and upward surging in the heart and chest.

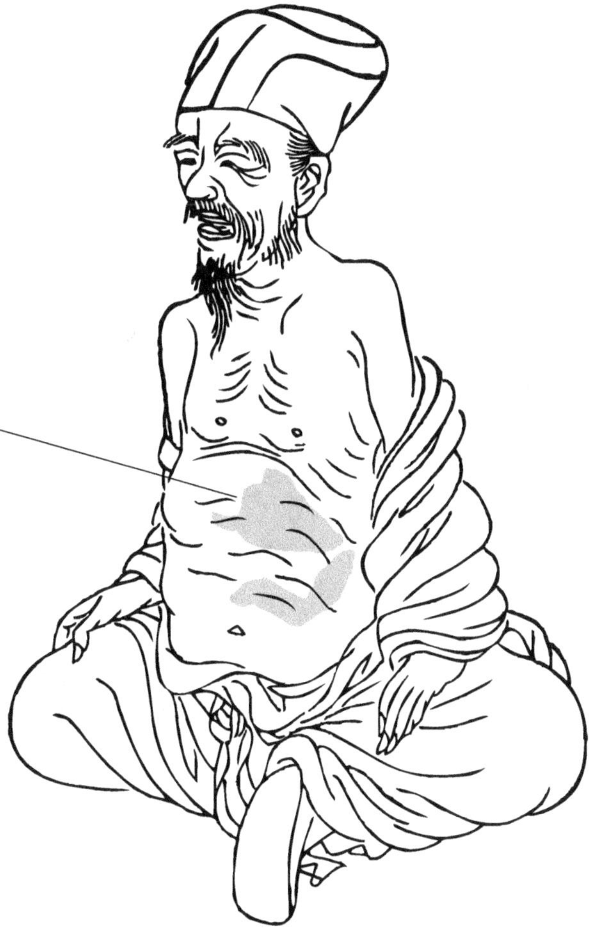

Fig. 61

則ち大建中湯の方
Dà Jiàn Zhōng Tāng

蜀椒（六分）・乾姜（一戔二分）・人參（八分、竹節）・飴（四戔六分）。

shǔ jiāo	蜀椒	6 fēn	
gān jiāng	乾薑	1 qián and 2 fēn	
rén shēn	人參	8 fēn	zhú jié rén shēn 竹節人參 [should be used]
yí táng	飴糖	4 qián and 6 fēn	

右四味、水一盞六分を以て、三味を煮て八分に取り、滓を去て飴を入れ六分にとり、一度に服す。

Boil the above four ingredients in one cup and six *fēn* of water [in the following manner]: boil [the first] three ingredients in eight *fēn* [of water], remove the residue, and add *yí táng* to make six *fēn* of the decoction. Take in a single dose.

同大建中湯之二圖
The Second Illustration for the Same Formula of Dà Jiàn Zhōng Tāng
大建中湯

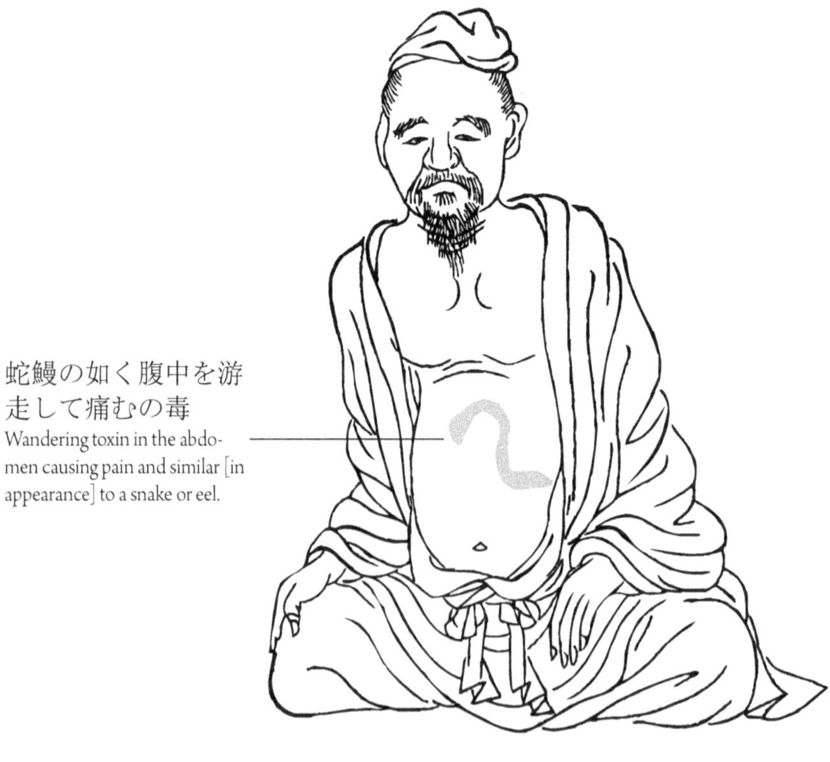
蛇鰻の如く腹中を游走して痛むの毒
Wandering toxin in the abdomen causing pain and similar [in appearance] to a snake or eel.

Fig. 62

圖の如く、時々蛇の如く、又た鰻の如きもの。腹中を游走して、頭かと思ふ處にて痛み、尾かと覺ふ處にていたみ、其の患へ、しのぶべからず。諸藥も効なし。其の餘の患ふる所、人々にして異なり、都べて此の方に非ざれば治せず。圖するが如く、その腹三狀あり。腹診を詳らかにして治療の効を奏すべし。

As shown in the illustration, the patient presents with [something in the abdomen that] occasionally resembles a snake or eel. It wanders about the inside of the abdomen, and there is pain present [in the region of where] the "head" [of the snake or eel] is and pain present [in the region] where the "tail" is; [the condition] causes insufferable pain. [In such cases,] all medicinals are ineffective. Other symptoms may differ from person to person, but all [cases] cannot be cured unless the present formula is used. As shown in the illustration, there are three lines on the abdomen. After the [abdominal pattern] has been elucidated through abdominal examination, the [present] treatment should be effective.

又た云ふ、此の症、まま旁らに下瘀血湯の症をあらはすことあり、考ふべし。則ち圖・方とも下に出だす。

Furthermore, [the physician] should consider that in this pattern, the patient may also present with a concurrent pattern for *Xià Yū Xuè Tāng*.[300] Here, [I shall] present [another] illustration [of the pattern] and its formula.

同大建中湯之三圖
The Third Illustration of [Another Pattern Corresponding to] the Same Formula of Dà Jiàn Zhōng Tāng 大建中湯

圖の如く、腹常に平穩にして、發する時は腹皮うごひて波の打ち來るが如き者。或るひは腹つねに之れを按して狀なく、發する時は忽ち塊物游走し、上下往來して疼み、手をふれ、近づくべからず。

As shown in the illustration, the abdomen is normally balanced and calm, but when an attack occurs, it appears as if there are waves in the abdominal skin that were made by

300. *Xià Yū Xuè Tāng* 下瘀血湯 (Jp: *Ge-Oketsu-Tō*; stasis-precipitating decoction) is discussed in its own section in this work.

hitting [the abdomen]. In some cases, when [the abdomen] is pressed, nothing can be felt, but when an attack occurs, a lump suddenly wanders up and down [the abdomen], causing pain that is exacerbated by the slightest touch of the hand.

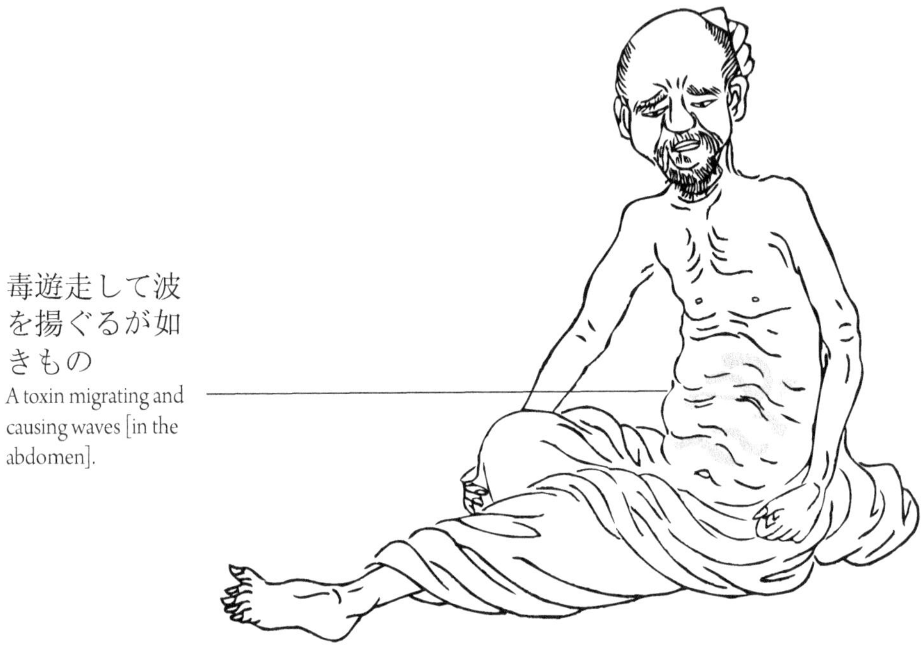

Fig. 63

又た云ふ、時として小さき嚢如きもの忽ち去りてなきが如く、又た來たる時は痛み忍びがたし。腹中に在るかと思へば、忽ち背に廻り、背に在るかと思へば、又た腹中に來たる。この三圖の腹診を詳らかにして、某々の病名にかかはらず、此の方を用ひて治せざることなし。

Furthermore, [the lump that] appears similar to a small sac, which often seems to quickly leave [the body, i.e., disappear]. When [the lump] comes [i.e., reappears], it causes unbearable pain. As soon as [the physician] believes that [the toxin] is in the abdomen, it suddenly moves to the back, and as soon as [the physician] believes that it is in the back, it again returns to the abdomen. [If the physician correctly] elucidates the abdominal patterns in these three illustrations without being swayed by the name of the disease that the patient may present with, there will be no [case] that remains uncured when these formulae are used.

腹證奇覽後篇卷之上終

End of Volume I of the second half[301] of *Fukushō-Kiran* 《腹證奇覽》 (Extraordinary Views of Abdominal Patterns)

301. This is the end of the third volume of the work.

腹證奇覽後編卷之下

Volume II of the second half[302] of *Fukushō-Kiran* 《腹證奇覽》 (Extraordinary Views of Abdominal Patterns)

湖南　稻葉克文禮父著

Master "Konan" Inaba "Katsu" Bunrei, Author

302. This is the fourth and final volume of the text.

十棗湯之證之圖

Illustration for the Shí Zǎo Tāng[303] [Pattern] 十棗湯

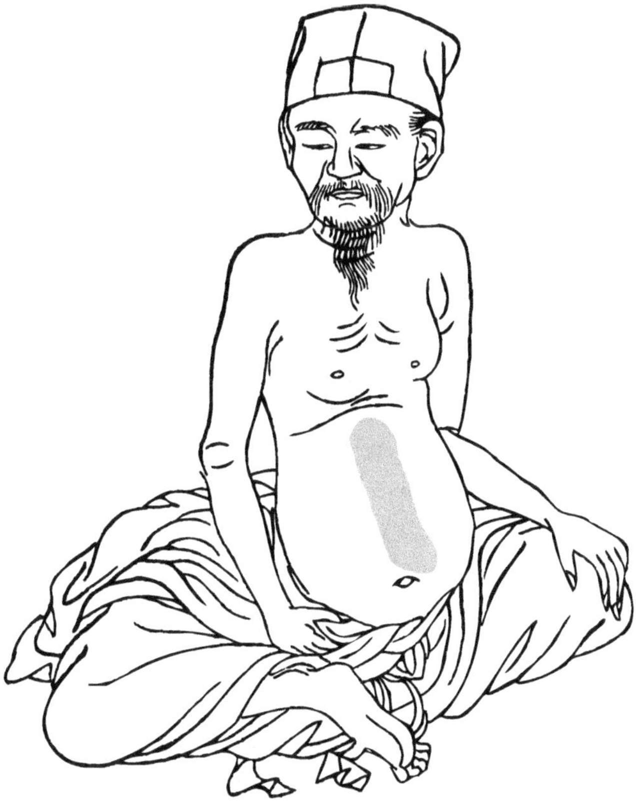

Fig. 64

圖の如く、腹中に堅塊有りて、その狀方長にして、之れを按してたゆまず。時々掣痛する者、此の症の準據とす。且つ堅塊の狀、之れを按すに、たとへば胸端より臍の邊まで長く、四、五寸ばかりの竹のふとさを按すが如く、或るひは胸より腹に至りて細長く引つぱり、或るひは短かくして脇下の傍に手に當たる物あり。

As shown in the illustration, the patient presents with a hard lump in the abdomen that is long and thin and does not slacken when pressed [with the hands]. Patients who occasionally experience [abdominal] pulling pain are indicated for this pattern. Furthermore, when this hard lump is pressed, it may feel similar to a bamboo stalk four or five *cùn*

303. The formula for *Shí Zǎo Tāng* 十棗湯 (Jp: *Jissō-Tō*; ten jujubes decoction) was originally found in *Jīn Guì Yào Lüè* and *Shāng Hán Lùn*. At present, this formula is not covered by the Japanese National Health Insurance program and is not commonly used in Japan.

thick from the end of the chest to the region surrounding the umbilicus. In some cases, there may be a sensation of something thin and long pulling at the abdomen from the chest. In other cases, [the lump] may feel short, and a pulling feeling may be felt with the hands under the rib-sides.

其の大小・長短によらず、只だ「掣痛」の二字を眼（がん）とすべし。「掣」は「引」なり、びくびくと引き痛むなり。凡そ痰飲有りて咳する者、或るひは四支、腰腹掣痛する者、その餘某々の患へをとはず、胸腹掣痛するの準據を以て、此の方を用ひて神効あることを知るべし。余、此の方を用ひ覺へて、その藥効の神なるを以て取ること有りて云ふ。

[The physician] should not be swayed by the size or length, but should simply focus on the two characters [comprising the expression] pulling pain [i.e., *chè tòng* 掣痛; Jp: *seitsū*]. The character for "pulling [i.e., *chè* 掣; Jp: *sei*]" [in this expression] is [the same meaning as the more common character used for] pulling [i.e., *yǐn* 引; Jp: *in*]. It refers to a pulling pain [accompanied by a] feeling of trembling. [Thus,] it can be understood that this formula has a divine efficacy not only in patients who cough up phlegm-rheum or have a pulling pain in the extremities, lumbus, or abdomen, but it is also indicated for any affliction in which pulling pain is present in chest or abdomen. I have used this formula and speak from experience concerning its divine efficacy.

大棗十戔、或るひは五、六戔を以て水一盞半入れ、六分に煎じ、滓を去りて甘遂の末を入れ、調和して頓服す。尤も効あり。但し甘遂末、病毒の淺深によりて分量の多少を考ふべし。或るひは二、三分、或るひは四、五、六分、甚だしきに至りては一戔。大いに瞑眩して吐下傾くるが如し。必ずしも恐るべからず。

Boil ten *qián* of *dà zǎo,* or in some cases five or six *qián,* in one and one-half cups of water to make six *fēn* of the decoction. Remove the residue, add *gān suì* powder, harmonize the ingredients, and take in a single dose. [The present formula] is most effective. However, depending on the depth of the toxin causing the disease, [the physician] may consider increasing or decreasing the quantity of *gān suì mò* [in the formula]. In some cases, two or three *fēn,* and in other cases four, five, or six *fēn* [may be administered]. In severe cases, up to one *qián* [may be administered. The patient] will experience severe dizziness [i.e., side effects] and bend down as if experiencing vomiting and diarrhea. There is no need to be frightened [by these signs].

則ち十棗湯の本方
Shí Zǎo Tāng

芫花・甘遂・大戟（ 各等分 ）・大棗（ 五分 ）。

yuán huā	芫花	equal amounts
gān suì	甘遂	equal amounts
dà jǐ	大戟	equal amounts
dà zǎo	大棗	5 fēn

右四味 、末丸となし 、水一盞二分を以て 、棗を煎じて六分に取り 、滓を去りて散一戔を入れ 、頓服す 。克按ずるに 、大棗五分東洞家省略の秤數にして用ひがたし 。今六戔を用ゆるに甚だ効あり 。

Powder the above four ingredients [and make] into pills. Boil [*dà*] *zǎo* in one cup and two *fēn* of water to make six *fēn* of the decoction. Remove the dregs and add one *qián* of the powder. Take in a single dose. I believe that [using] five *fēn* of *dà zǎo* is based on the [over]simplified calculations of the Tōdō family. [In my experience], using six *qián* is extremely effective.

又た右丸の方あり 、左に記す 。芫花（ 和物不可なり 。薩摩藤と稱するもの可也 ）・甘遂（ よく肥へたるもの可なり ）・大戟（ 和物不可なり 。綿大戟と號するもの可なり ）。右三味 、各等分末となし 、大棗のよく肥へたる肉を取りて 、之れを丸じ 、小豆の大きさのごとくす 。

Here, I shall list [the details of] the aforementioned formula of the pill. *Yuán huā*[304] (The Japanese variety is not acceptable. The variety known [in Japanese] as *satsuma-fuji* is acceptable),[305] *gān suì* (Extremely fat types are acceptable), *dà jǐ* (The Japanese variety is

304. There are several varieties of *yuán huā* 芫花 (Jp: *genka*; genkwa blossom), but the herb name generally refers to the dried flower buds of Daphne genkwa Sieb. et Zucc. (Thymelaeaceae). In any case, *yuán huā* is not used in any formula currently approved by the MHLW in Japan.
305. *Satsuma-fuji* 薩摩藤 usually refers to Dianthus japonicus, but is sometimes also used as an alternative name for *genkwa*. For this reason, it is unclear which is the Japanese variety that the author is referring to.

not acceptable. The type that is called *mián dà jǐ* is acceptable).[306] Make the three above ingredients into a powder using equal quantities of each ingredient. Take the pulp of *dà zǎo* (that has grown fat) to make round pills that are the size of adzuki beans.

半夏瀉心湯之圖

Illustration for the Bàn Xià Xiè Xīn Tāng[307] [Pattern] 半夏瀉心湯

圖の如く、心下痞鞕して、腸中雷鳴する者、此の方の症なり。余、按ずるに、久しく下痢止まず、腹痛の者、この症多し。或るひは大便閉して、時々腹痛する者、此の症間々あり。余が門、數々しば用ひて効ある毎に之れを信ず。或るひは心腹疼痛の者、此の症多し。

As shown in the illustration, when the patient presents with glomus and hardness in the region below the heart and thunderous rumbling in the intestines, it is the [right] pattern for this formula. I believe that many patients who present with enduring dysentery that does not cease and abdominal pain actually have this pattern. Patients who present with a fecal block and occasionally experience abdominal pain also have this pattern. My pupils have often used [the present formula] and have continued to deepen their trust in it each time that it has been effective. Many cases in which the patient presents with pain in the heart and abdomen are actually examples of this pattern.

306. There are several varieties of *dà jǐ* 大戟. *Dà jǐ* (Jp: *daigeki*; euphorbia root) generally refers to the root of Euphorbia pekinensis, but in Japan, other varieties may be used. *Mián dà jǐ* 綿大戟 (Jp: *men-daigeki*) generally refers to Stellera chamaejasme, but it is unclear which variety is the Japanese variety that the author is referring to. In any case, *dà jǐ* (*mián dà jǐ*) is not used in any formula currently approved by the MHLW in Japan.

307. The formula for *Bàn Xià Xiè Xīn Tāng* 半夏瀉心湯 (Jp: *Hange-Shashin-Tō*; pinellia heart-draining decoction) was originally found in *Jīn Guì Yào Lüè* and *Shāng Hán Lùn*. The extract preparation of the formula is covered by the Japanese National Health Insurance program as a prescription drug, and is also commonly sold in Japanese drug stores as an over-the-counter drug. It is currently indicated by the MHLW for: acute or chronic gastroenteritis, diarrhea, loose stools, dyspepsia, gastroptosis, neurotic gastritis, weak stomach, hangover, belching, heartburn, stomatitis, and neurosis in persons with moderate physical strength who have a feeling of a knot in the solar plexus, experience occasional nausea or vomiting, have decreased appetite, abdominal rumbling, or tend to have loose stools or diarrhea (體力中等度で、みぞおちがつかえた感じがあり、ときに惡心、嘔吐があり食欲不振で腹が鳴って軟便又は下痢の傾向のあるものの次の諸症：急・慢性胃腸炎、下痢・軟便、消化不良、胃下垂、神經性胃炎、胃弱、二日酔、げっぷ、胸やけ、口内炎、神經症).

又た按ずるに、下痢してのち心下痞鞕する者、此の症といへども、雷鳴せざる者あり。又た下痢の後といへども、未だ水氣つきずして雷鳴する者あり。是こに於いて腹診の術を失ふ。其の傳ありて云ふ、下痢の後、雷鳴せざる者は、毒の浮水の去るを以てなり。然りといへども、心下の底に痞鞕の毒は未だささらず。其の症の定極を知らんと欲せば、心下を按して病者嘔氣を覺ゆる者、是れなり。

Furthermore, I believe that some patients who present with glomus and hardness in the region below the heart after experiencing diarrhea have this pattern, even though [abdominal palpation] does not reveal any thunderous rumbling [in the intestines]. Other patients who present with this pattern experience thunderous rumbling due to the persistent water qì that remains after diarrhea [has stopped]. This is where [physicians] make a mistake in abdominal examination. One text explains that [the reason why] patients who do not present with thunderous rumbling after experiencing diarrhea is because the toxin has floated away through water [leaving the body]. However, this does not apply in cases in which the toxin causes glomus and hardness in the depths of the region below the heart. If [the physician] desires to thoroughly understand the

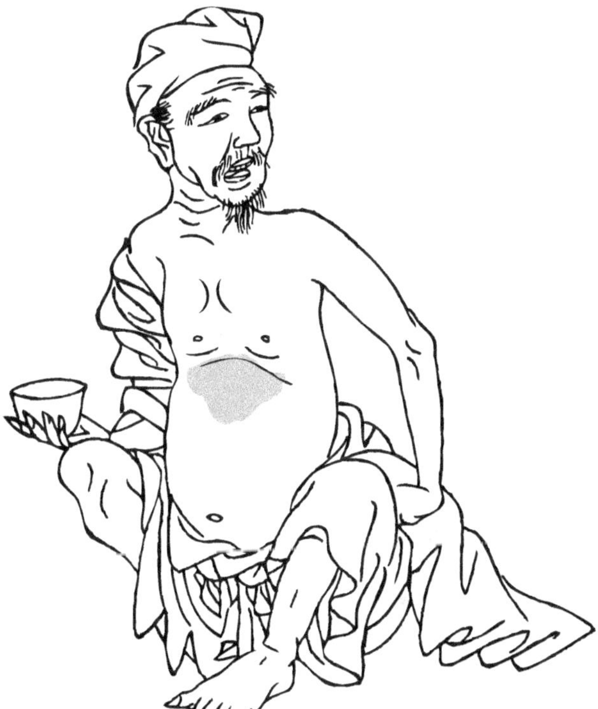

Fig. 65

pattern, [it can be defined as] the pattern in which the patient feels a desire to retch when the region below the heart is pressed.

又た云ふ、此の症に似たる者、三症有りて分別す。附子粳米湯、小柴胡湯、半夏瀉心湯なり。皆、時として腹痛することあり。其の別、半夏瀉心湯は心下痞して硬く、附子粳米湯は胸脇に逆滿して之れを按すに痛まず。小柴胡湯は胸脇苦滿なり。

Furthermore, [the patterns] that resemble this pattern can be divided into three different patterns: [the patterns for] *Fù Zǐ Gēng Mǐ Tāng*,[308] *Xiǎo Chái Hú Tāng*, and *Bàn Xià Xiè Xīn Tāng*. In all of these cases, the patient often experiences abdominal pain. [Signs] apart from [abdominal pain] are as follows: [in the pattern for] *Bàn Xià Xiè Xīn Tāng*, the region below the heart is hard due to glomus; [in the pattern for] *Fù Zǐ Gēng Mǐ Tāng*, the patient presents with counterflow fullness in the chest and rib-sides and there is no pain upon palpation. [The principal symptom for] *Xiǎo Chái Hú Tāng* is bitter fullness in the chest and rib-sides.

則ち半夏瀉心湯の方
Bàn Xià Xiè Xīn Tāng

半夏（九分）・黃連（一分半）・黃芩・乾姜・人參・大棗・甘草（各四分半）。

bàn xià	半夏	9 fēn
huáng lián	黃連	1.5 fēn
huáng qín	黃芩	4.5 fēn
gān jiāng	乾薑	4.5 fēn
rén shēn	人參	4.5 fēn
dà zǎo	大棗	4.5 fēn
gān cǎo	甘草	4.5 fēn

右七味、水二盞を以て一盞二分に煮とり、滓を去りて再び六分にとる。

308. *Fù Zǐ Gēng Mǐ Tāng* 附子粳米湯 (Jp: *Bushi-Kōbei-Tō*; aconite and rice decoction) is discussed separately in its own section in this work.

Boil the above seven ingredients in two cups of water to make one cup and two *fēn* of the decoction; remove the dregs and make six *fēn* of the decoction.

甘草瀉心湯之圖
Illustration for the Gān Cǎo Xiè Xīn Tāng[309] [Pattern]
甘草瀉心湯

圖の如く、半夏瀉心湯の症にして、心煩して心氣安からざる者、此の症の主なり。余、按ずるに、此こに心煩と云ふもの、甘草の症なり。甘草は急迫を弛める能あり。且つ腹を診察するに、心胸急迫して心煩するを知るべし。その心煩すること一ならず。

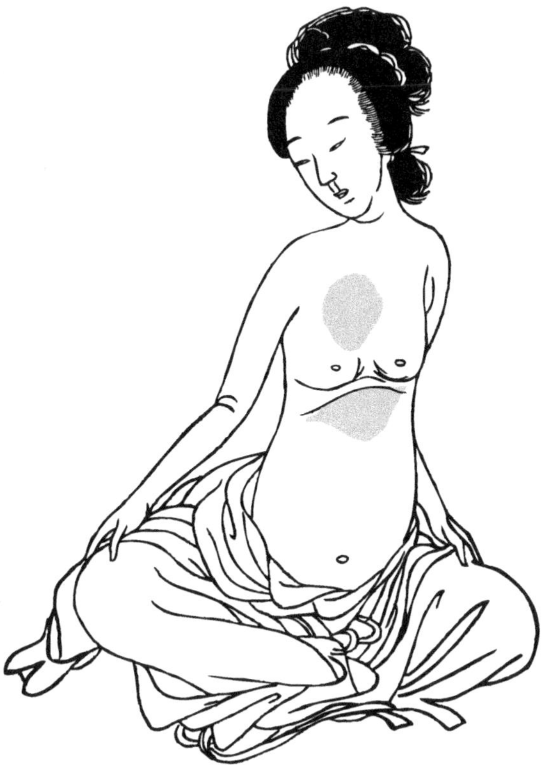
Fig. 66

As shown in the illustration, the patient presents with the pattern for *Bàn Xià Xiè Xīn Tāng* accompanied by heart vexation and disquieted heart qì. These are the primary [indications] for this pattern. I believe that what is meant here by heart vexation is a pattern [that is cured by] *gān cǎo*. *Gān cǎo* has the effect of relieving distress. Moreover, when performing the abdominal examination, the presence of distress in the heart and chest as well as heart vexation can be detected. [However,] the types of heart vexation are not uniform.

309. The formula for *Gān Cǎo Xiè Xīn Tāng* 甘草瀉心湯 (Jp: *Kanzō-Shashin-Tō*; licorice heart-draining decoction) was originally found in *Jīn Guì Yào Lüè* and *Shāng Hán Lùn*. The extract preparation of the formula may be sold in Japanese drug stores as an over-the-counter drug. It is currently indicated by the MHLW for: gastroenteritis, stomatitis, bad breath, insomnia, neurosis, and diarrhea in persons with moderate physical strength who have a feeling of a knot in the solar plexus and occasional irritation, diarrhea, nausea, or abdominal rumbling (體力中等度で、みぞおちがつかえた感じがあり、ときにイライラ感、下痢、はきけ、腹が鳴るものの次の諸症：胃腸炎、口内炎、口臭、不眠症、神經症、下痢).

或るひは苦満して心煩する者は、柴胡の症を考ふべし。只だ煩する者は、黄連の症としるべし。此の症、心胸引つぱり迫るを指頭に覺ふ。即ち急迫して心煩し安からざる者、是れなり。且つ外症は、その人、心重く眠りを好んで目を閉づること能はずして、起臥安からず。或るひは飲食を欲せず、又た食臭を聞ひて悪む。

When the patient presents with bitter fullness and heart vexation, it is a pattern [that is cured by] *chái hú*. When the patient presents with only vexation, it is the pattern [that is cured by] *huáng lián*. [When the patient has] this pattern, taut pulling can be felt with the fingertips in heart and chest [regions]. That is, the patient has distress, heart vexation, and [has] disquieted [heart qì]. Moreover, the external signs [of the pattern] are as follows: the patient has heaviness in the heart, is somnolent but unable to close the eyes, and has fidgetiness whether lying down or [sitting] up. In some cases, [the patient] has no desire for food or drink and has an aversion to the smell of food.

則ち甘草瀉心湯の方
Gān Cǎo Xiè Xīn Tāng

甘草（七分）・半夏（九分）・黄連（一分半）・黄芩・乾姜・大棗・人參（各四分半）。

gān cǎo	甘草	7 fēn
bàn xià	半夏	9 fēn
huáng lián	黄連	1.5 fēn
huáng qín	黄芩	4.5 fēn
gān jiāng	乾薑	4.5 fēn
dà zǎo	大棗	4.5 fēn
rén shēn	人參	4.5 fēn

右七味煎方、本方と同じ。

Decoct the above seven ingredients in the same manner as the base formula [i.e., *Bàn Xià Xiè Xīn Tāng*].

附子粳米湯之圖

Illustration for the Fù Zǐ Gēng Mǐ Tāng[310] [Pattern] 附子粳米湯

圖の如く、腹中雷鳴して胸脇へ逆滿し、之れを按してますます雷鳴して、絞痛切痛し嘔吐の者、此の症なり。余、按ずるに、腹中を按ずるに腹底暗然として自づから冷氣を覺ふ。且つつねの腹痛に非ず、その痛み絞り切るが如し。腹診を考ふるもの、忽諸せにすべからず。

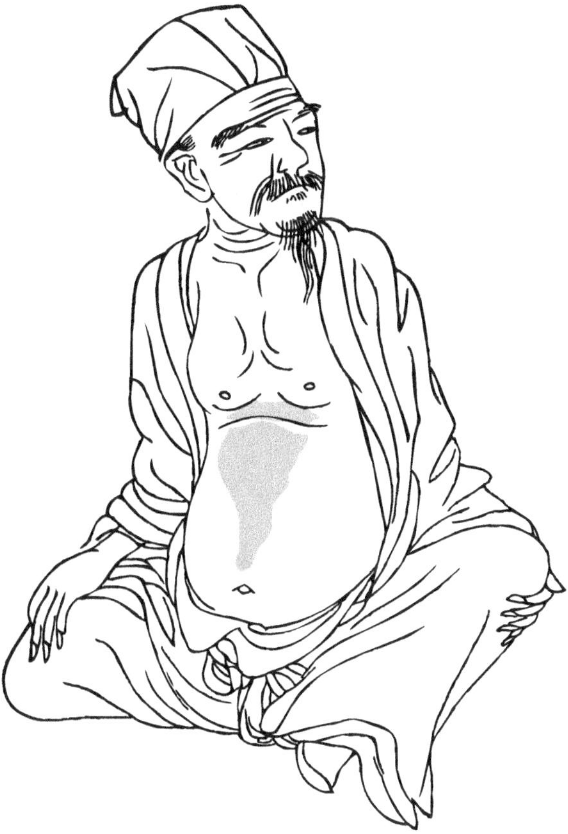

Fig. 67

As shown in the illustration, when the patient presents with thunderous rumbling in the abdomen that is exacerbated by palpation, counterflow fullness [that moves] into the chest and rib-sides, gripping pain, cutting pain, and retching and vomiting, this is the [right] pattern [that matches the present formula]. I believe that when palpating the abdomen [of a patient with this pattern], a cold qì can be subtly felt in the depths of the abdomen. Moreover, [in this pattern, the patient] does not present with ordinary abdominal pain, but a pain that feels like [the abdomen] is being gripped or cut. The person who is researching [pattern differentiation through] abdominal examination must not neglect [this point].

310. The formula for *Fù Zǐ Gēng Mǐ Tāng* 附子粳米湯 (Jp: *Bushi-Kōbei-Tō*; aconite and rice decoction) was originally found in *Jīn Guì Yào Lüè*. The extract preparation of the formula may be sold in Japanese drug stores as an over-the-counter drug. It is currently indicated by the MHLW for: stomach pain, abdominal pain, vomiting, acute and gastroenteritis in persons with weak physical strength who have a cold sensation in the abdomen accompanied by pain or abdominal rumbling (體力虛弱で、腹部が冷えて痛み、腹が鳴るものの次の諸症：胃痛、腹痛、嘔吐、急性胃腸炎).

則ち附子粳米湯の方
Fù Zǐ Gēng Mǐ Tāng

附子（ 四分強 ）・半夏（ 一錢一分 ）・甘草（ 二分 ）・大棗（ 五分 ）・粳米（ 二錢 ）。

fù zǐ	附子	a little more than 4 fēn
bàn xià	半夏	1 qián and 1 fēn
gān cǎo	甘草	2 fēn
dà zǎo	大棗	5 fēn
gēng mǐ	粳米	2 qián

右五味 、水一盞六分を以て 、六分に煮とる 。

Boil the above five ingredients in one cup and six *fēn* of water to make six *fēn* of the decoction.

甘麥大棗湯之圖
Illustration for the Gān Mài Dà Zǎo Tāng[311] [Pattern]
甘麥大棗湯

圖の如く 、腹皮攣急して 、これを按すに内實せず 。所謂藏躁急迫し 、大黄甘草湯の腹症に似て 、その人さはがしく 、眼するどく 、時々狂を發し 、數々欠伸して 、或るひは喜び 、或るひは悲しみ 、或るひは笑ひ 、或るひは泣き 、その狀 、狐狸の憑きたる如く 、又た俗に「 色狂ひ 」と云ふ者にも間々この症あり 。

As shown in the illustration, [the patient presents with] taut abdominal skin, and no internal repletion [can be felt] upon palpation [of the abdomen]. This is what as known

311. The formula for *Gān Mài Dà Zǎo Tāng* 甘麥大棗湯 (Jp: *Kan-Baku-Taisō-Tō*; licorice, wheat, and jujube decoction) was originally found in *Jīn Guì Yào Lüè*. The extract preparation of the formula is covered by the Japanese National Health Insurance program as a prescription drug, and may be sold in Japanese drug stores as an over-the-counter drug. It is currently indicated by the MHLW for: insomnia, pediatric nocturnal crying episodes, and convulsions in persons with moderate or weak physical strength who have neurologic hypersensitivity, are easily frightened, or have occasional bouts of yawning (體力中等度以下で 、神經が過敏で 、驚きやすく 、ときにあくびが出るものの次の諸症：不眠症 、小兒の夜泣き 、ひきつけ).

as visceral agitation and distress.[312] It appears similar to the abdominal pattern for *Dà Huáng Gān Cǎo Tāng*, in that the patient is boisterous, has a sharp eye, experiences occasional bouts of mania, and often yawns and stretches. [The patient is] sometimes happy, sometimes sad, sometimes laughing, and sometimes crying. Patients who have this pattern may also be what is colloquially known as "sex crazed," as if the patient were possessed by a fox [spirit].[313]

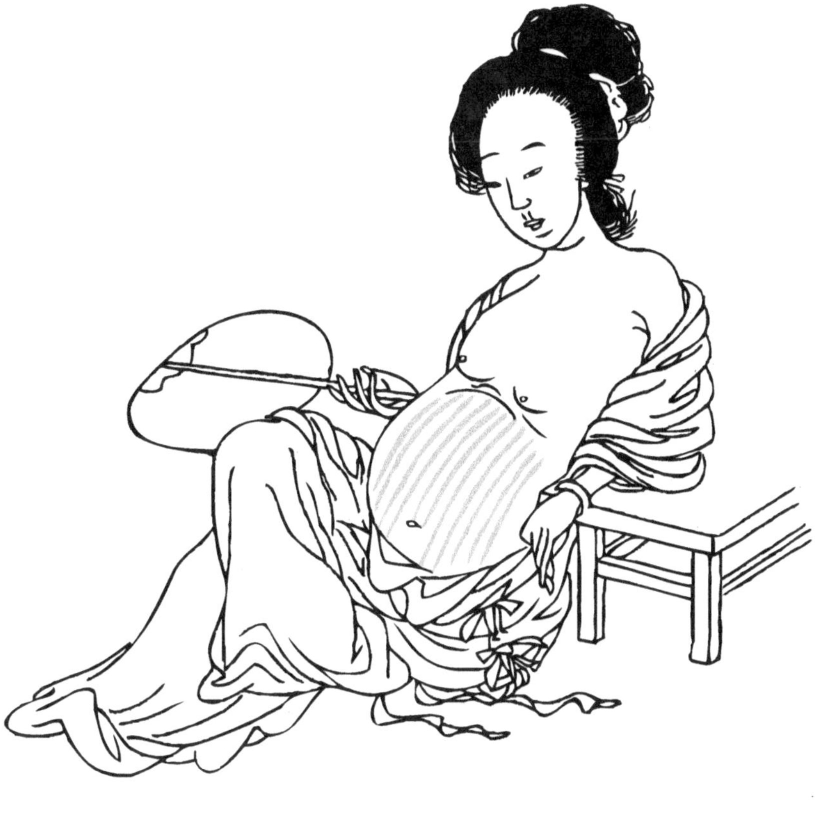

Fig. 68

312. Visceral agitation, also known as hysteria (Ch: *zàng zào* 臟躁; Jp: *zōsō*), refers to a paroxysmal mental disease marked by depression and melancholy, irritability, lack of control over emotions, sadness with an urge to weep, and sighing for no apparent reason.
313. In ancient Japan, foxes were viewed as supernatural creatures. Possession by the spirit of a demon fox, a condition referred to as *kitsune-tsuki* 狐憑き, was thought to be the cause of many types of psychiatric disorders, especially hypersexuality in women.

則ち甘麥大棗湯の方
Gān Mài Dà Zǎo Tāng

甘草（ 六分 ）・小麥（ 三戔二分 ）・大棗（ 五分 ）。

gān cǎo	甘草	6 fēn
xiǎo mài	小麥	3 qián and 2 fēn
dà zǎo	大棗	5 fēn

右三味 、水一盞二分を以て 、六分に煮とる 。

Boil the three ingredients in one cup and two *fēn* of water to make six *fēn* of the decoction.

余 、傳有りて云ふ 、發狂甚しき者は藥を服せず 。故に茶湯を止め 、此の方 、或るひは十貼 、二十貼をこく煎じて 、土瓶の類を以て渇する時ごとにかさね進めて服せしめ 、久くして治す 。

I have a text in which it is explained that patients who present with severe cases of mania do not [i.e., refuse to] take medicine. Thus, [in such cases] I prohibit the patient from drinking any tea, and make a concentrated decoction by decocting ten or twelve doses of the formula in an earthenware teapot.[314] When the patient feels thirsty, I give him the decoction, and [patient will be] cured after a long period of time.

甘草粉蜜湯之圖
Illustration for the Gān Cǎo Fěn Mì Tāng[315] [Pattern]
甘草粉蜜湯

圖の如く 、腹中に塊物ありて 、時々游走來去して存るが如く亡きが如く 、之れを按して捻りみるに 、長蟲數條を以て小菊に作れるが如く 、うざうざ動くことを指頭に覺ふ 。これ蚘蟲なり 。發する

314. The word dose here (Jp: *chō* 貼) is the Japanese counter word for doses of powdered medicine wrapped in paper packets.

315. The formula for *Gān Cǎo Fěn Mì Tāng* 甘草粉蜜湯 (Jp: *Kanzō-Fun-Mitsu-Tō*; licorice, processed galenite, and honey decoction) was originally found in *Jīn Guì Yào Lüè*. At present, this formula is not covered by the Japanese National Health Insurance program and is not commonly used in Japan.

時は涎沫を吐し、或るひは蟲を吐し、時々心痛・腹痛することあり、痛み忍び難し。

As shown in the illustration, the patient presents with a lump in the abdomen. [The lump] may sometimes feel as if it is wandering and arrives and departs [in the abdomen]. When [the lump] is palpated and twisted, a number of long wriggling insects in the shape of *kodemari* [i.e., spirea] can be felt with the fingertips. These are roundworms. When an attack occurs, the patient experiences drool foaming at the mouth, and in some cases, may sometimes eject an insect from the mouth or present with insufferable pain in the heart and abdominal regions.

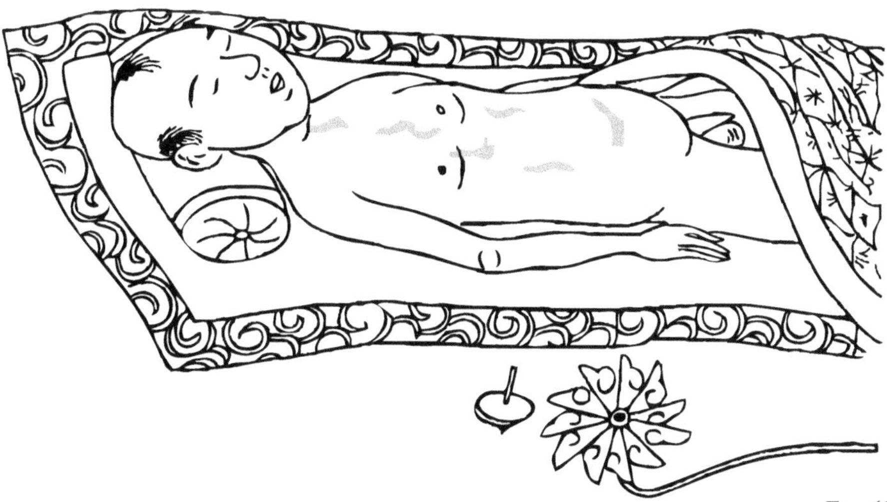

Fig. 69

余が門人、參州八名郡御園村の醫、稲垣某、大人・小人の蚘蟲を治するの家傳ありて、その國中の患ひを救ふこと數へがたし。余が爲に之れを傳與す。

One of my pupils, a certain physician with the [family] name of Inagaki who was from Misono Village, which is located in the Yana District of Sanshū, had a [secret] family formula to treat roundworms in adults and children. This formula has saved an untold number of patients in his province.[316] He passed on this [formula] to me.

316. Sanshū 參州 is the abbreviated name of Mikawa Province (Jp: *Mikawa-No-Kuni* 三河國). The province was located in the area that today forms the eastern half of Aichi Prefecture (Jp: *Aichi-Ken* 愛知縣).

則ち鷓胡菜丸の方
Zhè Hú Cài Wán[317]

海人草（一盞。[318]黒やき性を存す）・巴豆（五分。皮をさる）・大黄（八分）。

hǎi rén cǎo	海人草	burn until black without destroying its nature	1 qián
bā dòu	巴豆	remove the seed cover	5 fēn
dà huáng	大黄		8 fēn

右三味、末丸となし、三厘、五厘より三、四分に至る。その多少を分かち用ゆること考ふべし。右、大人・小兒蚘蟲の者、或るひは大便閉する者、みな此れを用ひて効あり。

Make the above three ingredients into powder pills from three to five *li,* up to three or four *fēn* in size.[319] [The physician] should consider the size [of the powder pills] to be used. The above [formula] is effective in all cases of roundworms in adults or children and in cases of fecal block.

又た云ふ、小兒の急腹痛、或るひは痘瘡まへの者、黄連・大黄を與へて三日、五日をへて、此の方を以て大ひに下す。その効、神の如し。

Furthermore, in cases of acute abdominal pain in children or [just] before pox sores [appear], *huáng lián* and *dà huáng* should be administered for three to five days, and then this

317. The original source of *Zhè Hú Cài Wán* 鷓胡菜丸 (Jp: *Shakosai-Gan*; Digenea Pill) is unclear, but the formula seems to have been popularized in Japan by *Meika-Hōsen*《名家方選》. Although not widely used in Japan at present, the extract preparation of the formula is approved by the MHLW to be sold in Japanese drug stores as an over-the-counter drug under the name *Zhè Gū Cài Tāng* 鷓鴣菜湯 (Jp: *Shakosai-Tō*; digenea decoction) or *Sān Wèi Zhè Gū Cài Tāng* 三味鷓鴣菜湯 (Jp: *Sanmi-Shakosai-Tō*; Three-Ingredient Digenea Decoction). It is currently indicated by the MHLW for: expulsion of ascaris. (Note: May be used regardless of physical strength) (回蟲の驅除 [注：體力に關わらず、使用できる]).

318. The original text uses the character for cup (Ch: *zhǎn* 盞; Jp: *san*), but this appears to be a mistake for *qián* (Ch: *qián* 戔 in this book, but more correctly written as 錢; Jp: *sen*).

319. *Lí* 厘 (also written as 釐; Jp: *rin*) was a traditional unit of measurement of length used in East Asia. The exact length varied depending on the time period and region in which it was used, but during the Meiji period in Japan, it was standardized as one one-hundredth of a *cùn* 寸 (Jp: *sun*), that is, 0.303mm.

formula should be used to greatly precipitate [the toxin]. The efficacy [of the formula] is divine.

則ち甘草粉蜜湯の方
Gān Cǎo Fěn Mì Tāng

甘草（ 二盞 ）・粉（ 一盞 ）・蜜（ 四盞 ）。

gān cǎo	甘草	2 qián
fěn	粉	1 qián
mì	蜜	4 qián

右三味 、水九分を以て 、先づ甘草を煮て六分にとり 、滓を去りて二味を入れ 、攪きまぜ和せしめ 、煎じ薄粥の如す 。

Boil the above three ingredients in nine *fēn* of water; first boil the *gān cǎo* to make six *fēn*, remove the dregs, and add the other two ingredients. Mix the ingredients and boil together until the decoction has the consistency of [rice] gruel.

余 、此の方に困苦して 、その効の有無を究むることありて云ふ 、此こに隊伍せし粉の品 。諸家の說多くして明らかならず 。『 千金方 』梁米粉に作る 。今試むるに功なし 。粉は鉛粉なり 。藥舗に唐の土と云ふもの 、是れなり 。然れども余 、一書に「 粉は輕粉 」と云ふに從ひ 、之れを用ひて妙効を得ること數々なり 。

[At first,] I struggled with [understanding] this formula, and having thoroughly investigated the efficacy [of the ingredients], I shall list here [the different] types of *fěn* [which have been used in the formula]. There are many different explanations [concerning what *fěn* is], and [the truth] has not yet been [completely] elucidated.[320] According to the *Qiān Jīn Fāng*,[321] *fěn* refers to *liáng mǐ fěn* 梁米粉. When I tried using [this formula], it was

320. *Jīn Guì Yào Lüè* simply lists *fěn* 粉 in the ingredient list of the formula, and there appears to have been no clear consensus concerning the correct crude drug to be used. Ancient and modern commentators have been split between the view of *fěn* as *qiān fěn* 鉛粉 (Jp: *enpun*; processed galenite), which was believed to work as a toxin to kill the roundworms responsible for roundworm abdominal pain, and the view of *fěn* as *mǐ fěn* 米粉 (Jp: *beifun*; rice powder), which was thought to stabilize roundworms and harmonize the stomach. The use of *qīng fěn* 輕粉 (Jp: *keifun*; calomel), as advocated by the author of this work, cannot be found in any extant text.

321. *Bèi Ji Qiān Jīn Yào Fāng* 《 備急千金要方 》(Essential Prescriptions Worth a Thousand

ineffective. [Some say that the] character *fěn* [in the formula] refers to *qiān fěn*. It is what is known as "Chinese earth" in pharmacies. However, one book that I have states that "*fěn* refers to *qīng fěn*." I used [*qīng fěn*] in accordance with [the explanation of the work] and have often obtained wondrous results [in my clinical practice].

舊に東都にある時、余が使ふ僕の兒三歳なるが、心腹痛を患へて止まざること半年ばかり。曾て衆醫大家の憐れみを受けて藥を服すといへども、皆、効なし。余、之れを診するに、かの蚘蟲有りて游走來去す。乃ち甘草粉蜜湯の本劑を以て之れをせむ。大ひに吐下して、數月の患へ、一時に去る。然れども又た顔赤く胸滿することあり。乃ち桂枝去芍藥湯を用ゆること五、六日にして、漸々快癒して志氣樂しみ、十日餘をへ、行歩することをえたり。

When I was traveling in the eastern capital [i.e., Edo], the three-year-old child of my servant suffered from unceasing pain in the heart and abdominal regions for approximately half a year. A multitude of physicians took pity on him and prescribed [various] medicinals, but they were all ineffective. When I examined him, I found that he had a roundworm that wandered [in the abdomen as if] arriving and departing. I subsequently used *Gān Cǎo Fěn Mì Tāng* as the base formula to attack [the toxin. The boy] experienced great vomiting and diarrhea, and the suffering that had continued for several months [finally] disappeared in an instant. However, his face sometimes became red and he experienced fullness in the chest. He used *Guì Zhī Qù Sháo Yào Tāng* for five or six days, whereupon he gradually recovered and his mind-qì became happier. After more than ten days, he became ambulant.

又た一女子、年十四才なるが、彼の小兒の妙効あるを聞きて、其の父、之れを背にして來たり、治を乞ふて止まず。之れを診するに、兩脚攣急して歩むことあたはず。又た坐すること能はず。臥す時は人に救はれ、木石を倒すが如し。此くの如く廢人たること四年ばかり。すなはち甘草粉蜜湯の正症なり。本方を以てかさね進む。大ひに瞑眩して吐下傾くるが如く、殆んど死せんとす。父母忍びず、大ひに哭す。余が云はく、「死生は天に在り。病毒を去らんと欲して何の恐るること有らんや。汝らをどろくこと勿れ」と云ひて歸る。翌日、快愈することを覺へて起つて歩むことを得たり。此くの如き類、余が門中に間々あり。諸君子、粉は輕粉を用ひて、その効いちじるしきことを知るべし。

in Gold For Every Emergency).

There was also one young woman, aged fourteen years, who heard about the wondrous effect [the drug had] on the child. Her father carried her on his back and brought her to me and unceasingly pleaded for me to treat [her]. When I examined her, she presented with hypertonicity in both legs and could not walk. She was also unable to sit down. When she [wanted to] lie down, she was assisted by other people, [who laid her down] like one might roll a log or stone. She had thus been a cripple for approximately four years. [This case] was the right pattern for *Gān Cǎo Fěn Mì Tāng*. [Hence,] I continued to use the formula. She experienced severe dizziness and bent over as if she were about to die, similar to a patient experiencing vomiting and diarrhea. Unable to bear [the sight of it], her father and mother wept loudly. I said to them, "Life and death are [decided by] heaven. The disease toxin is attempting to leave [the body], therefore what is there to fear? Do not be fearful!" Having said this, I returned home. The next day, the patient recovered: she could stand and became ambulant. The pupils in my school have experienced cases similar to this one. Esteemed readers, you should understand that when *qīng fěn* is used, the efficacy [of the formula] is remarkable.

桂枝去芍藥湯之圖
Illustration for the Guì Zhī Qù Sháo Yào Tāng[322] [Pattern]
桂枝去芍藥湯

圖の如く、腹中軟にして拘攣なく、胸滿して上衝し、又た腹中、力なくをぼふ。或るひは下劑を以て下してのち、必ず上衝・胸滿して、腹力なく覺ゆる者あり。此の方を用ゆれば腹中、和して快愈なるなり。凡そ大ひに下利するの後は、胸滿・上衝する者なり。

As shown in the illustration, the abdomen is soft and has no hypertonicity, but there is fullness in the chest that surges upward. Furthermore, it feels as if [the patient] has no abdominal strength. After [the toxin] has been precipitated through the use of a laxative, some patients invariably experience upward surging, fullness in the chest, and a lack of abdominal strength. If this formula is used, the abdomen will be harmonized, and [the patient] will experience a complete recovery. In general, patients present with fullness in the chest and upward surging, subsequent to experiencing great diarrhea or dysentery.

322. The formula for *Guì Zhī Qù Sháo Yào Tāng* 桂枝去芍藥湯 (Jp: *Keishi-Kyo-Shakuyaku-Tō*; cinnamon twig decoction minus peony) was originally found in *Jīn Guì Yào Lüè* and *Shāng Hán Lùn*. At present, this formula is not covered by the Japanese National Health Insurance program and is not commonly used in Japan.

余、此の方をしばしば用ひて効を得ること有り。然れども時に臨んで其の証をつまびらかにして、之れを治すべし。又た桂枝湯の症にして心痛する者、この方の正症なり。若し瘀血・衝逆せば、龍肝散を兼用すべし。

臍上動氣上りて心を衝き、胸満す。
Supraumbilical stirring qì that surges upward to the heart [as well as] fullness in the chest.

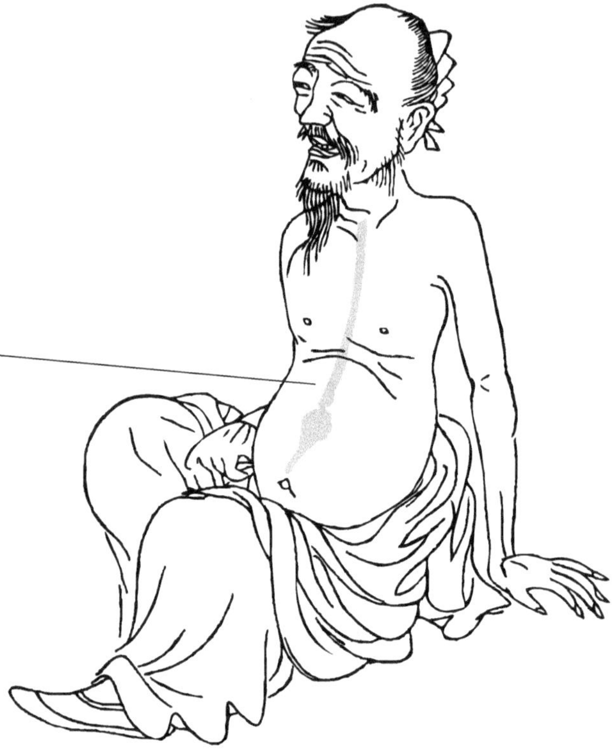

Fig. 70

I have often used this formula and obtained favorable results. However, [the condition] may [only] be treated after elucidating the pattern each time [i.e., for each individual case]. When the patient presents with the pattern for *Guì Zhī Tāng* and has heart pain, it is the right pattern for this formula. If [the patient] experiences blood stasis and a surging counterflow, *Lóng Gān Săn* may be used simultaneously.

凡そ下利の後、この方、或るひは小半夏加茯苓湯、あるいは桂枝湯、或るひは桂枝加苓朮湯、或るひは下利して心下痞鞕、雷鳴する者も、亦た雷鳴せざるものも、半夏瀉心湯の症、間々あり。その論、半夏瀉心湯の條下にあり。

After [the patient has experienced] diarrhea, he generally presents with the pattern for this formula, *Xiăo Bàn Xià Jiā Fú Líng Tāng, Guì Zhī Tāng*, or *Guì Zhī Jiā Líng Zhú Tāng.*[323]

323. The details of *Guì Zhī Jiā Líng Zhú Tāng* 桂枝加苓朮湯 (Jp: *Keishi-Ka-Ryō-Jutsu-Tō*;

In cases when the patient presents with diarrhea and glomus and hardness in the region below the heart with or without thunderous rumbling present [in the abdomen], it is the pattern for *Bàn Xià Xiè Xīn Tāng*. The details [of the formula] are listed in the section for *Bàn Xià Xiè Xīn Tāng*.

則ち桂枝去芍藥湯の方
Guì Zhī Qù Sháo Yào Tāng

桂枝・大棗・生姜(各九分)・甘草(六分)。

guì zhī	桂枝	9 fēn
dà zǎo	大棗	9 fēn
shēng jiāng	生姜	9 fēn
gān cǎo	甘草	6 fēn

右四味 、水一盞四分を以て 、六分に煮とる 。

Boil the above four ingredients in one cup and four *fēn* of water to make six *fēn* of the decoction.

cinnamon twig decoction plus poria and atractylodes) are not discussed in the present work. It appears that this formula may be a mistake or an adaption of *Keishi-Ka-Ryō-Jutsu-Bu-Tō* 桂枝加苓朮附湯 (Ch: *Guì Zhī Jiā Líng Zhú Fù Tāng*; cinnamon twig decoction plus poria, atractylodes, and aconite), an original formula of Yoshimasu Tōdō 吉益東洞. The extract preparation of *Keishi-Ka-Ryō-Jutsu-Bu-Tō* 桂枝加苓朮附湯 is covered by the Japanese National Health Insurance program as a prescription drug, and is also commonly sold in Japanese drug stores as an over-the-counter drug. It is currently indicated by the MHLW for: arthralgia and neuralgia in persons with weak physical strength who have cold extremities that feel stiff, oliguria, occasional palpitations, dizziness, or muscle twitching (體力虛弱で 、手足が冷えてこわばり 、尿量が少なく 、ときに動悸 、めまい 、筋肉のぴくつきがあるものの次の諸症 : 關節痛 、神經痛).

大黄硝石湯之圖

Illustration for the Dà Huáng Xiāo Shí Tāng[324] [Pattern]

大黄硝石湯

圖の如く、腹滿して心下より臍上まで之れを按すに實す。其の顏色、身體ことごとく黄を發し、時々自汗出でて、大便秘し、若しくは硬きもの、所謂黄疸病なるもの、是れなり。

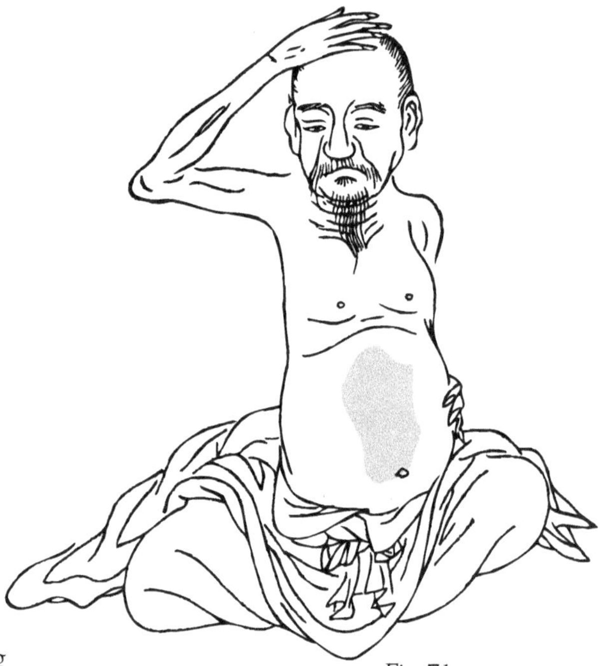

Fig. 71

As shown in the illustration, [the patient presents with] abdominal fullness and repletion that can be felt from the region located below the heart to the supraumbilical region upon palpation. When the patient presents with yellowing of the face and experiences spontaneous sweating accompanied by constipation or hard [stools], that is, [when the patient presents with] the disease that is known as jaundice, it is the [right] pattern [for this formula].

余、このしやうをしばしば療してかんがふるに、凡そその旁らに大柴胡湯の症、自若として備れり、且つ死する者多しといへども、生死は天工、治療は人事にして醫の與る所なり。余、尤も此の症の治に苦しむこと久し。

324. The details of *Dà Huáng Xiāo Shí Tāng* 大黄硝石湯 (Jp: *Daiō-Shōseki-Tō*; rhubarb and niter decoction) are not discussed in this work. The medicinal is composed of four ingredients (*dà huáng*, *xiāo shí*, *huáng bǎi*, and *shān zhī zǐ*) and has been traditionally used as a treatment for jaundice. The formula appears to have been copied from *Jīn Guì Yào Lüè*. However, some textual versions of *Jīn Guì Yào Lüè* substitute *huá shí* for *xiāo shí*, listing the formula as *Dà Huáng Huá Shí Tāng* 大黄滑石湯 (Jp: *Daiō-Kasseki-Tō*; rhubarb and talcum decoction). At present, the Japanese National Health Insurance program does not cover either formula and both appear to be rarely used in Japan.

I have often treated this pattern and considered [the best way to treat it]: I have found that in general, patients [who present with the pattern] naturally have the comorbid pattern for *Dà Chái Hú Tāng*. Furthermore, although many [of these] patients die, life and death are the work of [i.e., are decided by] heaven. Hence, physicians [can only] do all that is humanly possible to provide treatment. I had struggled to [find a] cure for this pattern for the longest time.

近ごろ、游歴中に富岳に上りて降路に迷ひ、怪しき寺に投じて、甲斐の徳本の『十九方』を得たり。その方中に「磁石丸」と云ふ奇方有りて、黄疸・黄肝病に兼用すること毎夜二戔。その効いちじるし。乃ち前篇に磁石丸の圖竝びに治論を記す。此こに又たその方法を記す。

During my recent travels climbing Mt. Fuji, I lost my way as I was descending the mountain. I happened upon a strange [Buddhist] temple, where I obtained a copy of [*Tokuhon-Ō-*]*Jūku-Hō*, written by Tokuhon of Kai Province.[325] The book contains a wondrous formula named *Jishaku-Gan*, of which a simultaneous dose of two *qián* is to be administered each night for the treatment of jaundice (yellow liver disease). The efficacy [of the formula] is remarkable. I have included an illustration and explanation of *Jishaku-Gan* in a previous volume. Here, I shall write again the method [to prepare the formula].

則ち磁石丸の方
Jishaku-Gan

磁石（二戔）・浮石・滑石（各三戔）・大黄（四戔）。

cí shí	磁石	2 qián
fú shí	浮石	3 qián
huá shí	滑石	3 qián
dà huáng	大黄	4 qián

右四味、木丸となし、毎夜一戔五分、或るひは二戔を白湯を以て送下す。

325. As earlier explained, the authenticity of the received version of *Tokuhon-Ō-Jūku-Hō*《徳本翁十九方》is disputed. The author apparently obtained a copy of the book from a monk at a Zen Buddhist temple located in Kai Province (Jp: *Kai-No-Kuni* 甲斐國), now Yamanashi Prefecture (Jp: *Yamanashi-Ken* 山梨縣).

Make the above four ingredients into a powder pill, and take one *qián* and five *fēn*, or up to two *qián* with hot water each night.

且つ黄疸病及び五疸を治するの方法は徳本翁の傳、一にして止まず。その餘の諸病、みな、十九方を以て、先後の取舍・交錯の妙術あり。然れども文多きが故に此こに記せず。他日を待つて三編に出ださんと欲す。

Moreover, according to text [written by] the venerable Tokuhon, the method to treat "yellow" jaundice or [any of] the five jaundices is to [use this formula] by itself without ceasing.[326] With regard to all other diseases, wondrous techniques for the selection of order and combination [of formulae] can be found in *Tokuhon-Ō-Jūku-Hō*. However, because the text is long, I shall omit it here.[327] I hope to publish it in a third volume at a future date.[328]

326. There are various definitions of the five jaundices (Ch: *wǔ dàn* 五疸; Jp: *go-tan*) in traditional Chinese texts. Although the author does not refer to any single definition, it can be assumed that as part of the Ancient School (Jp: *Kohō-Ha* 古方派) of Kampō medicine, he followed the definition as laid out in *Jīn Guì Yào Lüè*. According to the "Symptom Complex and Treatment of Jaundice Chapter (Ch: *Huáng Dǎn Bìng Mài Zhèng Bìng Zhì* 黄疸病脈證並治; Jp: *Ōdan-Byō-Myakushō-Hei-Chi*)," the five jaundices are as follows: *huáng dàn* 黄疸 (Jp: *ō-dan*; yellow jaundice), *gǔ dàn* 谷疸 (Jp: *koku-tan*; grain jaundice [i.e., jaundice due to dietary irregularities]), *jiǔ dàn* 酒疸 (Jp: *shu-tan*; liquor jaundice), *nǚ láo dàn* 女勞疸 (Jp: *jorō-tan*; sexual taxation jaundice), and *hēi dàn* 黑疸 (Jp: *koku-tan*; black jaundice).

327. The section on yellowing disease (*ōbyō* 黄病)/five jaundices in Volume I of the received text of *Tokuhon-Ō-Jūku-Hō* is as follows:

黄疸病。汗、衣を染むるが如きもの、発陳湯及び磁石丸兼服して可なり。心煩する者、解毒丸を兼用すべし。身黄黑、腹脹、大便黑く、時々下痢する者、磁石丸・順氣丸兼服して可なり。不治ものは、清済子を用ふべし。腹滿胸躍り、大便硬きもの、解毒丸・瀉心圓兼服して可なり。水を飲まんと欲し、小便不利者、容平丸・解毒丸兼服す。總べて黄病、其の証を不別、如何ともすることなきもの、磁石丸・解毒丸合方を用ひて可なり。

Yellow jaundice diseases: When [profuse] sweat appears to stain the clothing, *Hatchin-Tō* (Ch: *Fā Chén Tāng*; oldness-diffusion decoction) and *Jishaku-Gan* may be concomitantly used. When the body is yellowish black, the abdomen is distended, stools are black, and [the patient] often presents with dysentery, *Jishaku-Gan* and *Junki-Gan* may be concomitantly administered. When [the patient is] not cured, *Seisaishi* (*Qīng Jì Zǐ*; Clearing-Salvation) [Powder] may be used. When the abdomen is full, the chest [feels as if it were] leaping, and stools are hard, *Gedoku-Gan* and *Shashin-En* may be concomitantly administered. When [the patient] desires to drink water and urination is inhibited, *Yōhei-Gan* (*Róng Píng Wán*; Countenance-Calming Pill) and *Gedoku-Gan* are to be concomitantly administered. In all cases of a yellowing disease, regardless of the pattern, when nothing else can be done, *Jishaku-Gan* and *Gedoku-Gan* may be used in combination.

328. This is the final volume of the present work, which was published in 1800. Subsequent to publication of the work, the author became bedridden and died in 1805. For this reason, Wakuda

鶴丸之圖

Illustration for the Kaku-Gan[329] [Pattern] 鶴丸

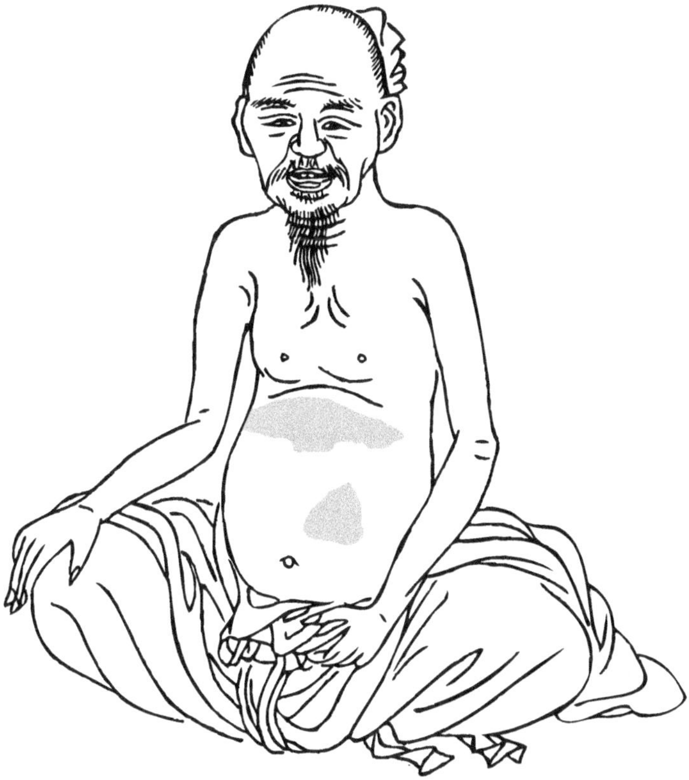

Fig. 72

圖の如く、胸膈痞塞若しくは腹中に血塊有りて、之れを按せば痛み、或るひは心下痞鞕し、心煩急迫して、時々胸腹いたみ、或るひは上りて心をつき、食すること能はず。或るひは大便の通じがたき者、此の方の主る處なり。

As shown in the illustration, the patient presents with glomus and hardness in the chest and diaphragm or a blood clot in the abdomen that causes pain upon palpation. In some

Yoshitora was entrusted by the author to carry out further research of abdominal patterns; his findings were subsequently published as *Fuku-Shō-Kiran-Yoku* (The Wings to Extraordinary Views of Abdominal Patterns). Most published versions of this work include the *Fuku-Shō-Kiran-Yoku* as a set.

329. As implied by the name, *Kaku-Gan* 鶴丸 (Ch: *Hè wán*; Kaku's pill) is a secret formula from the school of Kaku Taiei 鶴泰榮. Hence, it was probably never widely used and is largely unknown in Japan.

cases, the patient presents with glomus and hardness in the region below the heart, heart vexation, and distress. The patient may often experience chest or abdominal pain, and in some cases [qì] surges up into the heart and the patient is unable to eat. This formula governs [the pattern] in which the patient presents with fecal stoppage.

然りといへども、すべて丸・散・圓を用ゆることは、皆、兼用にして本劑を詳らかにして用ひざれば、たとひ治すと云ふとも、偶れ中たりにして、其の治に非ずのそしりを免れず。凡そ此の鶴丸を兼用すべき症は、桂枝人參湯、あるひは小柴胡湯の類、或るひは心下痞鞕脇下鞕滿結實するもの。其の餘積聚家、みな腹診と現症とを詳らかにして、本劑を用ひて、ままこの鶴丸一錢五分、或るひは一錢を兼用して効あり。

However, when simultaneously using any type of pill, powder, or other drug, unless the [efficacy of] the base formula is elucidated, even if the patient is cured, it will be impossible to avoid the accusation that the cure was by chance and not due to [the effects of] the treatment. This *Kaku-Gan* may be simultaneously used for patterns such as [the patterns for] *Guì Zhī Rén Shēn Tāng*, *Xiǎo Chái Hú Tāng*, or [patterns in which] the patient presents with glomus and hardness in the region below the heart and hard fullness and bound repletion in the rib-sides. For all other cases of accumulations and gatherings, this drug should be used after the abdominal patterns and current symptoms have been elucidated through examination; the simultaneous use of one *qián* and five *fēn* or one *qián* of this *Kaku-Gan* is effective.

則ち鶴丸の方
Kaku-Gan

大黃（七錢）・芒硝（五錢）・甘草（二錢）・人參・黃連（各一錢半）。

dà huáng	大黃	7 qián
máng xiāo	芒硝	5 qián
gān cǎo	甘草	2 qián
rén shēn	人參	1.5 qián
huáng lián	黃連	1.5 qián

右五味、末となし糊丸す。

Grind the above five ingredients to make flour and water paste pills.

この一方は、先師鶴先生より傳ふる所なり。故に鶴丸と稱す。即ち千金硝石大圓の變方、當歸を以て黄連に代へ藥製も亦た異なり。余、この丸を數年用ひえて、効あるをしれり。故に稱すること能はずして此こに出だせり。

This formula was passed down from my teacher, Kaku-Sensei. Hence, [I] call [this pill] *Kaku-Gan*. It is a modified formula of *Xiāo Shí Dà Wán*, [a formula] from *Qiān Jīn* [*Fāng*]; [in this formula,] *dāng guī* is substituted for *huáng lián*, and the method of preparation also differs.[330] I have used this pill for several years and experienced its efficacy. I have listed it here without being able to give it a [proper] name.

330. As explained in the text, the formula for *Xiāo Shí Dà Wán* 硝石大丸 (Jp: *Shōseki-Dai-Gan*; niter large pill) was originally found in *Bèi Jí Qiān Jīn Yào Fāng*. As implied from the name, *xiāo shí* (Jp: *shōseki*; niter) or *pò xiāo* (Jp: *bokushō*; impure mirabilite) should be used instead of *máng xiāo*, but it is unclear if the use of *máng xiāo* in *Kaku-Gan* is deliberate or a mistake. The text of *Bèi Jí Qiān Jīn Yào Fāng* is as follows: "治十二症瘕、及婦人帶下、絕產無子、並欲服寒食散而腹中有症瘕實者、當先服大丸下之、硝石(六兩、朴硝亦得)、大黃(八兩)、人參、甘草(各二兩)." ([This formula] treats not only the twelve concretions and conglomerations, but also vaginal discharges, female infertility, and childlessness; when the patient desires to take the powder cold and presents with abdominal concretions and conglomerations, *Xiāo Shí Dà Wán* should be first administered to precipitate them. [The formula is as follows:] *xiāo shí* [6 *liǎng*; *pò xiāo* may also be used], *dà huáng* [8 *liǎng*], *rén shēn*, *gān cǎo* [2 *liǎng* each].)

桃核承氣湯小腹急結之圖

Illustration for the Táo Hé Chéng Qì Tāng[331] [Pattern] 桃核承氣湯 [in the Case of a] Tense Bound Smaller Abdomen[332]

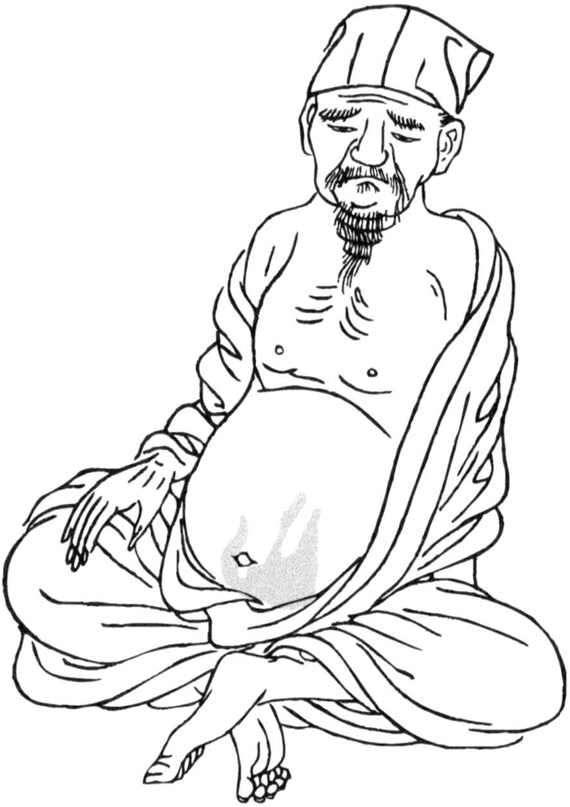

Fig. 73

331. The formula for *Táo Hé Chéng Qì Tāng* 桃核承氣湯 (Jp: *Tōkaku-Jōki-Tō*; peach kernel qì-infusing decoction) was originally found in *Shāng Hán Lùn*. The extract preparation of the formula is covered by the Japanese National Health Insurance program as a prescription drug, and may be sold in Japanese drug stores as an over-the-counter drug. It is currently indicated by the MHLW for: irregular menstruation, dysmenorrhea, menstrual pain, menstrual or postpartum anxiety, low back pain, constipation, simultaneous symptoms of hypertension (headache, dizziness, stiff shoulders), hemorrhoids, and bruises in persons with moderate or strong physical strength who have hot flashes and tend to experience constipation (體力中等度以上で、のぼせて便祕しがちなものの次の諸症：月經不順、月經困難症、月經痛、月經時や產後の精神不安、腰痛、便祕、高血壓の隨伴症狀「頭痛、めまい、肩こり」、痔疾、打撲症).

332. As later explained in the present section, according to traditional Chinese abdominal examination theory, this should be *shào fù* 少腹 (Jp: *shōfuku*; lesser abdomen) instead of *xiǎo fù* 小腹 (Jp: *shōfuku*; smaller abdomen).

前編に圖するところの桃軍圓は臍上急結して胸脇に逆滿するもの所謂血癪あるひは肝積などいふものに多し。此の圖はただちに小腹急結の甚だしきものを擧ぐ。是れ亦たしらずんばあるべからず。前編の圖說と併せ見るべし。

In the illustration [of the pattern] for *Tō-Gun-En* in the previous volume, the supraumbilical region is tense bound,[333] and the patient presents with counterflow fullness in the chest and rib-sides. It is common in patients who present with [conditions] such as the so-called blood or liver accumulations.[334] This illustration is an example of a rapidly [appearing] severe case of tense bound smaller abdomen. [The physician] must also understand this [pattern]. Refer to the illustration and explanation listed in the previous volume for a comparison [of the patterns matching *Tō-Gun-En*].

圖の如く、小腹に急結有りて上衝して惡血深し。もろもろ久病を患ふる者に此の症多くあり。數多の病名にかかはらず、只だ此の腹症を眼がんとして此の方を本劑ときはめ、小腹急結の病毒を攻むるなり。

As shown in the illustration, the patient presents with a tense bound smaller abdomen, upward surging, and malign blood that runs deep. Patients who are suffering from various enduring diseases often present with this pattern. Regardless of whichever of the many [possible] diseases that the patient may present with, [the physician should] simply focus on this abdominal pattern and resolve to administer the present formula as the base formula to attack the toxin [that is causing] the tense bound lesser abdomen.

その毒あさき者は、此の一方にして治することも有れども、毒ふかき者は日を追ふて重ね進むる時は、其の毒うごき變じて諸症交はり起こるもの也。その時、怠らず兼用してかたはらの諸症を去りて後、又た本劑に復してかさね進む。此くの如くにして月を重ね年をへる時は、いかなる難病・痼疾たりとも、治せずと云ふことなし。

333. Tense bind (Ch: *jí jié* 急結; Jp: *kyūketsu*) in the smaller or lesser abdomen generally refers to lower abdominal cramp, that is, a subjective sensation of distention and fullness of the lower abdomen, usually with difficult urination.

334. The original text actually says blood *shaku* (Jp: *kesshaku* 血癪), but it seems that this may be a mistake for blood accumulation (Ch: *xuè jī* 血積; Jp: *kesseki*).

When the toxin is shallow, this formula may occasionally be used to treat [the pattern], but when the toxin is deep and has progressed over many days, the toxin stirs and undergoes transmutation, causing various confluent patterns. When this happens, simultaneous treatment should be performed tirelessly, and after one of the confluent patterns has been eliminated, administration of the base formula may be resumed and continued. In this way, when [treatment] continues over a period of months or years, even intractable or longstanding diseases will be cured.

然れども、又たその方法、是れのみに限らず、ことごとく腹中を探り知りて、毒の狀（かたち）に依りて天然自得の腹診あり。是れ余が臆見短智を以て知るものに非ず。實に力を盡し功をつみて得るところ也。諸君子、狐疑することなく、此の術に深く志し、つとめて以てその自得なることを知るべし。且つ經文に云ふ、「但だ小腹急結の者は乃ち之れを攻む可し」と云々。

However, not limited to only this case, the method [of performing treatment] is to completely explore and understand the abdomen [of the patient]: by performing an abdominal examination, a natural [cure based on] examination of the form of the toxin [can be obtained]. I know this not based on my own conjectures or limited wisdom, but from accumulation of the successes that I have experienced through making all efforts in actual [clinical practice]. Esteemed gentlemen [i.e., readers], if you deeply aspire after this technique [of abdominal examination] and put it into practice without any doubts in your minds, you will naturally come to understand it. The text [of *Shāng Hán Lùn*] states: "this [formula] may be used to attack [the patterns of] patients who present with only a tense bound smaller abdomen."[335]

余、按ずるに、此の十字の語、天然自得の腹診にして、病毒を去るの妙術を教ゆることをしれり。然るゆえんは皆、余が諸州游歴に二十餘年のあひだ、竝びに門人もこの腹診を以て病痾を治すること、舉げてかぞへがたきを以てなり。

335. The original text as found in the "On Identification of Pulse, Symptom Complex, and Treatment of Greater Yáng Diseases Chapter (Ch: *Biàn Tài Yáng Mài Zhèng Bìng Zhì* 辨太陽病脈證并治; Jp: *Ben-Taiyō-Byō-Myakushō-Hei-Chi*)" is as follows: 外解已、但少腹急結者、乃可攻之、宜桃核承氣湯方 (When the exterior is resolved, *Táo Hé Chéng Qì Tāng* should be used to attack [the patterns of] patients who present with only a tense bound smaller abdomen). Although the original text of *Shāng Hán Lùn* uses the term *shào fù* 少腹 (lesser abdomen), the author of this book uses *xiǎo fù* 小腹 (smaller abdomen) in keeping with his policy not to distinguish these two traditionally different abdominal regions.

I believe that [based on] this phrase of ten [Chinese] characters [in the text], we can understand that [the author] is teaching [us] about abdominal examination, a natural [method] to be learned from experience. It is through this wondrous method [that we can] remove disease toxins from the body. For this reason, during my travels across various provinces over a period of twenty years, my pupils and I have used [the method] abdominal examination to [diagnose and] treat an untold number of long-standing diseases.

則ち桃核承氣湯の方
Táo Hé Chéng Qì Tāng

大黄（ 一戔 ）・芒硝（ 六分 ）・桃仁・桂枝・甘草（ 各五分 ）。

dà huáng	大黄	1 qián
máng xiāo	芒硝	6 fēn
táo rén	桃仁	5 fēn
guì zhī	桂枝	5 fēn
gān cǎo	甘草	5 fēn

右五味、水一盞半を以て、六分に煮とり、滓を去りて芒硝を入れ、一度に服す。且つ云ふ、前編の桃軍圓は本劑承氣にして、大黄・芒硝、君たるを以て服することを難しとせず。故に之れを略す。最も効あり。

Boil the above five ingredients in one and one-half cups of water to make six *fēn* of the decoction. Remove the dregs, add *máng xiāo,* and administer [the decoction] in a single sitting. Furthermore, *Tō-Gun-En,* mentioned in the previous volume, is a qì-coordinating decoction. *Dà huáng* and *máng xiāo* are the sovereign [ingredients] of the formula, and [the formula] is not difficult [for patients] to take. Therefore, I will omit [the details here]. It is the most effective [medicinal for the pattern described here].

則ち桃軍圓の略方
Tō-Gun-En

大黄（ 十戔 ）・芒硝（ 六戔 ）・桃仁・桂枝・蕎麥（ 各五戔 ）。

dà huáng	大黄	10 qián
máng xiāo	芒硝	6 qián
táo rén	桃仁	5 qián
guì zhī	桂枝	5 qián
qiáo mài	蕎麥	5 qián

右五味 、細末となし 、蜜を以てねる 。此の方 、永久に用ひざれば沈痾を治すること能はず 。故に之れを丹となす 。

Grind the above five ingredients into a fine powder and mix with honey. If this formula is not administered over a long period of time, heavy [i.e., severe] diseases cannot be cured. It is for this reason that this [medicinal] is called an elixir.

千金甘草湯之圖
Illustration for the [Qiān Jīn] Gān Cǎo Tāng[336] [Pattern]
《千金》甘草湯

圖の如く 、腹中拘攣急迫し 、或るひは腹滿して時々いきだはしく上衝し 、又た息ぎれすることを覺ゆる者 、此の症の眼なり 。此こに「 拘攣 」と云ふは 、腹中に物ありて指頭に拘はり 、引つぱる如く覺ゆるを云ふ 。又た「 急迫 」は 、「 引きつりせまる 」義なり 。「 急 」は腹皮にて弓の弦を按してたゆまざる如くをぼふ 。「 迫 」は 、をし付けらるる如く 、或るひは胸 、或るひは腹 、いきたはしく息ぎれのする如く覺ゆるなり 。

336. There are several formulae with the name *Gān Cǎo Tāng* 甘草湯 (Jp: *kanzō-tō*; licorice decoction). As seen from the title, this version was taken from *Bèi Jí Qiān Jīn Yào Fāng*. At present, this formula is not covered by the Japanese National Health Insurance program and is not commonly used in Japan. Moreover, in Japan, *Gān Cǎo Tāng* generally refers to the formula containing only *gān cǎo* that is found in *Shāng Hán Lùn*.

As shown in the illustration, the patient presents with hypertonicity and distress in the abdomen. In some cases, the patient has abdominal fullness and occasional upward surging that causes a choking [i.e., stuffy] feeling, and the patient may experience loss of breath. [These symptoms] are the indications of this pattern. Here, what is meant by "hypertonicity" is [the feeling of] something in abdomen causing tension that can be felt with the fingertips, as if [the abdomen] is being pulled. The word "distress" means being forcibly pulled.[337] *Jí* 急 [i.e., the first character of the word "distress"] refers to the feeling of the abdominal skin being pulled taut, similar to [the feeling of] a bow string [being pulled]. *Pò* 迫, [i.e., the second character], refers to the sensation of being forcibly pressed in the chest or in the abdomen, causing a choking feeling of breathlessness.

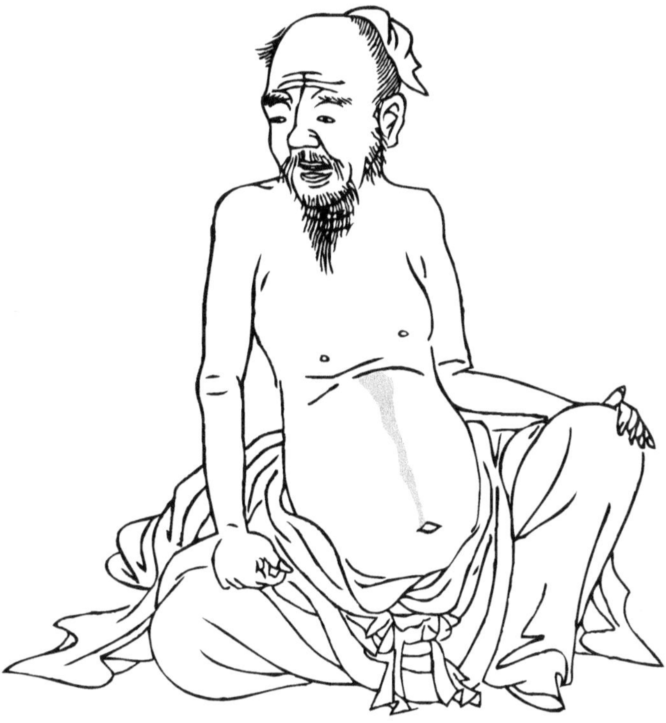

Fig. 74

又たこの症は口中かわき、手足冷ゆるもの多し。或るひは唇の乾くこともあり。本文に云ふ、「産乳餘血不盡、逆しまに、心胸を搶き、手足逆冷・唇乾き・腹脹り・短氣」とあり。

Furthermore, many patients who have this pattern present with dry mouth and cold extremities. In some cases, the lips are also dry. In the main text [of *Bèi Jí Qiān Jīn Yào Fāng*],

337. There are a number of different words in Chinese that are commonly translated as distress. The word used in this section is *jí pò* 急迫 (Jp: *kyūhaku*).

it is stated that "[*Gān Cǎo Tāng*] treats postpartum persistent flow of blood, counterflow prodding the heart and chest [regions], counterflow cold of the extremities, dry lips, abdominal distention, and shortness of breath."[338]

則ち甘草湯の方
[Qiān Jīn] Gān Cǎo Tāng

甘草・桂枝・芍藥・阿膠（ 各八分 ）・大黄（ 一錢 ）。

gān cǎo	甘草	8 fēn
guì zhī	桂枝	8 fēn
sháo yào	芍藥	8 fēn
ē jiāo	阿膠	8 fēn
dà huáng	大黄	1 qián

右五味 、東流水（ 漢土は川多く東に流る 。本邦にては南へ流る川の水にても可也 ）二盞四分を以て 、一盞に煮とり 、滓を去りて阿膠を入れ 、一度に服す 。

Boil the above five ingredients in two cups and four *fēn* of water [from a river] that flows in an easterly direction (most rivers in China flow toward the east, but in this country [i.e., Japan], water from a river that flows in a southerly direction may be used) to make one cup of the decoction.[339] Remove the residue, add *ē jiāo*, and take [the decoction] in a single dose.

余 、この方と前に記する桃軍圓を久しく用ひをぼへて 、癲癇を治することと間々あり 。然れども此の二方に限りて治すと云ふにも非

338. The original text as found in the "Formulae for Women, Part II Chapter (Ch: *Fù Rén Fāng Zhōng* 《 婦人方中 》; Jp: *Fujin-Hō-Chū*)" is as follows: 甘草湯 、治產乳餘血不盡 、逆搶心胸 、手足逆冷 、唇乾 、腹脹 、短氣方.
339. In ancient China, water flowing in an easterly direction from rivers to the sea was a common symbol of the natural order of the world. In the "*Xú Wú Guǐ* 徐無鬼 (Jp: *Jo-Mu-Ki*) Chapter" of *Zhuāng Zǐ* 《 莊子 》 it is explained that "海不辭東流 、大之至也" (...when the sea does not reject the streams that flow into it in their eastward course, we have the perfection of greatness). This thinking can also be seen in some ancient medical texts such as *Jīn Guì Yào Lüè*: in the details of the formula for *Zé Qī Tāng* 澤漆湯 (Jp: *Takushitsu-Tō*; sun spurge decoction), it is recommended to use five *dòu* of easterly flowing water (original text: 以東流水五斗).

ず。世上、多くは癲癇と云ふ病名になづみ、名方・妙藥・禁祕の方など云ふものを以て療すれども、彼治して、是れ治せざること多し。方症相對せざるが故なり。只だその腹症を詳らかにして毒のある處を明察し、その毒つきるまで攻めていかなる難病たりとも治せずと云ふことなし。是れ天然の方法なり。

I have long used this formula and the previously-mentioned *Tō-Gun-En* [in clinical practice], and seen [both formulae] cure [cases of] withdrawal and epilepsy. However, this does not mean that treatment [of this condition] is limited to these two formulae. [Physicians] of the world are too focused on the diagnosis of "withdrawal and epilepsy," and attempt to treat the condition with all sorts of famous, "wondrous," or secret formulae; in some cases [the condition is] cured, but in others not.[340] This is because these formulae were not matched to the pattern. [The physician must] simply elucidate the abdominal pattern [in order to] clearly identify the location where the toxin resides and attack said toxin until it disappears. [When treatment is performed in this way,] any intractable disease will not remain uncured. This is the natural method [of treatment].

余、かつて京師に在つて、寺町新竹屋町邊に住する匠人嘉七と云ふ者を療せり。其の者、癲癇を患ふること歳久し。その時に二十七、八也。時として病發するときは人事をしらず、百藥効なし。夫婦相なくの外すべきことなし。然れども、發せざる時は、平人の如くその業をつとむ。近ごろに至りて、病毒深く加して日夜をこらざることなし。夜にして發する時は水火をさけず、或るひは唇をかみやぶり、或るひは舌をかみ、殆んど死せんとす。

When I was in the capital region [i.e., Kyōto],[341] I treated an artisan named Kashichi who lived near the Shinchikuya area of Tera-Machi.[342] He suffered from withdrawal and epilepsy for many years. At that time, he was twenty-seven or twenty-eight [years old]. When an [epileptic] attack occurred, the patient would lose consciousness, and the hundred medicinals were ineffective [to cure his disease]. He had no spouse, and there was nothing else that could be done [to support him]. However, when he did not

340. Although *dian xián* 癲癇 (Jp: *tenkan*) has been literally translated as "withdrawal and epilepsy," most Japanese texts, including the present work, do not differentiate the two conditions, and the expression is used to refer to any type of epilepsy.

341. Jīng shī 京師 (Jp: keishi) refers to the capital region where the emperor resided. Although Edo (now Tōkyō) was the de facto capital of Japan during the Edo period, the emperor continued to reside in Kyōto.

342. Tera-Machi (literally, "temple town") is a street that runs north-south in Kyōto. A large number of temples and shops are located along the street.

experience an attack, he could work normally like a healthy person. In recent years, the disease toxin had grown deeper, and there was no day or night in which an attack did not occur. When attacks occurred at night, [the patient] was unable to avoid [dangerous things such as] water or fire. In some cases, he would bite his lips to the point of injury, and in other cases he would bite his tongue; it appeared as if he were largely on the verge of death.

余、之れを診するに、その腹、別にこばむことなし。胸脇苦滿及び實して小腹急結す。之れを按していたみ、兩眼つねに引きつり、白眼にして人を睨むが如し。乃ち大柴胡湯の本劑を與ふること日に三たび。毎夜、桃軍圓を雞卵の大ひさほど空心に用ゆ。時々、先天滅毒丸、五分を兼用す。かくの如く重ね進めて、毎夜、合掌の灸を四十餘日して、全く治して平人の如し。然れどもかく早く治するは甚だ少なし。多くは一年、或るひは一年半、二年。早く治すと云ふも、半年ばかりなり。

When I examined him, there was no region of his abdomen that refused [palpation, i.e., no impediments in the abdomen were felt. He presented with] bitter fullness and repletion in the chest and rib-sides as well as a tense bound smaller abdomen. When I pressed [these regions], the patient experienced pain and both eyes rolled back (as if they were being pulled) to show the whites of his eyes; it appeared as if he was giving a menacing look. I therefore administered the base formula of *Dà Chái Hú Tāng* three times per day. Each night, I had him [also] take *Tō-Gun-En* pills the size of chicken eggs on an empty stomach. From time to time, I also simultaneously used five *fēn* of *Metsu-doku-Gan.*[343] While continuing to administer [the drug] as written here, I performed moxibustion using a clasped-hand technique each night for more than forty nights. The patient subsequently made a full recovery and became a healthy person. However, it is extremely rare [for such a condition] to be cured so quickly. In many cases, [treatment] takes one, one and one-half, or two years. Even in cases in which [the condition] is quickly cured, [the treatment still] takes approximately a half year [until completion].

343. *Metsudoku-Gan* 滅毒丸 was a Kaku family secret recipe. See Volume 1, Footnote 48 for a more detailed explanation.

癲癇治不治之圖
Illustrations of Curable and Incurable Cases of Withdrawal and Epilepsy

下へすじあるもの全く治す。
When there are lines running inferior [to the pupil, the condition] can be completely cured.

上へすじあるもの治せず。
When there are lines running superior [to the pupil, the patient] cannot be cured.

難治
Intractable [case]

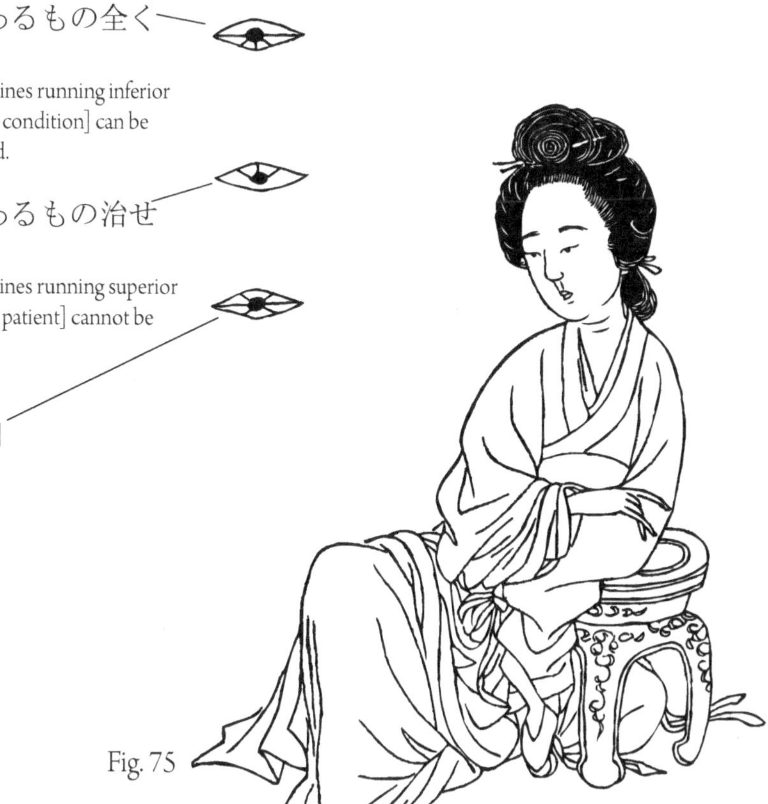

Fig. 75

相州佐竹の醫、豐浦某家祕の方。癲癇を治するの妙劑也と云ひ、「混元丹」と號す。

There is a secret family formula of a certain physician named Toyoura[344] who lives in the Satake region of Sōshū.[345] Saying that it is a wondrous formula to treat withdrawal and epilepsy, he named it *Kongen-Tan*.[346]

344. No information concerning this individual is available.
345. Sōshū 相州 is the abbreviated name of Sagami Province (Jp: *Sagami-No-Kuni* 相模國), which was located in what is today the central and western regions of Kanagawa Prefecture (Jp: *Kanagawa-Ken* 神奈川縣).
346. As stated in the text, *Kongen-Tan* 混元丹 (Ch: *Hùn Yuán Dān*; placenta elixir) is a secret

則ち方：

The formula is as follows:

混元衣（ 六戔 、黒やき ）・天南星・附子・銀朱（ 各三戔 、光明朱也 ）・牛黄・雞舌（ 各一戔五分 、丁子なり ）。

hùn yuán yī	混元衣	charred	6 qián
tiān nán xīng	天南星		3 qián
fù zǐ	附子		3 qián
yín zhū	銀朱	bright yín zhū [is to be used]	3 qián
niú huáng	牛黄		1 qián and 5 fēn
jī shé [xiāng]	雞舌[香]		1 qián and 5 fēn
dīng zǐ*	丁子		

* *Jī shé xiāng* 雞舌香 (Jp: *keizetsukō*; clove fruit) refers to fructus caryophylli, but *dīng zǐ* 丁子 (Jp: *chōji*; clove blossom) generally refers to flos caryophylli. It is unclear to which part of the plant Caryophyllus aromaticus the author is referring.

右大味 、各々別に末となし糊丸す 。但し混元衣 、男の病ひには女を用ひ 、女の病ひには男を用ゆと云ふ 。下 、之れに倣へ 。

Grind each of the above ingredients into a powder separately to make flour and water paste pills. However, in the case of *hùn yuán yī*, it is said that a female [placenta] should be used for diseases in men, and a male [placenta] should be used for diseases in women. Follow this [principle] when using the [formula] below.

又た安鎮丸の方
Anchin-Gan[347]

（ 主治 、上に同じ ）

The indications [for this drug] are the same as above:

formula and was probably never widely used in Japan. There is a medicinal with the name *Kongen-Tan* 混元丹 that can be bought online in Japan, but the formula is completely different from the formula listed here.

347. The source of the formula for *Anchin-Gan* 安鎮丸 (Ch: *Ān Zhèn Wán*; quieting and settling pill) is unclear. It also appears to be a secret formula and was likely never well known in Japan.

混元衣（ 一兩 ）・蒟蒻根（ かげぼしにして ）・鹿角屑・甘草（ 各七分 ）。

hùn yuán yī	混元衣		1 liǎng
jǔ ruò gēn	蒟蒻根	dried in the shade	7 fēn
lù jiǎo xiè	鹿角屑		7 fēn
gān cǎo	甘草		7 fēn

右四味 、黒焼きにし 、別に末とし合して 、更に生甘草の末・麝香（ 各二分 ）を加へ 、再び合して之れを和し七服となし 、日に一貼を服し 、七日にして盡す 。もし愈ゆるや否やを知らんと欲せば 、蒟蒻根の生末一錢を服すべし 。病未だつきざれば 、忽ち發す 。

Char the above four ingredients, grind each into a powder separately, and mix together. Add *gān cǎo* and *shè xiāng* (two *fēn* each) and mix [the ingredients] together again and divide into seven doses. Administer once daily for seven days until [the drug] is used up. If [the physician] desires to know if the patient will be cured or not, he should administer one *qián* of *jǔ ruò gēn* (raw flakes). While the disease has not yet completed its course, [symptoms] will suddenly reappear.

一方：

[Here is] another formula:

欝金（ 六兩 ）・苦參・枯礬（ 各三兩 ）。

yù jīn	鬱金	6 liǎng
kǔ shēn	苦參	3 liǎng
kū fán	枯礬	3 liǎng

右三味 、水煎或るひは糊丸 。

Decoct the three above ingredients in water or make flour and water paste pills.

豐浦子云ふ 、「 世に癲癇の妙方・奇藥ありといへども 、みな 、方症相對するを以てよく治する也 。然らざれば 、彼治して是れ治せず 」と 。此の言 、甚だ信なり 。

Dr. Toyoura [once] said, "Even all of those so-called wondrous formulae and extraordinary medicinals that are used to treat withdrawal and epilepsy can only cure [the condition] if the formula has been [correctly] matched to the pattern. If [formula-pattern matching] is not performed, some patients will be cured and others will not be cured." This saying is indeed true!

余、諸州を游歴中に名家累代舊傳の妙藥・奇方と稱するものを受け得たり。其の數、凡そ二百五十餘なり。時々、之れを用ひ試みるに、少しの効を得ることありといへども、全く治することまれ也。或るひは彼治すれども是れ治せず。その準縄（すみかね）定めがたし。故に捨ててもちひず。

During my travels across various provinces, I have collected wondrous medicinals and extraordinary formulae found in the ancient texts [written by] the famous physicians of successive generations. In total, I have collected more than 250 [formulae]. On occasion, I have attempted to use [the formulae], and although a slight effect was observed in some cases, [the medicinals] did not completely cure [the diseases]. Some cured [the diseases] and others did not. It was difficult to establish a level-line [i.e., a standard for pattern identification and treatment]. Hence, I have ceased to use them.

然りといへども、此に記する所の五方は、豐浦子の奇方にして、妙効あること余が舊友之れをいへり。故に之れを得て余に傳ふ。且つ余も亦た腹診の術を以て癲癇を治すること間々あり。故に此にならべ記す。學ぶ者、ゑらび用ひて、某々の効を詳らかにして極め知りて、天下後世に傳へのこさば、廢疾をすくふの一助ともならんか。

However, my old friend once said that these five extraordinary formulae from Dr. Toyoura (that are listed here in this [work]) have wondrous efficacy. For this reason, he obtained [the formulae] and passed them on to me. I also have used [the formulae in accordance with] the techniques for abdominal examination to cure cases of withdrawal and epilepsy. Thus, I have listed [the formulae] here. As the student [of abdominal patterns] selects and uses the formulae after elucidating and thoroughly understanding their respective indications and passes them on to future generations, it will be a great help in saving patients from crippling diseases.

下瘀血湯之圖

Illustration for the Xià Yū Xuè Tāng[348] [Pattern] 下瘀血湯

Fig. 76

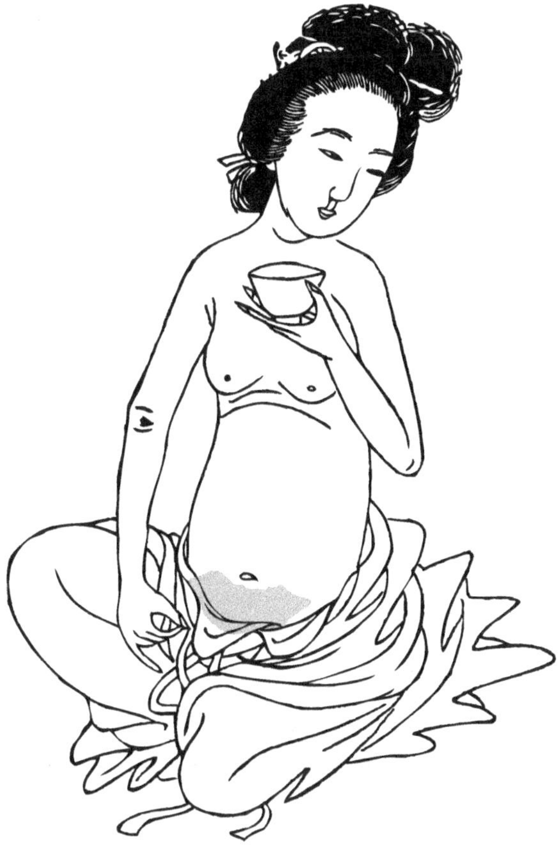

圖の如く、臍下に瘀血有りて、小腹急痛忍ぶべからず。甚だしきは手も近づくべからず。本方の主るところとす。又た凡そ劑を投ずるに、臍下の診を以て分別する者、八、九あり。詳らかなることは下に記す。此の症は臍下をさぐりみるに、その指頭にこたへ堅きものあるを覺へ、時に急に痛むもの、此の方の正症なり。

As shown in the illustration, the patient presents with blood stasis in the subumbilical region and insufferable acute pain in the smaller abdomen. In severe cases, [the patient] is unable to bear even the slightest touch of the hand [during abdominal examination].

348. The formula for *Xià Yū Xuè Tāng* 下瘀血湯 (Jp: *Ge-Oketsu-Tō*; stasis-precipitating decoction) was originally found in *Jīn Guì Yào Lüè*. At present, this formula is not covered by the Japanese National Health Insurance program and is not commonly used in Japan.

This formula governs [the pattern]. Moreover, when administering the medicinal, differentiation of the pattern can be made by examination of the subumbilical region in eight or nine [out of ten cases]. I shall write my elucidated findings below. When [the physician] searches around the subumbilical region and the fingertips feel hardness that springs back and acute pain is present [on palpation], it is the right pattern for this formula.

余、考ふるに、是れ大血症にして、婦人は經水通ぜず、男子も亦た血症のものに多し。その人或るひは腰痛久しく止まず、或るひは淋疾・痔・脫肛などの患ひある者あり。或るひは大建中湯の症を發する者、間々此の證あり。

I believe that this is a great blood pathocondition in which a woman presents with inhibited menstrual flow. However, male patients also often present with blood pathoconditions. These [male] patients may present with enduring lumbar pain that does not cease, and others suffer from strangury disease, hemorrhoids, or prolapse of the rectum. When [such] patients present with the pattern for *Dà Jiàn Zhōng Tāng*, it is the right pattern [for this formula].

則ち下瘀血湯の方
Xià Yū Xuè Tāng

大黄（四戔）・桃仁・䗪蟲（各二戔五分）。

dà huáng	大黄	4 qián
táo rén	桃仁	2 qián and 5 fēn
zhè chóng	蟅蟲	2 qián and 5 fēn

右三味、細末にして蜜を以てねり四丸となし、酒八分を以て一丸を六分に煎じ取りて、一度に服す。

Grind the above three ingredients into a fine powder and mix with honey to make four pills. Boil one pill in eight *fēn* of sake to make six *fēn* of the decoction. Take in a single dose.

余、舊に東都にある時、一男子三十四、五歳、大腹痛にて臍下痛むこと三年、百療効なしと云ふ。余、之れを診するに、暗然として冷氣を覺ふ。腹皮強急して頭足あるが如し。乃ち大建中湯を與へ、一月許りにして漸々愈ゆ。又た臍下痛むを覺ふ、忍び難し。乃ち下瘀血湯を與ふ。數日にして全く愈ゆ。

I once was in the eastern capital [i.e., Edo], where I encountered a man of the age of thirty-four or thirty-five. He presented with great abdominal pain, [especially] pain in the subumbilical region, for three years; he said that the hundred treatments [i.e., various types of treatment] were ineffective [in curing his condition]. When I examined him, I felt a subtle cold qì [in the abdomen]. He presented with taut abdominal skin that appeared similar to a cephalopod. I administered *Dà Jiàn Zhōng Tāng* to him, and he gradually recovered over a period of approximately one month. He subsequently felt unbearable pain in the subumbilical region. [Therefore, I] administered *Xià Yū Xuè Tāng* [to him]. The patient was completely cured within several days.

土瓜根散之圖

Illustration for the Tǔ Guā Gēn Sǎn[349] [Pattern] 土瓜根散

圖の如く、臍旁小腹滿拘攣するもの有りて、婦人は經水利せず、或るひは白物を下し、或るひは帶下の患へあり。男子は血症にして、時として腹痛する者に此の症間々あり、且つ小腹拘急することあるを考ふべし。

As shown in the illustration, the patient presents with fullness and hypertonicity in the regions beside the umbilicus and in the smaller abdomen. In the cases of women, menstrual flow is inhibited and in some cases the patient may present with a white discharge or [other types of] vaginal discharge. This pattern is [the true] pattern for men who present with a blood pathocondition and often experience abdominal pain. [*Tǔ Guā Gēn Sǎn*] may also be considered in cases of hypertonicity of the smaller abdomen.

349. The formula for *Tǔ Guā Gēn Sǎn* 土瓜根散 (Jp: *Dokakon-San*; cucumber gourd root powder) was originally found in *Jīn Guì Yào Lüè*. At present, this formula is not covered by the Japanese National Health Insurance program and is not commonly used in Japan.

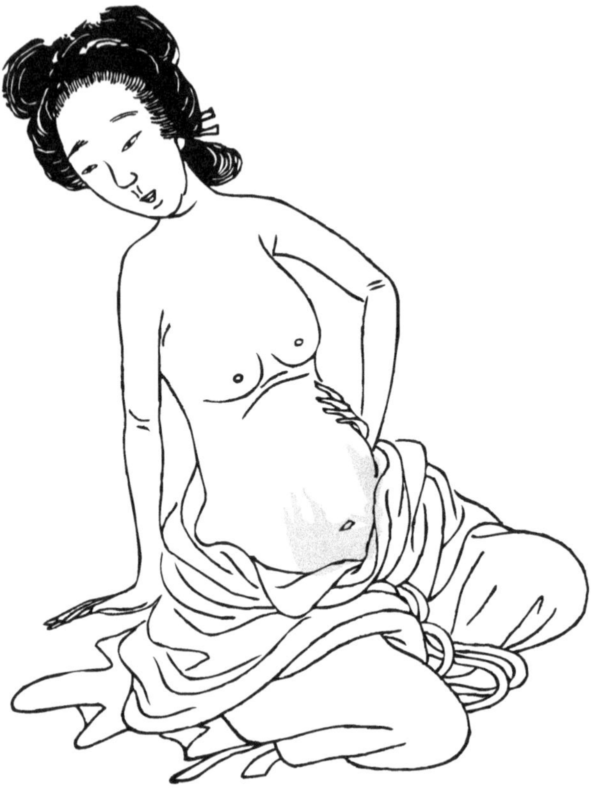

Fig. 77

則ち土瓜根散の方
Tǔ Guā Gēn Sǎn

土瓜根・芍藥・桂枝・䗪蟲（ 各等分 ）。

tǔ guā gēn	土瓜根	equal amounts
sháo yào	芍藥	equal amounts
guì zhī	桂枝	equal amounts
zhè chóng	蟅蟲	equal amounts

右四味 、細末にして酒を以て 、一戔五分を服す 。日々に三貼を用ゆ 。

Grind the above four ingredients into a fine powder, mix with sake, and administer one *qián* and five *fēn* [of the drug] three times daily.[350]

350. Some modern Japanese sources recommend 3g of each ingredient, but there appears to be no consensus regarding the exact quantities to be used.

遠州濱松の士、和久田某、蟅蟲の考に曰く、「字彙に「之」、「夜」の切、音「柘」。蟲の名、一に曰く、「蝗」の類。一に曰く、「鼠婦」。按ずるに、本草化生蟲の部に出づ。字彙に蝗の類とすること尤も據りどころあり。

A certain scholar of Hamamatsu [City] in Enshū[351] named Wakuda[352] said that "according to the *Zì Huì*,[353] the [first] character of the word *zhè chóng* 蟅蟲 (Jp: *sha-chū*; ground beetle) should be pronounced using the pronunciation of the characters *zhī* 之 (Jp: *shi*) and *yè* 夜 (Jp: *ya*), according to the *fǎnqiè* method; the pronunciation is the same as the character *zhè* 柘 (Jp: *sha*). [*Zhè chóng* is defined as] the name of an insect; one source says that it is similar to a grasshopper (Jp: *inago* 蝗; Ch: *huáng*), and another source says that it is [similar to] a wood louse (Ch: *shǔ fù* 鼠婦; Jp: *sofu*)." I believe that the Transformation and Engenderment of Insects Chapter in *Běn Cǎo* [*Gāng Mù*] is the source [of this information].[354] The claim by the *Zì Huì Dictionary* that it is similar to a grasshopper is the most reliable [view].

今、字義を審らかにして之れを按ずるに、蟅蟲と蝗と本一物にして、其の化生するに隨ふて、名を殊にするならん。蓋し「蟅」の字、「庶」に從ふ。衆多の義に取るものならん。

By elucidating the meaning of the character, it can be seen that *zhè chóng* and *inago* are originally the same creature, and only differ in name based on their respective transformations and engenderments.[355] The [meaning of the] character for *zhè* 蟅 can be

351. Enshū 遠州 is the abbreviated name of Tōtōmi Province (Jp: *Tōtōmi-No-Kuni* 遠江國), which today forms the western region of Shizuoka Prefecture (Jp: *Shizuoka-Ken* 靜岡縣).
352. Wakuda Yoshitora 和久田叔虎 (1768–1824 CE) was the pupil of the author and the author *Fuku-Shō Kiran-Yoku*《腹證奇覽翼》(The Wings to Extraordinary Views of Abdominal Patterns), the follow-up work to the present work.
353. *Zì Huì*《字彙》(Jp: *Jii*; Lexicon) is a Chinese dictionary, edited by Méi Yīngzuò 梅膺祚 (Jp: Bai Yōso; ca. late *Míng* dynasty) and published in 1615. The work is divided into fourteen volumes and contains a total of 33,179 Chinese characters. It was the first dictionary to introduce the modern radical-stroke system using the system of 214 radicals commonly used today.
354. *Běn Cǎo Gāng Mù*《本草綱目》(Jp: *Honzō-Kōmoku*; Herbal Foundation Compendium), the most complete and comprehensive traditional Chinese compendium of materia medica, was written by Lǐ Shízhēn 李時珍 (Jp: Ri Jichin; 1518–1593 CE) and published posthumously in 1593. The book appears to have been widely read among physicians in Japan during the Edo period. There does not appear to be a "Transformation and Engenderment of Insects (Ch: *Huà Shēng Chóng* 化生蟲; Jp: *Kasei-Chū*) Chapter" in *Běn Cǎo Gāng Mù*: the author may be referring to the chapter in *Wakan-Sansai-Zue*《和漢三才圖會》(Sino-Japanese Illustrated Compendium of the Three Talents) .
355. This section explains the opinion of the author that *zhè chóng* 蟅蟲 used in China and the

understood from [the right component] *shù* 庶 (Jp: *sho*).[356] The meaning [of *shù*] can be taken as "multitude."

今、華舶のせ來たる所の物をみるに、本草の簸箕蟲と云ふ者、その形よく似たり。地鼈と云ふものも亦た少しく似たり。

When observing the creatures brought [to Japan] on Chinese ships,[357] they appear similar to the *bò jī chóng* 簸箕蟲 (Jp: *haki-chū*) that are [described] in *Běn Cǎo Gāng Mù*. They also appear slightly similar to a creature called *dì biē* 地鼈 (Jp: *chibetsu*).[358]

之れを我が邦に產する所の物に考ふるに、即ち水田の泥中、或るひは池澤の中にすむ甲蟲、その形相似たり。俗呼んで、「盛長蟲」と云ふ。此の蟲、五、六月の比、黍粒の如き小卵數十を生みて背にをふ。稻禾長ずるを待ちて、禾の本に其の卵を附けて去る。この卵、風化して蝗を生ず。

When considering [the insects for crude drug use] that are produced in Japan, their appearance is similar to that of a Japanese rhinoceros beetle (Jp: *kabuto-mushi* 甲蟲; Ch: *jiǎ chóng*), which lives in the mud in [rice] paddy fields or in ponds or marshes. [In

inago 蝗 commonly found in Japan not only have similar effects, but are in fact derived from the same source; his reasoning is largely based on the pre-modern Chinese theory of engendering transformation (Ch: *shēng huà* 生化; Jp: seika), similar to equivocal generation. *Zhè chóng* (Jp: *sha-chū*; ground beetle), also known as *tǔ biē chóng* 土鱉蟲 (Jp: *dobetchū*), generally refers to Eupolyphaga sinensis, a species of wingless, flightless cockroach native to Western China and Mongolia. The dried body is used in traditional Chinese medicine. *Inago* (Ch: *huáng*; grasshopper) generally refers to any one of the several species of the genus Oxya in the family Catantopidae. It was common for Japanese physicians to substitute native Japanese materials for elusive Chinese crude drugs, but the efficacy of the Japanese substitutes was not always clear. Furthermore, because Chinese crude drugs are now easily obtained in Japan, and formulae containing insect-derived crude drugs are currently not approved by the Japanese government for use as prescription drugs, there has been little interest in verifying the claim of the author.

356. The original text uses the alternate character 䗪, but there is no difference in meaning from the more commonly used 蟅.

357. During the Edo period, the Tokugawa shogunate technically enforced a policy of isolationism (Jp: *sakoku* 鎖國) in Japan, but trade with China, Korea, Holland, and the Ryūkyū Kingdom was allowed to continue in Kyūshū 九州 at specified ports. Thus, it was possible, albeit difficult and expensive, for Japanese physicians to obtain crude drugs and medicinals from China. It can be surmised that for this reason, the author recommended the use of *inago*, which were easier to find in Japan.

358. In *Běn Cǎo Gāng Mù*, *bò jī chóng* 簸箕蟲 and *dì biē* 地鼈 are both listed as alternate names of *zhè chóng* 蟅蟲. Hence, it is unclear what insects the author is referring to.

Japan,] these [insects] are colloquially called "*mori-naga-mushi* 盛長蟲" [literally, "exuberantly long insect"]. In the fifth or sixth month [of the traditional lunisolar Japanese calendar], this insect lays several dozen small eggs approximately the size of broomcorn millet seeds and carry them on its back. They wait for the rice plants to grow tall, and then lay the eggs on the bases of the plants. The eggs undergo efflorescence and are transformed into *inago*.

蝗の形たる方首青身・兩鬚・六足。後の二脚長くしてよく跳る。羽あれども、飛ぶこと能はず。背に黑文あり。形は「王」の字に似たり。「蝗」の字、「皇」に從ふこと、之れを以てなり。

The *inago* has a square head, a green-blue body, two whiskers, and six legs. The two posterior legs are long, and [as a result,] it can jump well. Although it has wings, it cannot fly. There is a black marking on the backside [of the insect]. The shape [of the marking] appears similar to the Chinese character for king [i.e., *wáng* 王; Jp: *ō*]. The Chinese character for *inago* 蝗 contains the radical for emperor [i.e., *huáng* 皇; Jp: *kō*], thus, the name [of the animal] is derived from this fact.[359]

短き者は五、六分、長きものは一寸許り。稲禾を食ふて害をなす。霜降の後、色赤くなりて死す。即ち民間に呼んで「伊那古」と云ふ者、是れなり。是れ蝗の親は蟅蟲にして、其の子を生ずること衆多なるを以て、「蟅」と名づくるならん。本草に土鼈、簸箕の名を辨ずといへども、「蟅」字の義を詳らかにせず。又た蝗を生ずることを知らず。或るひは甲ありと云ひ、或るひは甲なく鱗ありと云ふ。見るべし、其の物を究極せざることを。

Short ones are five or six *fēn* in length, but long ones [can reach] approximately one *cùn* in length. They eat and cause damage to rice plants. After the frost begins to fall, they become red in color and die. This is why [the insects are] popularly called "*inago*."[360] The parents of *inago* are *zhè chóng* 蟅蟲, and [the character] *zhè* 蟅 in the name is derived from the fact that [these insects] lay many eggs. Although the author of *Běn Cǎo* [*Gāng*

359. This appears to be a false etymology of the word. It is now commonly accepted that *huáng* 蝗 is a phono-semantic compound character (Ch: *xíng shēng wén zì* 形聲文字; Jp: *keisei-moji*) with the phonetic element of *huáng* 皇, rather than a compound ideograph (Ch: *huì yì wén zì* 會意文字; Jp: *kaii-moji*) as the author suggests.

360. In Japanese, *inago* may also be colloquially written using the Chinese characters 稲子, which literally means "rice plant child."

Mù] differentiated the names of *dì biē* 地鼈 and *bò jī* [*chóng*] 簸箕[蟲], he did not elucidate the meaning of the character *zhè* 蟅. Furthermore, [the author] did not know that *inago* are born [from these insects. The text simply] states that according to one [physician, *zhè chóng*] have a shell, but according to another [physician,] they lack a shell and instead have scales.[361] Thus, it can be seen that it is necessary to analyze the names [of insects] more fully.

其の功能を論ずるに及んでは、「蟅」、「蝗」同根性、故に其の功亦た同じ。且つ華產の物尤も高價なり。又た真贋審らかならず。故に多く用ひて經驗するもの少し。今、水田中にある蟅蟲も、亦た采り得ること易からず。蝗は甚だ多し、取り得ること尤も易し。七、八月の間、稻禾中に在るを取り、火に炙りて殺し、日に干して之れを貯ふ。此を蟅蟲に易へ用ゆること、古人も未だ發明せず、仙石伯州刺史の醫、中川友三と云ふ者、鶴先生の門に在りて、予が師稻葉翁の先輩也。始めて蝗を以て蟅蟲に易へ用ゆることを知りて、其の效驗を極む。予因つて諸家の說を參考して、以て此こに記す。

When discussing the functions [of these insects, it should be kept in mind that] both *zhè* [*chóng*] and *inago* share the same source. Therefore, their efficacy is the equivalent. Chinese products are the most expensive, but their authenticity cannot be confirmed. For this reason, I have used many [varieties], but have little experience with [the varieties of *zhè chóng* from China]. The *zhè chóng* that inhabit paddy fields are also by no means easy to catch. [By contrast,] *inago* are exceedingly abundant and are the easiest to catch. During the seventh and eighth months [of the lunisolar calendar], collect [*inago*] that live in rice plants, fry them with fire to kill them, dry in the sun, and store [the materials]. Even the ancients did not discover that *zhè chóng* may be substituted. It was Nakagawa Tomozō[362] (the physician of the provincial governor of the Sengoku region of

361. The original text as found in *Běn Cǎo Gāng Mù*《本草綱目》is as follows:「弘景曰、形扁如鱉、有甲不能飛...恭曰...狀似鼠婦，而大者寸余，形小似鱉，無甲而有鱗」(According to [Táo] Hóngjǐng [陶]弘景 [Jp: (Tō) Kōkei; 456–536 CE], [*zhè chóng* 蟅蟲] has a flat shape similar to [*dì*] *biē* [地]鼈, has a shell, and cannot fly...According to Sū Gōng 蘇恭 [599–674 CE; Jp: So Kyō]...it has an appearance similar to *shǔ fù* 鼠婦. Large ones can grow to be more than a cun in size. [*Zhè chóng*] has a small shape similar to [*dì*] *biē*, [but] does not have a shell and [instead] has scales...).

362. There are no details concerning Nakagawa Tomozō. Furthermore, the name 友三 could be read as Tomozō, Tomomitsu, or Yūzō. Because the correct reading is unclear, the most popular reading of Tomozō has been selected here.

Hakushū)[363] who first discovered that *inago* may be substituted for *zhè chóng*, and deeply explored the efficacy [of the formula]. I have referred to the explanations of various specialists and shall list [illustrations of the findings] here.

華產䗪蟲腹面圖
Illustration of the Abdomen of Chinese Zhè Chóng 蟅蟲

世俗大師出と稱するものこれなり 。
This type is colloquially referred to as "the great master."

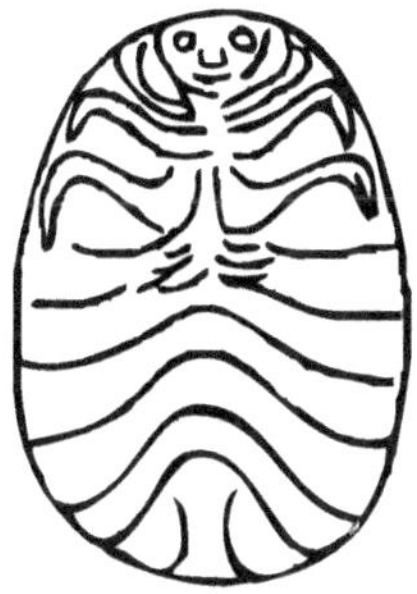

Fig. 78

本邦蝗の圖
Illustration of Japanese Inago 蝗

Fig. 79

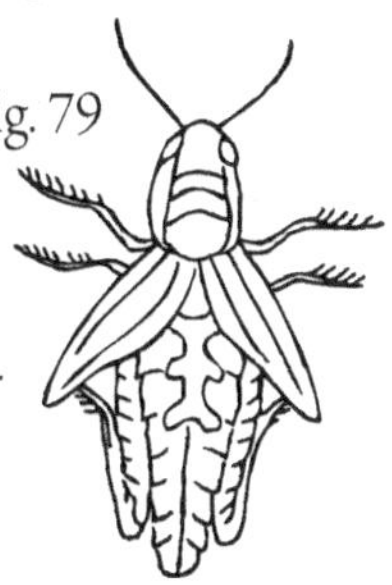

背に「 王 」字あるもの是れなり 。
This type has the [Chinese] character for king (i.e., *wáng* 王) on its back.

363. Hakushū 伯州 is the abbreviation of Hōki Province (Jp: *Hōki-No-Kuni* 伯耆國), the area that is today the western part of Tottori Prefecture (Jp: *Tottori-Ken* 鳥取縣).

八味丸之圖

Illustration for the Bā Wèi Wán[364] [Pattern] 八味丸

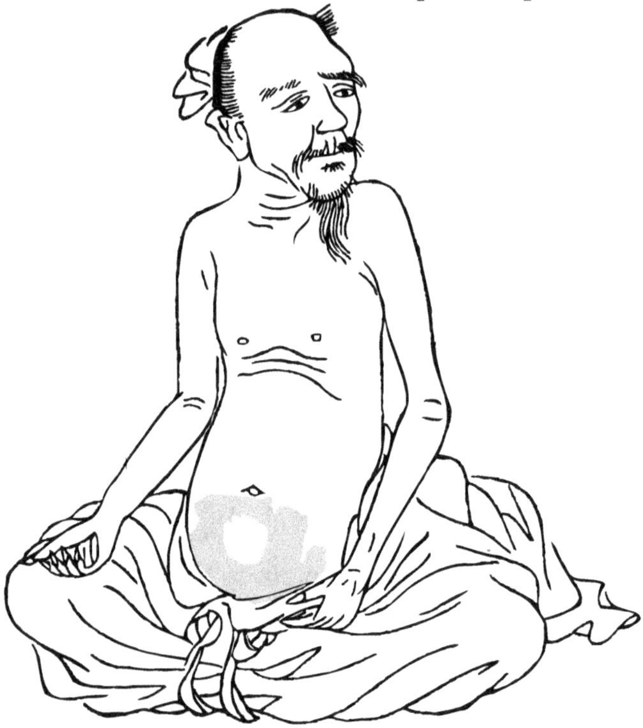

Fig. 80

小腹不仁若しくは拘急。凡そ不仁は其の處、我が身のごとく覺へざるものを云ふ。又た按ずるに皮薄く綿絮の如く軟弱なるもの亦た不仁。

364. The formula for *Bā Wèi Wán* 八味丸 (Jp: *Hachimi-Gan*; eight-ingredient pill) was originally found in *Jīn Guì Yào Lüè* under the name of *Cuī Shì Bā Wèi Wán* 崔氏八味丸 (Jp: *Sai-Shi-Hachimi-Gan*; Cuī's eight-ingredient pill). In Japan, is more commonly known as *Bā Wèi Dì Huáng Wán* 八味地黄丸 (Jp: *Hachimi-Jiō-Gan*; eight-ingredient rehmannia pill). The extract preparation of the formula is covered by the Japanese National Health Insurance program as a prescription drug, and is also commonly sold in Japanese drug stores as an over-the-counter drug. It is currently indicated by the MHLW for: leg pain, low back pain, numbness, geriatric blurred vision, itching, painful urination, sensation of incomplete bladder emptying, nocturia, frequent urination, edema, various symptoms associated with hypertension (stiff shoulders, dull headache, tinnitus), and mild incontinence in persons with moderate or weak physical strength who are easily fatigued, tend to have cold extremities, oliguria or polyuria, or occasional dry mouth (體力中等度以下で、疲れやすくて、四肢が冷えやすく、尿量減少又は多尿で、ときに口渇があるものの次の諸症：下肢痛、腰痛、しびれ、高齢者のかすみ目、かゆみ、排尿困難、殘尿感、夜間尿、頻尿、むくみ、高血壓に伴う隨伴症狀の改善（肩こり、頭重、耳鳴り）、輕い尿漏れ)。

[This is a case of] insensitivity or hypertonicity in the smaller abdomen. Regions of insensitivity are generally [numb] regions that the patient does not feel are part of his body. Furthermore, when [abdominal] palpatory findings reveal that the patient has thin skin that is weak as a thread, it is also a case of insensitivity.[365]

圖の如く、臍下不仁、或るひは小腹不仁して、小便不利の者。又た一症、手足煩熱し、腰痛、小腹拘急し、小便不利の者。又た一症、不仁するにあらずして、小腹拘急の者。又た臍の四邊堅大にして盤の如く、之れを按して陰莖・陰門に徹し痛む者。痳病・血症の者にこの症多し。

As shown in the illustration, the patient presents with insensitivity of the subumbilical region or the smaller abdomen and inhibited urination. In another pattern [that matches the formula for *Bā Wèi Wán*], the patient presents with vexing heat in the extremities, lumbar pain, hypertonicity in the smaller abdomen, and inhibited urination.[366] In another pattern [that matches the formula for *Bā Wèi Wán*], the patient does not present with [abdominal] insensitivity, but has hypertonicity in the smaller abdomen. Furthermore, some patients present with a large hard [lump], which appears similar to a dish, around the four sides of the umbilicus. Upon palpation [of the lump], pain penetrates to the penis [in men] or yīn door [i.e., vulva, in women]. This pattern is common in patients who present with strangury disease or a blood pathocondition.

則ち八味丸の方
Bā Wèi Wán

地黄（八戔）・山茱萸・薯蕷（各四戔）・茯苓・牡丹皮・澤瀉（各三戔）・桂枝・附子（各二戔）。

dì huáng	地黄	8 qián
shān zhū yú	山茱萸	4 qián
shǔ yù*	薯蕷	4 qián
fú líng	茯苓	3 qián

365. As explained in the text, lower abdominal insensitivity (Ch: *xiǎo fù bù rén* 小腹不仁; Jp: *shōfuku-fujin*) refers to numbness or a loss of sensation in the lower abdominal region.
366. Vexing heat in the extremities (Ch: *shǒu zú fán rè* 手足煩熱; Jp: *shusoku-hannetsu*) refers to a subjective feverish feeling in the palms and soles.

mǔ dān pí	牡丹皮	3 qián
zé xiè	澤瀉	3 qián
guì zhī	桂枝	2 qián
fù zǐ	附子	2 qián

* *Shǔ yù* 薯蕷 (Jp: shoyo) is commonly referred to as *shān yào* 山藥 (Jp: *sanyaku*) in Japan.

右八味、末となし、蜜を以て丸ず。

Grind the eight ingredients into a powder and use honey to make pills.

余、此の方を用ひ知りて云ふ、臍下及び小腹不仁と云ふ者、指頭にて按ずるに、ずぶりと凹み力なく、その人、心ぼそく便りなくをぼふ。不仁なること知るべし。且つ小便不利、或るひは腹底に暗然として少しの冷氣を覺ふ。心を沈めて之れを察すべし。もし其の冷氣なくして、附子の症あらんと疑ふ時は、背を見るべし。必ず手の裏ほどの冷氣あらば、附子の症としるべし。又たこの症にして、或るひは悸し、或るひは手足冷ゆるもの、みな、これ八味丸の正症なり。

In my experience using this formula, I have found that patients who present with what is referred to as insensitivity in the subumbilical region and smaller abdomen have deep pitting [in the abdominal region] and a lack of [abdominal] strength that can be felt upon palpation using the fingertips. The patient feels helpless and incapable [of becoming well]. This is how [the physician] can know [what is meant by] insensitivity. Furthermore, the patient may present with inhibited urination or a slight cold qì that can be subtly felt in the depths of the abdomen. [The physician] should quiet his heart and examine [the patient]. If [the patient presents with] no cold qì and a pattern for *fù zǐ* is suspected, the back [of the patient] should [also] be visually examined. If the patient has a cold qì in the backs of the hands, it is the indication for a pattern [that is matched to] *fù zǐ*. Moreover, any case in which the patient presents with this pattern and has palpitations or cold extremities is the right pattern for *Bā Wèi Wán*.

瘡毒家陰莖腐落之圖
Illustration of a Patient Who Presents with Sore-Toxins and Putridity of the Penis

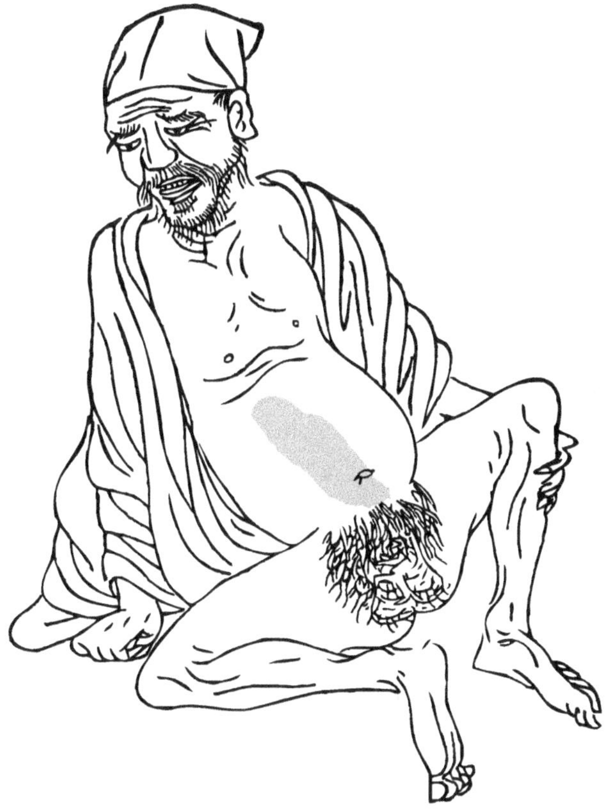

Fig. 81

圖の如く、陰莖腐り落ちて、その狀、肉臠のただれたるが如くにして、疼痛忍びがたし。其の腹も亦た圖のごとく、堅塊有りて臍下より鳩尾に至り、之れを按すに自若として動かず。その人羸瘦して、時々寒熱往來し、手足のうら熱して、大便閉し不食す。此れ大承氣湯の症なり。瘡毒とのみ心得て治療するゆへに愈へず。この症のみに限らず、凡そ瘡毒と云ふも、みな腹底に毒あるを以てなり。

As shown in the illustration, the penis has putrefied: it appears similar to a rotten piece of meat and causes pain that is hard to bear. The abdomen of the patient is also shown in the illustration: [palpatory findings reveal] a hard lump that extends from the subumbilical region to *Jiū Wěi* (CV-15). When pressed, [the lump] remains unperturbed and does not move. The patient presents with marked emaciation, [generalized] alternating heat [effusion] and [aversion to] cold, heat [effusion] in the palms and soles, fecal block, and the inability to eat. This is the pattern for *Dà Chéng Qì Tāng.* [If the physician] cares only [about curing] the sore-toxin, [the patient] will not recover. This [principle] is not limited only to this pattern: in all cases of sore-toxins, the patient has a toxin in the depths of the abdomen.

俗に「古濕」と號して、瘡毒の治しがたく、或るひは鼻梁落ち、或るひは耳しひ、或るひは目盲し、生質に非ずして、五體不具なるもの、みな腹症に本づき、舊染の毒を去ることをしらずして、みだりに輕粉劑、或るひは山歸來劑などを用ひて攻むるが故なり。

All cases of intractable sore-toxins that are colloquially referred to as [being due to] "old [i.e., long-standing] dampness" are difficult to cure; in some cases, the patient presents with falling off of the nose beam [i.e., the stem of the nose], deafness, or blindness (that is, any noncongenital disability of the five body constituents). All [such cases] are based on this abdominal pattern, [but physicians] do not understand [the importance of] eliminating the old transmitted toxin, and carelessly attack [the pattern] by using *Qīng Fěn Jì* or *Shān Guī Lái Jì.*[367]

余、舊に東都にある時、内田某なる人、ひろく醫書に渉り、又たよく治療をなせり。余が腹診を唱ふるを聞きて、厚く信じて門に入らんことを乞ふ。余、その厚く醫に志して、深く此の術を好むをよみして、ついに腹診の術をつたふ。一日一病客をたずさへ來たり診をこふて云はく、「此の人瘡毒を患へて、世にいはゆる『蠟蠋下疳』と號するものになれり。前に、瘍醫に托して治をうくれども、數月効なくして、ついに陰莖腐落し疼み忍びがたし」。

I was once traveling in the eastern capital [i.e., Edo], when I met a certain person [with the family name of] Uchida who widely read [i.e., was well-versed in] medical texts, and was skilled in performing medical treatment. He had heard of my advocacy of abdominal examination and deeply believed in [the art]. Therefore, he entreated [me] to enter

367. The details of the formulae for *Qīng Fěn Jì* 輕粉劑 (Jp: *Keifun-Zai*; calomel preparation) and *Shān Guī Lái Jì* 山歸來劑 (Jp: *Sankirai-Zai*; smooth greenbrier preparation) are unclear. At present, neither formula is covered by the Japanese National Health Insurance program and both appear to be unknown in Japan.

[my] school. I commended his strong dedication to [the way of] medicine and his deep love of this art. For this reason, I subsequently passed on the techniques for abdominal examination to him. One day, he brought a patient to me and requested me to treat him saying, "This person has been suffering from a sore-toxin and has what is commonly known as 'wax candle lower body *gān*.'[368] I previously asked a surgeon to treat him, but after several months there has been no effect, and his penis has become putrid and [appears to be] falling off, causing him insufferable pain. I attempted to attack [the toxin] with *Xiǎo Chái Hú Tāng* and Tokuhon's *Shashin-En*, but there was no effect, so I would like to ask you to perform a diagnosis."

余、小柴胡湯をよび徳本家の瀉心圓を以て攻むれども、その効なきを以て、先生に托して診を乞ふ」と云ふ。余、これを診するに、腹底に堅塊ありて臍下より鳩尾に至り自若として動かず。「是れ大承氣の正症なり」と云ふ。内田子異しんで云はく、「予かつてもろもろの醫書をよみ、數々衆醫に會して奇說を聞くといへども、未だ先生の診する所の如きをきかず。厚く先生を信ずといへども、是に於て疑ひを發せざること能はず」と云ふ。余が云く、「子も亦た後世學の惑ひいまだ脱せざるが故なり。此の病客の如きは大承氣のほか他症なし」と。乃ち之れを與ふること數月にして全く治せり。

When I examined the patient, there were hard lumps that did not stir located in the depths of the abdomen from the subumbilical region to *Jiū Wěi* (CV-15). I said, "this is the true pattern for *Dà Chéng Qì* [*Tāng*]." Mr. Uchida marveled and responded, "I have read all kinds of medical books, met a number of physicians, and listened to their extraordinary stories, but I have never heard of a method of diagnosis such as the one that you perform. Sensei, I deeply believe you, but I am not without my doubts." I replied, "This is because you also have been unable to remove the confusion of the latter generations. Patients such as this present with, do not [match the pattern for] *Dà Chéng Qì Tāng* or other patterns." After administering [the formula] to the patient over several months, he was completely cured.

368. In this context, *gān* 疳 (Jp: *kan*) refers to progressive sores or ulceration.

則ち大承氣湯の方
Dà Chéng Qì Tāng

厚朴（ 二戔四分 ）・枳實（ 一戔五分 ）・大黄（ 一戔二分 ）・芒硝（ 六分 ）。

hòu pò	厚朴	2 qián and 4 fēn
zhǐ shí	枳實	1 qián and 5 fēn
dà huáng	大黄	1 qián and 2 fēn
máng xiāo	芒硝	6 fēn

右四味 、水三盞を以て一盞二分に煎じ 、厚朴・枳實の滓を去りて大黄を入れ 、六分に煎じ 、又た滓をさりて芒硝を入れて 、一度に服す 。日に三たび服す 。

Boil the above four ingredients in three cups of water to make one cup and two *fēn* of the decoction. Remove the dregs of *hòu pò* and *zhǐ shí,* add *dà huáng,* and boil again to make six *fēn* of the decoction. Remove the dregs again, add *máng xiāo,* and take [all of the decoction] in a single dose. [The decoction should be] administered three times per day.

司瘡家骨節疼痛之圖
Illustration of a Patient with Sores [Who Presents] with Joint Pain

圖の如く 、身體羸瘦して 、行歩すること能はず 、手足疼痛して發する時は忍びがたし 。その腹も亦 、圖の如く 、心下に毒結衆して 、之れを按して疼み 、腹底に暗然として冷氣を覺ふ 。時に上衝頭痛し 、寒熱往來 、或るひは惡風・惡寒す 。是れ桂枝加附子湯の正症なり 。毎夜 、芎黄散二戔を兼用し 、四 、五日して毎夜 、七寶丸六分を用ゆること三日にして 、又た故の如く芎黄を用ゆ 。此くの如く二 、三次 、或るひは五 、六 、七次して 、毒の淺深により之れを攻むべし 。毒淺き者は一 、二次にして愈ゆるもの間々あり 。毒深き者は六 、七次にしていゆ 。時に臨んで考ふべし 。

As shown in the illustration, the patient presents with generalized emaciation and weakness, is nonambulatory, and has insufferable pain in the extremities. Furthermore, as seen in the illustration of the abdomen, the toxin binds and gathers in the region below the heart. When [the region is] pressed, pain is present, and a cold qì can be subtly felt in the depths of the abdomen. The patient often experiences headaches associated with upward surging and alternating heat [effusion] and [aversion to] cold. In some cases, the patient presents with an aversion to wind and cold. This is the right pattern for *Guì Zhī Jiā Fù Zǐ Tāng*. Two *qián* of *Xiōng Huáng Săn* should be given simultaneously each night for four or five nights, [followed by a regimen of] six *fēn* of *Shichihō-Gan* each night for three nights,[369] and then *Xiōng Huáng Săn* should be used again. Depending on the depth of the toxin, this cycle should be repeated two or three or even up to five, six, or seven times to attack [the pathotoxin]. When the toxin is shallow, the patient will recover after one or two cycles. When the toxin is deep, [the patient] will recover after six or seven cycles. [The number of cycles to be used] should be considered based on the circumstances.

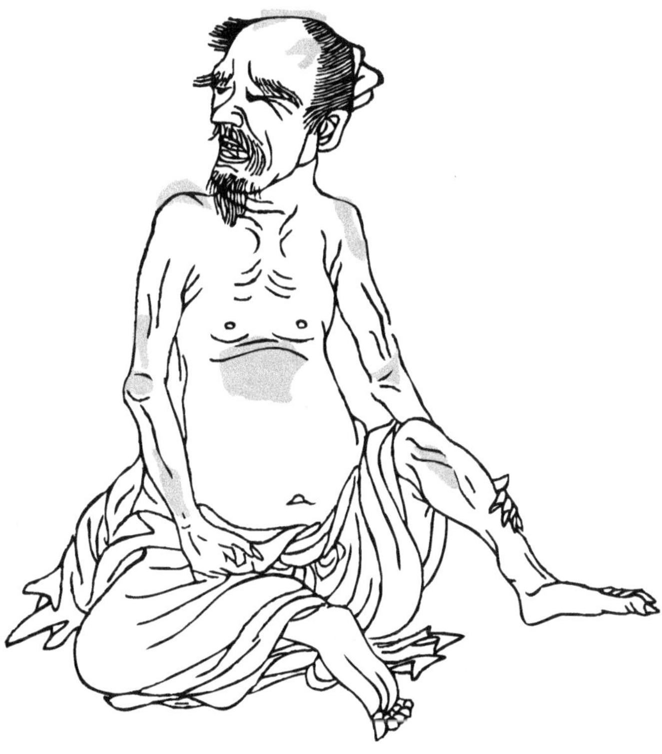

Fig. 82

369. Although there are several different formulae with the name *Shichihō-Gan* 七寶丸 (Ch: *Qī Bǎo Wán*; seven-jewel decoction), this particular version is an original formula of Yoshimasu Tōdō 吉益東洞, and is found in *Tōdō-Sensei-Kajuku-Hō* 《東洞先生家塾方》(Master Tōdō's Family Formulary). At present, this formula is not covered by the Japanese National Health Insurance program and is not commonly used in Japan.

傳に云はく、「或るひは惡浮腫の者、礬黄丸、可なり。羸瘦して骨節疼痛の者、七寶丸、可なり」。若しくは瘡毒家、或るひは二、三分より四、五分に至る。大いに下るものは兼用をやめ、本劑のみ用ゆること二、三日して、又た梅肉散を兼用すること。此くの如く一、二次、六、七次、前の如く毒の淺深に隨つて考ふべし。

[One] text states that "when the patient presents with malign puffy swelling, *Ban-Ō-Gan* may be used.[370] When the patient presents with marked emaciation and joint pain, *Shichihō-Gan* may be used." In the case of a patient who presents with a sore-toxin, two or three *fēn*, or up to four or five *fēn* [of the drug may be administered]. If the patient has precipitation [i.e., diarrhea], discontinue the simultaneous use [of other drugs] and use only the base formula for two or three days. *Bainiku-San* may also be simultaneously used.[371] In this way, [the drug] may be considered for administration in one, two or up to six or seven cycles according to the depth of the toxin, as previously mentioned.

凡そ輕粉劑を用ゆるの傳、初め四、五日下劑を用ひ、下利してのち用ゆべし。否らざれば輕粉の毒、口中にあたりただれて、他日食すること能はず。余、この劑を數用數効して、病者をして苦惱せしめんことを恐れて、此くの如く熟するものなり。

Texts concerning the use of formulae that include *qīng fěn* generally recommend using a laxative for four or five days at first and using [*qīng fěn*] after the patient has [started to] experience diarrhea. Unless [treatment is performed in] this way, the toxicity of *qīng fěn* will cause putrid [ulceration] of the mouth, and [the patient] will be unable to eat for days. I have used this formula seen its efficacy a number of times. Because I feared causing patients pain and distress, I became adept at [using] the formula as written here.

370. Although *Ban-Ō-Gan* 礬黄丸 (calcined alum and rhubarb pill) shares the same name with the more popular Chinese formula *Fán Huáng Wán* 礬黄丸 (alum and yellow wax pill), the formulae greatly differ. As explained in the section for *Guì Jiāng Zǎo Cǎo Huáng Xīn Fù Tāng* 桂薑棗草黄辛附湯, this version is associated with the Tōdō family, but the exact source is unclear. At present, no version of this formula is covered by the Japanese National Health Insurance program, and none is commonly used in Japan.

371. There are several different formulae with the name *Méi Ròu Sǎn* 梅肉散, but this version of *Bainiku-San* 梅肉散 (Ch: *Méi Ròu Sǎn*; mume powder) seems to have been copied from *Meika-Hōsen*《名家方選》(Selected Formulae of Distinguished Masters) and popularized by Yoshimasu Tōdō 吉益東洞, although the quantities of ingredients used by the author slightly differ from those used in the traditional version. At present, this formula is not covered by the Japanese National Health Insurance program and is not commonly used in Japan.

則ち桂枝加附子湯の方
Guì Zhī Jiā Fù Zǐ Tāng

桂枝・芍藥・大棗・生姜（ 各七分 ）・附子（ 六分 ）・甘草（ 五分 ）。

guì zhī	桂枝	7 fēn
sháo yào	芍藥	7 fēn
dà zǎo	大棗	7 fēn
shēng jiāng	生薑	7 fēn
fù zǐ	附子	6 fēn
gān cǎo	甘草	5 fēn

右六味 、水一盞半を以て 、六分に煮とる 。

Boil the six ingredients in one and one-half cups of water to make six *fēn* of the decoction.

七寳丸の方
Shichihō-Gan

牛膝・輕粉（ 各四戔 ）・土茯苓（ 三戔 ）・大黄（ 二戔五分 ）・丁子（ 一戔 ）。

niú xī	牛膝	4 fēn
qīng fěn	輕粉	4 fēn
tǔ fú líng	土茯苓	3 qián
dà huáng	大黄	2 qián and 5 fēn
dīng zǐ	丁子	1 qián

右五味 、末となして糊丸す 。右の治に云はく 、痼疾・沈痾の毒及び瘡毒にて骨節疼痛する者は 、みな 、之れを兼用して可なり 。

Grind the above five ingredients into a powder to make flour and water paste pills. The above treatment may be used simultaneously for any patient who presents with a toxin causing an intractable or heavy disease or a sore-toxin and has joint pain.

礬黄丸の方
Ban-Ō-Gan

枯礬（ 十五箋 ）・大黄（ 十箋 ）・輕粉（ 五箋 ）。

kū fán	枯礬	15 qián
dà huáng	大黄	10 fēn
qīng fěn	輕粉	5 qián

右三味、末となして糊丸す。右の治に云はく、無名の惡浮腫・骨節疼痛、及び疥癬・白癜風、一切の惡瘡に兼用して、みな大効あり。余、數年來用ひ得て經驗すること、擧げてかぞふべからず。

Grind the above three ingredients into a powder to make flour and water paste pills. The above-mentioned treatment is highly effective when used simultaneously for cases of innominate malign puffy swelling, joint pain, scabs and lichen, white patch wind, or any type of malign sore. I have used this formula for several years and experienced its efficacy in innumerable cases.

梅肉散の方
Bainiku-San

梅肉（ 鹽梅・核ともに黒燒き ）・山梔子（ 各三箋、黒燒き ）・巴豆（ 一箋、皮を去る ）・輕粉（ 八分 ）。

méi ròu	梅肉	salted mumes, charred complete with the kernel*	3 qián
shān zhī zǐ	山梔子	charred	3 qián
bā dòu	巴豆	remove the outer seed coat	1 qián
qīng fěn	輕粉		8 fēn

* In Japan, mumes (Jp: *ume* 梅) are commonly pickled in salt and dried to make the popular Japanese food *umeboshi* 梅干し.

右四味、末となし湖丸す。一、二分より四、五分まで用ゆ。小兒の頭瘡、或るひは無名の惡瘡を發するもの、赤子より五、六歳の者は、一、二厘より四、五厘に至る。毒深き者は一分、一分五厘に至る。或るひは婦人の乳岩・乳腫などにみな用ひて大効あり。

Grind the above four ingredients into a powder to make flour and water paste pills. [The formula] should be used in doses of one or two *fēn,* or up to four or five *fēn.* [In the case of] head sores or innominate malign sores in pediatric patients (infants up to children aged five or six years), one or two, or up to four or five *li* [of the pills] may be used. In cases when the toxin is deep, up to one *fēn* or one *fēn* and five *li* [may be used]. The formula is also extremely effective when used in women for cases of mammary rocks, swelling of the breasts, etc.

湖南稻葉意仲克文禮著

Written by Konan Inaba Ichū Katsu Bunrei

浪華岡熊岳畫

Illustrations by Oka Yūgaku of Naniwa[372]

腹證奇覽後編卷之下終

End of the final volume of *Fukushō-Kiran*《 腹證奇覽 》
(Extraordinary Views of Abdominal Patterns)

372. Oka Yūgaku 岡熊岳 (1762–1833 CE) was a famous artist of the Edo period.

People

Zhāng Zhòngjǐng	張仲景	Chō Chūkei	150-219 CE	4, 131
Zhū Sù	朱橚	Shu Shuku	1361–1425 CE	174

Places

Banshū	播州	Harima Province (Harima-No-Kuni 播磨國)	186
Bishū	尾州	Owari Province (Owari-No-Kuni 尾張國)	102
Bushū	武州	Musashi Province (Musashi-No-Kuni 武藏國)	75
Chikuzen-No-Kuni	筑前國	Chikuzen Province	51
Doshū	土州	Tosa Province (Tosa-No-Kuni 土佐國)	48
Edo	江戸	Tōkyō Metropolis (Tōkyō-To 東京都)	xxv, 4–9, 28–49, 64, 76–87, 105–106, 127–159, 214, 231–258
Enshū	遠州	Tōtōmi Province (Tōtōmi-No-Kuni 遠江國)	241
Fukuoka-Ken	福岡縣	Fukuoka Prefecture	51
Gōshū	江州	Ōmi Province (Ōmi-No-Kuni 近江國)	132
Hakushū	伯州	Hōki Province (Hōki-No-Kuni 伯耆國)	84, 245
Kanagawa-Ken	神奈川縣	Kanagawa Prefecture	75, 233
Kibi-No-Kuni	吉備國	Kibi Province	105
Kōshū	甲州	Kai Province (Kai-No-Kuni 甲斐國)	xxiv, 63
Kyōto	京都		xx–xxvi, 49, 105, 231
Kyūshū	九州		51, 242
Mikajima	三ヶ島	part of Tokorozawa City (Tokorozawa-Shi 所澤市)	75–76
Mount Fuji			xxiv
Nan-A	南阿	Southern Awa Province (Awa-No-Kuni 阿波國)	133
Naniwa	浪華	former name of Ōsaka 大阪	xx, 92, 132–133, 258
Saitama-Ken	埼玉縣	Saitama Prefecture	75
Sanshū	參州	Mikawa Province (Mikawa-No-Kuni 三河國)	211
Settsu-No-Kuni	攝津國	Settsu Province	xx
Sōshū	相州	Sagami Province (Sagami-No-Kuni 相模國)	233
Tanimachi			92
Washū	和州	Yamato Province (Yamato-No-Kuni 大和國)	105

Cited Texts

Single Medicinals

Pinyin	Chinese	Japanese	Common Name	Latin Name	
ài yè	艾葉	gaiyō	mugwort	folium artemisiae argyi	121
bā dòu	巴豆	hazu	croton	fructus crotonis	11, 51, 212, 256
bài jiàng	敗醬	haishō	patrinia	herba patriniae	90–93, 123–124
bái jiè zǐ	白芥子	hakugaishi	white mustard	semen sinapis albae	117
bái jiǔ	白酒	hakushu	white liquor	spiritus granorum incolor	28–30, 104–111
bái mì	白蜜	shiromitsu	honey	mel	116, 175
bái táo huā	白桃花	hakutōka	white peach flower	flos persicae albae	21, 110, 186–187
bái zhú	白朮	byakujutsu	white atractylodes	rhizoma atractylodes macrocephalae	113, 140
bàn xià	半夏	hange	pinellia	rhizoma pinelliae	16, 66, 108–119, 149–161, 179–186, 202–217
bèi mǔ	貝母	baimo	fritillaria	bulbus fritillariae	127
cāng zhú	蒼朮	sōjutsu	atractylodes	rhizoma atractylodis	139–140, 158–180
chái hú	柴胡	saiko	bupleurum	radix bupleuri	xxiv, 5–19, 35–36, 56, 92–109, 126, 155, 182–183, 204–206, 219–232, 251
chén pí	陳皮	chinpi	tangerine peel	pericarpium citri reticulatae	113
chén xiāng	沉香	jinkō	aquilaria	lignum aquilariae resinatum	57
chuān xiōng	川芎	senkyū	chuanxiong	rhizoma chuanxiong	81, 110–121, 147–152
cí shí	磁石	jiseki	loadstone	magnetitum	30, 112, 219
dà huáng	大黄	daiō	rhubarb	radix et rhizoma rhei	xxii, 9–69, 81–84, 100–125, 141, 154–192, 209–238, 252–256
dà jǐ	大戟	taigeki	euphorbia	radix euphorbiae pekinensis	43–51, 117, 201–202

gé gēn	葛根	kakkon	pueraria	radix puerariae	29, 60–63, 83, 104, 118, 147–152, 172–173
gēng mǐ	粳米	kōbei	non-glutinous rice	semen oryzae	204–208
guā lóu rén	栝蔞仁/瓜蔞仁	karonin	trichosanthes seed	semen trichosanthis	111–118, 147
guā zǐ/ dōng guā zǐ	瓜子/冬瓜子	kashi/ tōgashi	wax gourd seed	semen benincasae	122
guǎng dōng rén shēn	廣東人參	kanton-ninjin	American ginseng	radix panacis quinquefolii	156
guì pí	桂皮	keihi	thin cinnamon bark	cortex cinnamomi tenuis	152
guì xīn	桂心	keishin	shaved cinnamon bark	cortex cinnamomi rasus	147–153
guì zhī	桂枝	keishi	cinnamon twig	ramulus cinnamomi	1–16, 39–48, 67, 104–123, 143–180, 214–255
hǎi rén cǎo	海人草	kaininsō	digenea	digenea	212
hòu pò	厚朴	kōboku	officinal magnolia bark	cortex magnoliae officinalis	69, 114–120, 252
hǔ pò	琥珀	kohaku	amber	succinum	39
huá shí	滑石	kasseki	talcum	talcum	121, 218–219
huái shí	槐實	kaijitsu	sophora fruit	fructus sophorae	
huáng bò	黄檗	ōbaku	phellodendron	cortex phellodendri	100
huáng là	黄蠟	ōrō	yellow wax	cera flava	254
huáng lián	黄連	ōren	coptis	rhizoma coptidis	xxii, 9, 64–66, 117–119, 141, 179–192, 204–223
huáng qín	黄芩	ōgon	scutellaria	radix scutellariae	9, 57, 108–109, 141–159, 179–192, 204–206
huáng tǔ	黄土	ōdo	loess	loess	157–159
hùn yuán yī	混元衣	kongen'i	placenta	placenta hominis	234–235
jī shé/ jī shé xiāng	雞舌/雞舌香	keizetsu/ keizetsukō	clove fruit	fructus caryophylli	234
jiāo yí/ yí tāng	膠飴/飴糖	kōi/ itō	malt sugar	maltosum	115, 194
jú pí	橘皮	kippi	tangerine peel	pericarpium citri reticulatae	32, 112

qiān fěn/ hēi xī	鉛粉/黑錫	enpun/ kokushaku	processed galenite	galenitum praeparatum	213–214
qiān niú zǐ	牽牛子	kengoshi	morning glory	semen pharbitidis	43
qiáo mài	蕎麥	kyōbaku	buckwheat	semen fagopyri	24, 111, 228
qīng fěn	輕粉	keifun	calomel	calomelas	50–51, 84, 213–215, 250–256
rén shēn	人參	ninjin	ginseng	radix ginseng	8–21, 67, 104–119, 142–206, 222–223
sāng bái pí	桑白皮	sōhakuhi	mulberry bark	cortex mori	152
shān guī lái	山歸來	sankirai	smooth greenbrier	rhizoma smilacis glabrae	250
shān zhī zǐ	山梔子	sanshishi	gardenia	fructus gardeniae	125, 218, 256
shān zhū yú	山茱萸	sanshuyu	cornus	fructus corni	247
shāng lù	商陸	shōriku	phytolacca	radix phytolaccae	39, 60
sháo yào	芍藥	shakuyaku	peony	radix paeoniae	2–15, 48–59, 74, 107–123, 138–140, 152–189, 214–217, 230–240, 255
shè xiāng	麝香	jakō	musk	moschus	235
shēng jiāng	生薑/生姜	shōkyō	fresh ginger	rhizoma zingiberis recens	3–11, 48, 100–118, 149–175, 217, 255
shí gāo	石膏	sekkō	gypsum	gypsum fibrosum	67, 176
shǔ jiāo	蜀椒	shokushō	zanthoxylum	pericarpium zanthoxyli	194
shǔ yù	薯蕷	shoyo	dioscorea	rhizoma dioscoreae	247–248
shuǐ yín	水銀	suigin	mercury	hydrargyrum	11, 50–51
shuǐ zhì	水蛭	suitetsu	leech	hirudo	124–125
táo huā	桃花	tōka	peach flower	flos persicae	20–21, 110, 179–187
táo rén	桃仁	tōnin	peach kernel	semen persicae	111–125, 154, 227–238
tiān nán xīng	天南星	tennanshō	arisaema	rhizoma arisaematis	234
tián qī/ sān qī	田七/三七	denshichi/ sanshichi	notoginseng	radix notoginseng	156
tíng lì	葶藶	teireki	lepidium/descurainiae	semen lepidii seu descurainiae	54, 116–117

Formulas

guì zhī jiā fù zǐ tāng	桂枝加附子湯	keishi-ka-bushi-tō	160–163, 253–255
guì zhī jiā guì zhī tāng	桂枝加桂枝湯	keishi-ka-keishi-tō	4
guì zhī jiā líng zhú fù tāng	桂枝加苓朮附湯	keishi-ka-ryō-jutsu-bu-tō	217
guì zhī jiā líng zhú tāng	桂枝加苓朮湯	keishi-ka-ryō-jutsu-tō	216
guì zhī jiā zào jiá tāng	桂枝加皂莢湯	keishi-ka-sōkyō-tō	4
guì zhī jiā zhú fù tāng	桂枝加朮附湯	keishi-ka-jutsu-bu-tō	160
guì zhī qù sháo yào tāng	桂枝去芍藥湯	keishi-kyo-shakuyaku-tō	2–5, 48, 214–217
guì zhī rén shēn tāng	桂枝人参湯	keishi-ninjin-tō	8, 67, 104, 178, 222
guì zhī tāng	桂枝湯	keishi-tō	1–4, 16, 107, 145–160, 216
gǔn tán wán	滚痰丸	kontan-gan	57
hè jiā gān suì táo huā tāng	鶴家甘遂桃花湯	kaku-ka-kanzui-tōka-tō	21, 185
hè wán	鶴丸	kaku-gan	15, 221
hòu pò sān wù tāng	厚朴三物湯	kōboku-sanmotsu-tō	69, 120
hǔ pò tāng	琥珀湯	kohaku-tō	39
huáng lián tāng	黄連湯	ōren-tō	64–66, 119
huáng lián táo huā sǎn	黄連桃花散	ōren-tōka-tō	187
huáng tǔ tāng	黄土湯	ōdo-tō	157–158
hùn yuán dān	混元丹	kongen-tan	233
jiāng fù tāng	薑附湯	kyō-bu-tō	175
jiě dú wán	解毒丸	gedoku-gan	9
jú pí dà huáng máng xiāo tāng	橘皮大黄芒硝湯	kippi-daiō-bōshō-tō	32, 112
kòng xián dān	控涎丹	kōzen-tan	117
lǐ zhōng jiā fù zǐ tāng	理中加附子湯	richū-ka-bushi-tō	167–168
lǐ zhōng tāng	理中湯	richū-tō	104, 167
líng guì gān zǎo tāng	苓桂甘棗湯	ryō-kei-kan-sō-tō	81
líng guì zhú gān tāng	苓桂朮甘湯	ryō-kei-jutsu-kan-tō	77–81, 122, 155
líng jiāng zhú gān tāng	苓薑朮甘湯	ryō-kyō-jutsu-kan-tō	34, 78–85
liù jūn zǐ tāng	六君子湯	rikkunshi-tō	33–35, 113
lóng gān sǎn	龍肝散	ryū-kan-san	159, 216

General

The Chinese Medicine Database

www.cm-db.com

The Chinese Medicine Database has been organized around one central principle -- translation of Classical Asian texts, and dissemination of that information.

There are thousands of Asian medicine texts that have never been translated. We have compiled a small list on our website of the ones that we have found, but we believe that there are tens of thousands of documents that span from the *Hàn* Dynasty to pre-Republican times. Most of these documents will never be read by people in the West, simply because of lack of translation.

We have created a vehicle, that allows interested practitioners, students, institutions, and scholars to help support and fund the translation of these documents, and then mine and synthesize the data that is gained from these texts.

The Database contains:

Monographs on:

- 690 Single Herbs
- 1510 Formulas
- Mayway's Patents
- ITM's Formulations
- Golden Flowers Formulations
- Classical Pearls Formulations by Heiner Fruehauf
- OBGYN Modifications to Formulas
- Single Points: the 361 Regular Points
- Time Line of the History of Chinese Medicine

Beer Hall Lecture Series:

Watch videos from our monthly Beer Hall lecture series with guest speakers such as: Arnaud Versluys, Subhuti Dharmananda, Jason Robertson, Craig Mitchell, Michael Max, Lorraine Wilcox, and Ed Neal.

CEU/ PDA/ Livestreaming Lectures:

We now have a stand alone video system which allows people to watch lectures without being a subscriber. These lectures feature top quality lecturers speaking on classical Chinese medicine and medicinals. This can be found at: http://cm-db.com/xstreaming.php

Play STORT:

Play our free online game STORT where you can learn Chinese while having a bit of fun (www.cm-db.com/stort).

A Chinese-English dictionary:

Containing over 105,000 terms, including the Eastland and the WHO term sets.

Our Translation Tools:

A pop-up translation system using the terminology in our books, as well as our Chinese-English dictionary system. This allows the user to translate their own documents out of Chinese.

Translations:

Shāng Hán Lái Sū Jí	傷寒來蘇集	Renewal of Treatise on Cold Damage
Qí Jīng Bā Mài Kǎo	奇經八脈考	Explanation of the Eight Vessels of the Marvellous Meridians
Shāng Hán Míng Lǐ Lùn	傷寒明理論	Treatise on Enlightening the Principles of Cold Damage
Wú Jū Tōng Yī Àn	吴鞠通医案	Case Studies of Wú Jūtōng
The Nàn Jīng	難經	The Classic of Difficulties
The Zàng Fǔ Biāo Běn Hán Rè Xū Shí Yòng Yào Shì	臟腑標本寒熱虛實用藥式	Viscera and Bowels, Tip and Root, Cold and Heat, Vacuity and Repletion Model for Using Medicinals
Wēn Rè Lún	温熱論	Treatise on Warm Heat Disease
Shāng Hán Shé Jiàn	傷寒舌鑒	Tongue Mirror of Cold Damage
Xǔ Shì Yī Àn	許氏醫案	Case Histories of Master Xǔ
Fǔ Xìng Jué Zāng Fǔ Yòng Yào Fǎ Yào	輔行決臟腑用藥法要	Secret Instructions for Assisting the Body: Essential Methods for the Application of Drugs to the Viscera & Bowels
Biāo Yōu Fù	標幽賦	Indicating the Obscure
Liú Juān Zǐ Guǐ Yí Fāng	劉涓子鬼遺方	Liu Juanzi's Formulas Inherited from Ghosts
Shèn Jí Chú Yán	慎疾芻言	Precautions in Illness: My Humble Thoughts
Yào Zhèng Jì Yí	藥症忌宜	Medicinals & Patterns Contraindications & Appropriate [Choices]
Fù Kē Wèn Dá	婦科問答	Questions and Answers in Gynecology
Nèi Jīng Zhī Yào	内經知要	Essential Knowledge from the Nèijīng
Běn Cǎo Bèi Yào	本草備要	The Essential Completion of Traditional Materia Medica
Bǎi Zhèng Fù (Jù Yīng)	百症賦《聚英》	Ode of the Hundred Diseases from The Great Compendium of Acupuncture-Moxibustion

Benefits:

Subscribers to the Database receive a 10% discount on our published books when they are in pre-release.

Published Books:

2008 Bèi Jí Qiān Jīn Yào Fāng 備急千金要方:
Essential Prescriptions Worth a Thousand Gold Pieces For Emergencies. vol. 2-4
by Sūn Sīmiǎo 孫思邈
Translated by Sabine Wilms.
ISBN 978-0-9799552-0-4
Permanently Out of Print

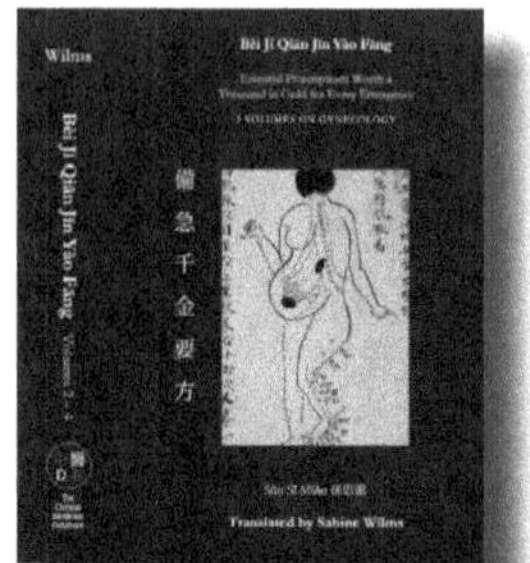

2010 Zhēn Jiǔ Dà Chéng 針灸大成:
The Great Compendium of Acupuncture & Moxibustion vol. I
by Yáng Jìzhōu 楊繼洲
Translated by Sabine Wilms.
ISBN 978-0-9799552-2-8

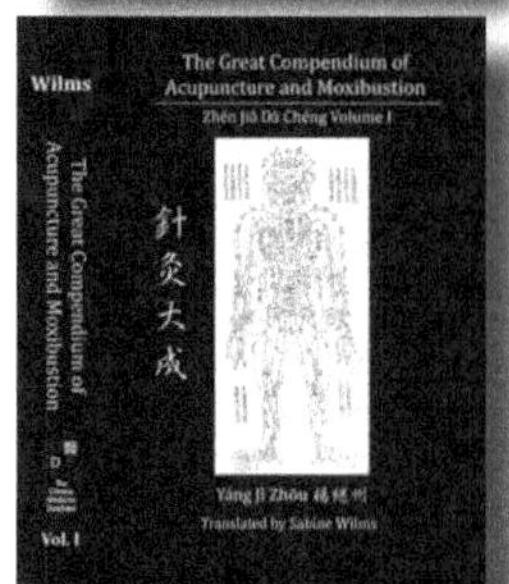

2010 Zhēn Jiǔ Dà Chéng 針灸大成:
The Great Compendium of Acupuncture & Moxibustion vol. V
by Yáng Jìzhōu 楊繼洲
Translated by Lorraine Wilcox.
ISBN 978-0-9799552-4-2

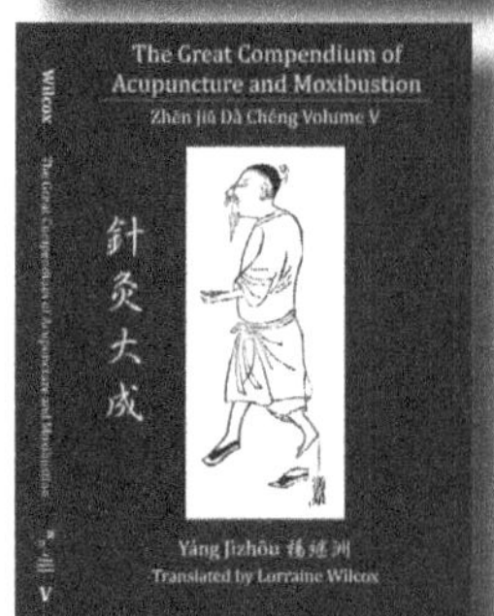

2010 Jīn Guì Fāng Gē Kuò 金匱方歌括:
Formulas from the Golden Cabinet with Songs vol. I - III
by Chén Xiūyuán 陳修園
Translated by Sabine Wilms.
ISBN 978-0-9799552-5-9

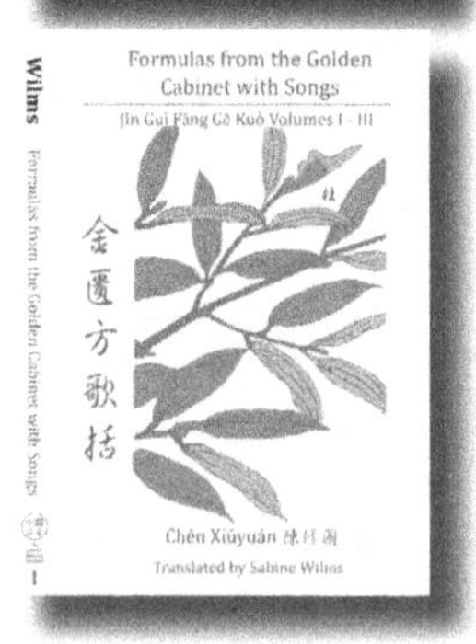

2011 Zhēn Jiǔ Dà Chéng 針灸大成:
The Great Compendium of Acupuncture & Moxibustion vol. VIII
by Yáng Jìzhōu 楊繼洲
Translated by Yue Lu.
ISBN 978-0-9799552-7-3

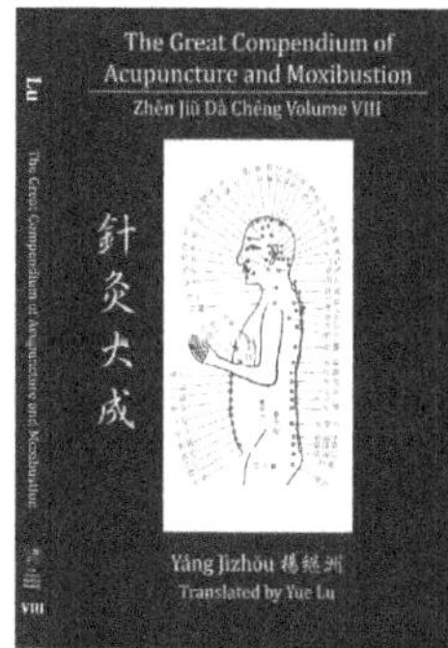

2011 Zhēn Jiǔ Dà Chéng 針灸大成:
The Great Compendium of Acupuncture & Moxibustion vol. IX
by Yáng Jìzhōu 楊繼洲
Translated by Lorraine Wilcox.
ISBN 978-0-9799552-6-6

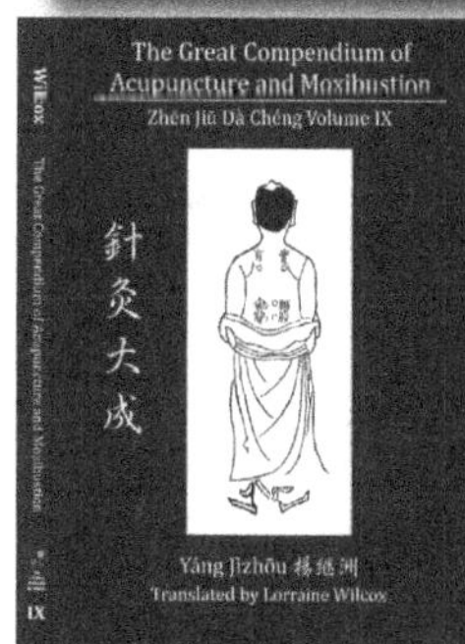

2012 Raising the Dead and Returning Life: Emergency Medicine of the Qīng Dynasty
by Bào Xiāng'áo 鮑相璈
Translated by Lorraine Wilcox.
ISBN 978-0-9799552-3-5

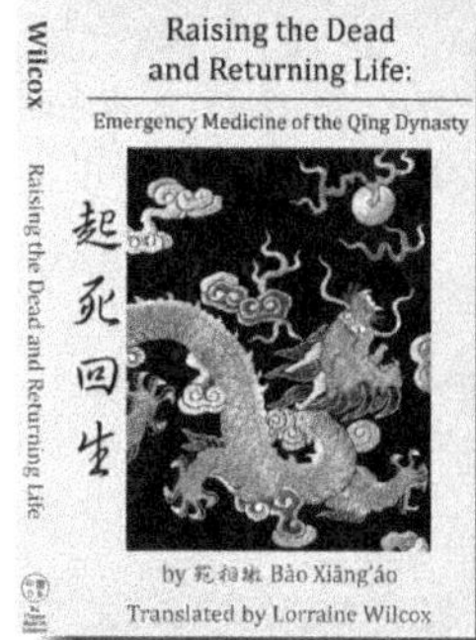

2014 Zhēn Jiǔ Zī Shēng Jīng 針灸資生經:
The Classic of Supporting Life with Acupuncture and Moxibustion Vol. I-III
by Wáng Zhízhōng 王執中
Translated by Yue Lu.
ISBN 978-0-9799552-1-1

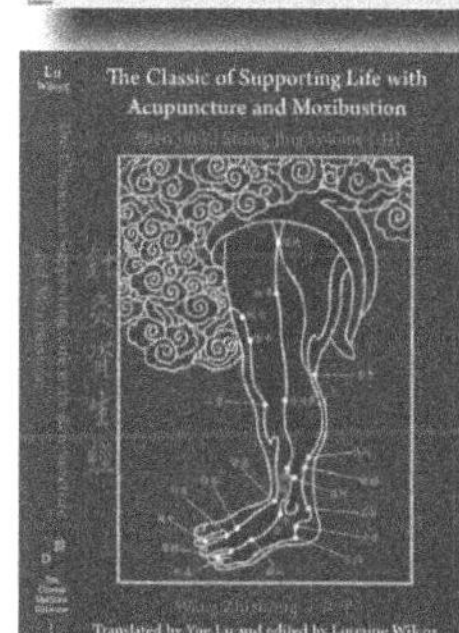

2014 Jīn Guì Fāng Gē Kuò 金匱方歌括:
Formulas from the Golden Cabinet with Songs
vol. IV - VI
by Chén Xiūyuán 陳修園
Translated by Eran Even.
ISBN 978-0-9799552-8-0

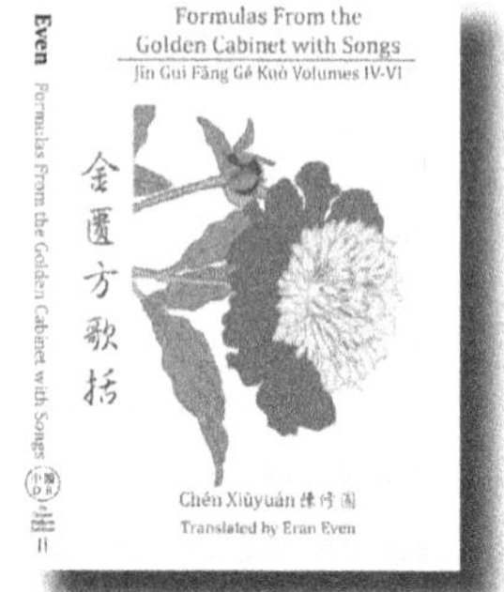

2015 Zhēn Jiǔ Zī Shēng Jīng 針灸資生經:
The Classic of Supporting Life with Acupuncture and Moxibustion
Vol. IV-VII
by Wáng Zhízhōng 王執中
Translated by Yue Lu.
ISBN 978-0-9799552-9-7

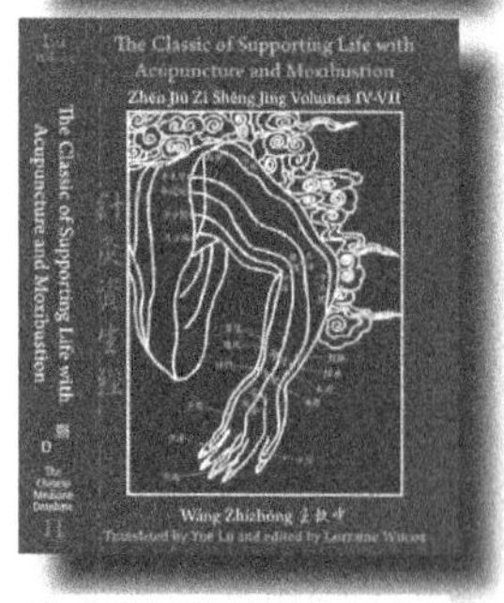

2015 Nǚ Yī Zá Yán 女醫雜言:
Miscellaneous Records of a Female Doctor
by Tán Yǔnxián 談允賢
Translated by Lorraine Wilcox.
ISBN 978-0-9906029-0-3

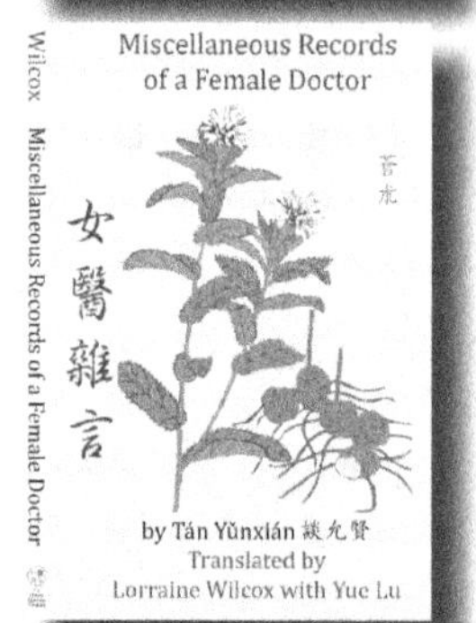

2016 Nǚ Kē Cuō Yào 女科撮要:
Outline of Female Medicine
by Xuē Jǐ 薛己
Translated by Lorraine Wilcox.
ISBN 978-0-9906029-1-0

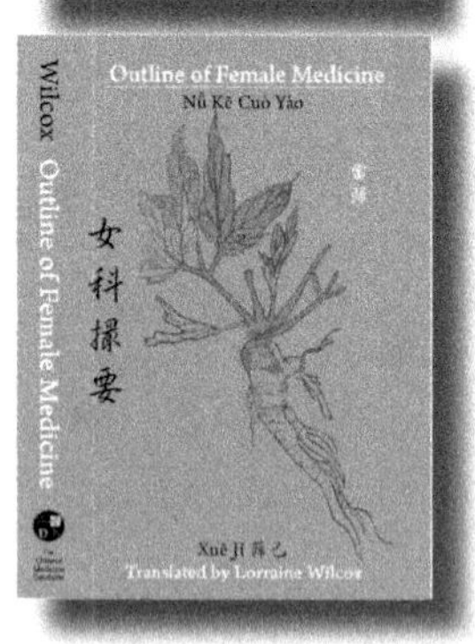

2016 Shén Nóng Běn Cǎo Jīng Dú 神農本草經讀:
Reading of the Divine Farmer's Classic of Materia Medica
by Chén Xiūyuán 陳修園
Translated by Corinna Theisinger.
ISBN 978-0-9906029-2-7

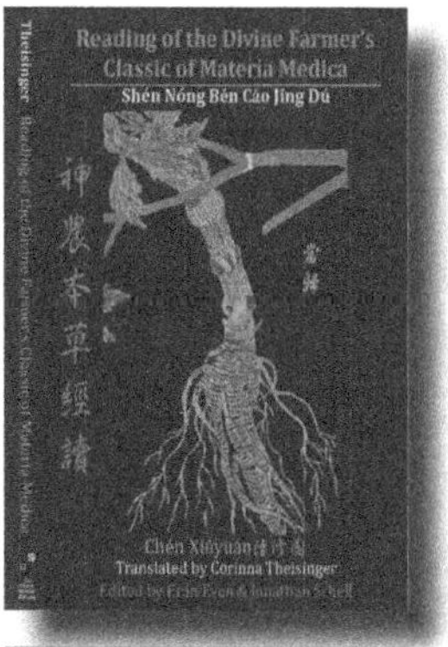

2017 Zhèng Tǐ Lèi Yào 正體類要:
Categorized Essentials of Repairing the Body
by Xuē Jǐ 薛己
Translated by Lorraine Wilcox.
ISBN 978-0-9906029-3-4

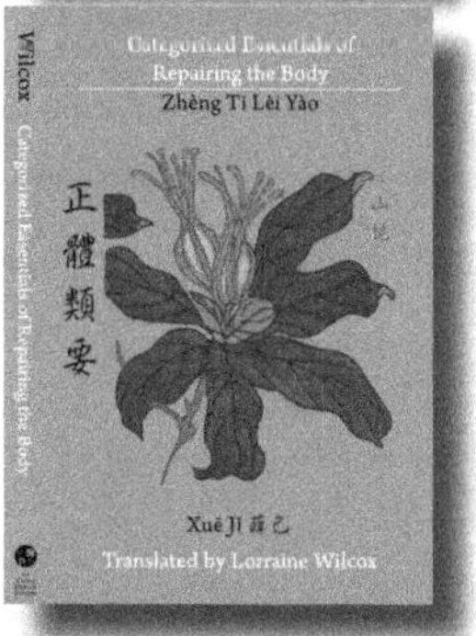

2018 Zhù Jiě Shāng Hán Lùn 注解傷寒論:
Commentary On The Discussion of Cold Damage With Annotations
by Chéng Wújǐ 成無己
Translated by Jonathan Schell L.Ac..
ISBN 978-0-9906029-4-1

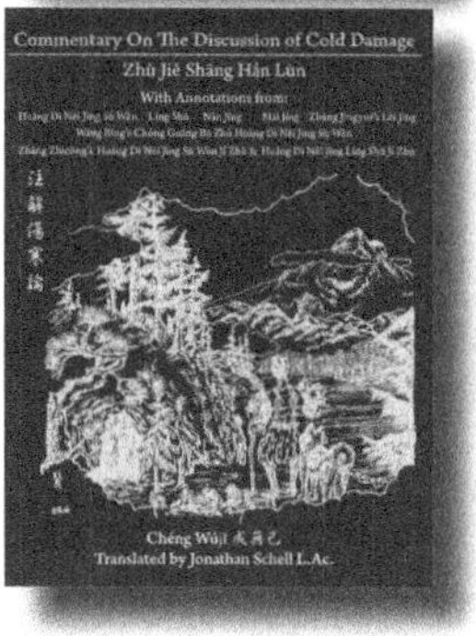

www.ingramcontent.com/pod-product-compliance
Lightning Source LLC
LaVergne TN
LVHW052249200926
848481LV00002B/316
9780990602958